TOP TRAILS™

Maui

MUST-DO HIKES FOR EVERYONE

Written by

Sara Benson

WILDERNESS PRESS *. . . on the trail since 1967*

Top Trails Maui: Must-Do Hikes for Everyone

1st EDITION 2011

Front cover photos copyright © 2011 by Debra Behr/Alamy *(main)*;
Michael Connolly, Jr. *(inset)*
Interior photos by Sara Benson and Michael Connolly, Jr.
Maps: Sara Benson and Lohnes+Wright
Cover and interior design: Frances Baca Design and Larry B. Van Dyke
Layout: Larry B. Van Dyke
Editor: Laura Shauger

ISBN 978-0-89997-625-9

Manufactured in the United States of America

Published by: **Wilderness Press**
Keen Communications
2204 First Avenue South, Suite 102
Birmingham, AL 35233
(800) 443-7227
info@wildernesspress.com
www.wildernesspress.com
Visit our website for a complete listing of our books and for ordering information.

Distributed by Publishers Group West

Cover photo: Sliding Sands Trail in Haleakala National Park *(main)*;
bromeliad, Keanae Arboretum *(inset)*

SAFETY NOTICE: Although Wilderness Press and the author have made every attempt to ensure that the information in this book is accurate at press time, they are not responsible for any loss, damage, injury, or inconvenience that may occur to anyone while using this book. You are responsible for your own safety and health while in the wilderness. The fact that a trail is described in this book does not mean that it will be safe for you. Be aware that trail conditions can change from day to day. Always check local conditions, know your own limitations, and consult a map.

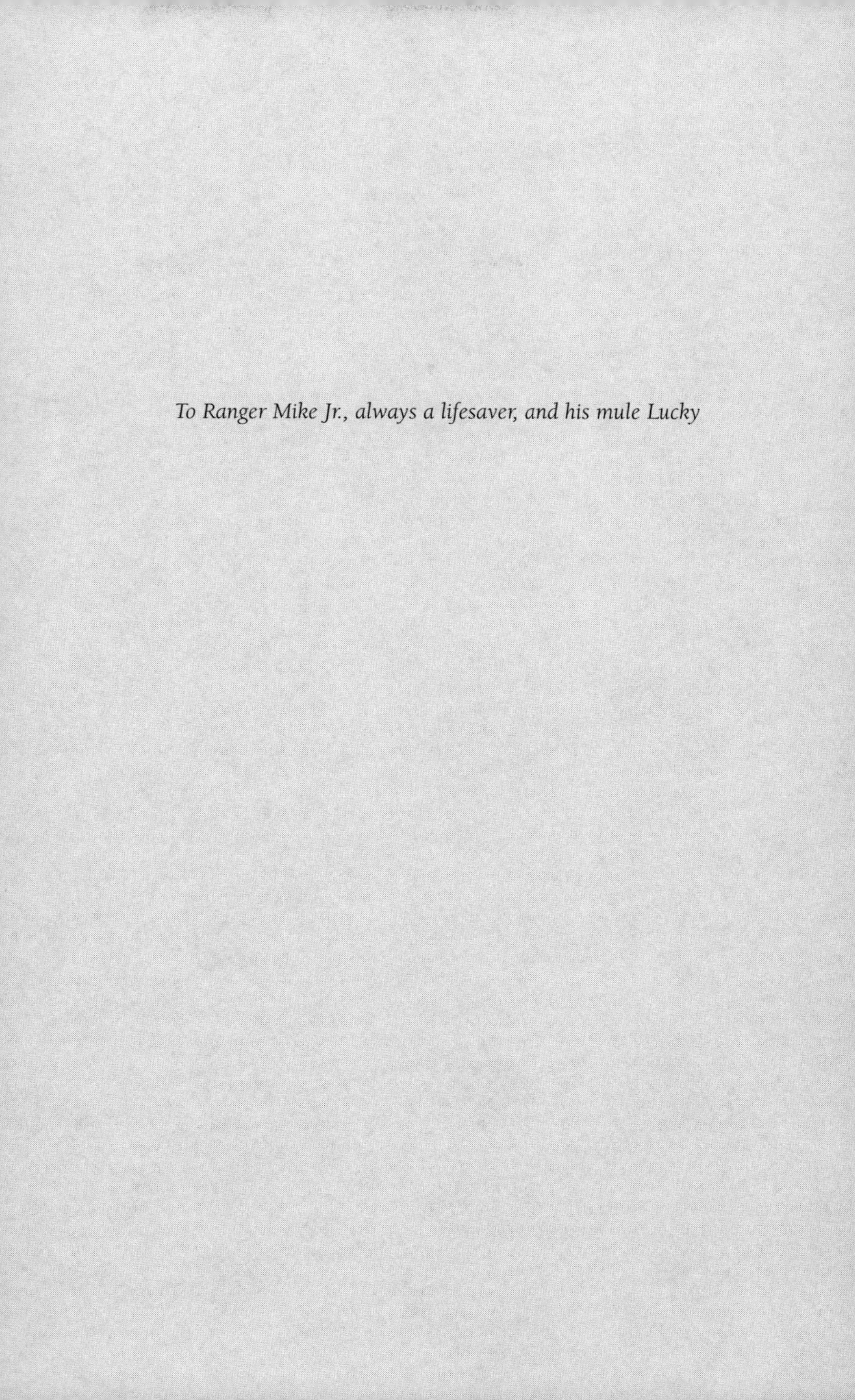

To Ranger Mike Jr., always a lifesaver, and his mule Lucky

The Top Trails™ Series

Wilderness Press

When Wilderness Press published *Sierra North* in 1967, no other trail guide like it existed for the Sierra backcountry. The first print run sold out in less than two months, and its success heralded the beginning of Wilderness Press. Since we were founded more than 40 years ago, we have expanded our territories to cover California, Alaska, Hawaii, the U.S. Southwest, Pacific Northwest, Midwest, Southeast, New England, Canada, and Baja California.

Wilderness Press continues to publish comprehensive, accurate, and readable outdoor books. Hikers, backpackers, kayakers, skiers, snowshoers, climbers, cyclists, and trail runners rely on Wilderness Press for accurate outdoor adventure information.

Top Trails

In its Top Trails guides, Wilderness Press has paid special attention to organization so that you can find the perfect hike each and every time. Whether you're looking for a steep trail to test yourself on or a walk in the park, a romantic waterfall or a city view, Top Trails will lead you there.

Each Top Trails guide contains trails for everyone. The trails selected provide a sampling of the best that the region has to offer. These are the "must-do" hikes, walks, runs, and bike rides, with every feature of the area represented.

Every book in the Top Trails series offers:

- The Wilderness Press commitment to accuracy and reliability
- Ratings and rankings for each trail
- Distances and approximate times
- Easy-to-follow trail notes
- Map and permit information

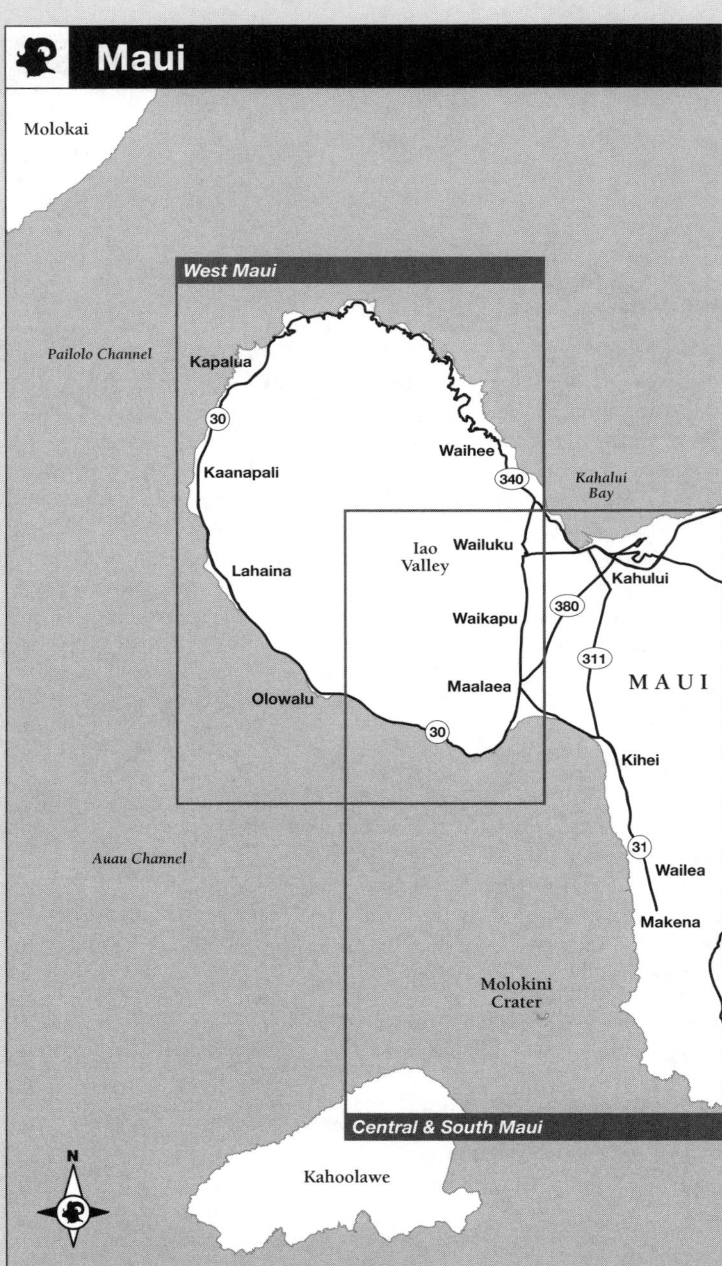
Maui
Molokai
West Maui
Pailolo Channel
Kapalua
30
Kaanapali
Waihee
340
Kahalui
Bay
Iao
Valley
Wailuku
Lahaina
Kahului
380
Waikapu
311
Maalaea
MAUI
Olowalu
30
Kihei
Auau Channel
31
Wailea
Makena
Molokini
Crater
Central & South Maui
N
Kahoolawe

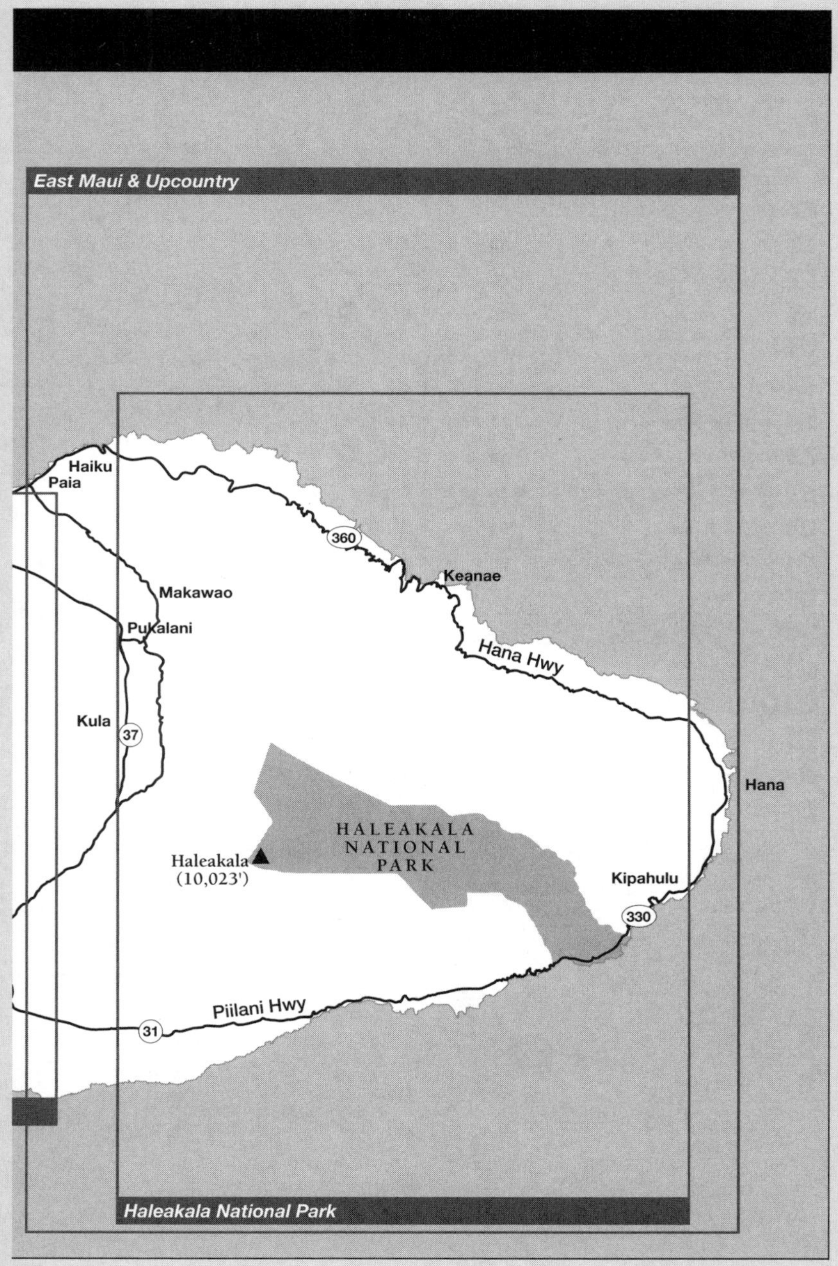
East Maui & Upcountry
Haiku
Paia
360
Keanae
Makawao
Pukalani
Hana Hwy
Kula
37
Hana
HALEAKALA NATIONAL PARK
Haleakala (10,023')
Kipahulu
330
Piilani Hwy
31
Haleakala National Park

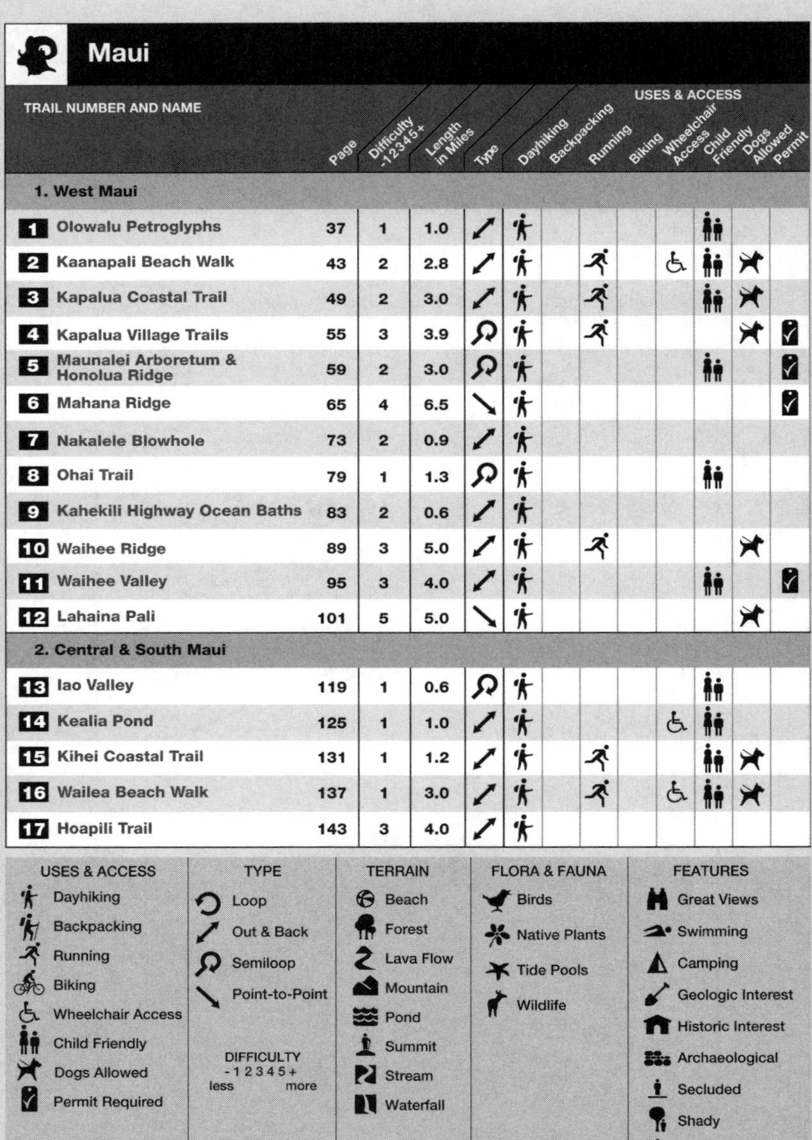

Maui

TRAIL NUMBER AND NAME	Page	Difficulty -12345+	Length in Miles	Type	Dayhiking	Backpacking	Running	Biking	Wheelchair Access	Child Friendly	Dogs Allowed	Permit
1. West Maui												
1 Olowalu Petroglyphs	37	1	1.0	Out & Back	✓					✓		
2 Kaanapali Beach Walk	43	2	2.8	Out & Back	✓		✓		✓	✓	✓	
3 Kapalua Coastal Trail	49	2	3.0	Out & Back	✓		✓			✓	✓	
4 Kapalua Village Trails	55	3	3.9	Semiloop	✓		✓				✓	✓
5 Maunalei Arboretum & Honolua Ridge	59	2	3.0	Semiloop	✓					✓		✓
6 Mahana Ridge	65	4	6.5	Point-to-Point	✓							✓
7 Nakalele Blowhole	73	2	0.9	Out & Back	✓							
8 Ohai Trail	79	1	1.3	Semiloop	✓					✓		
9 Kahekili Highway Ocean Baths	83	2	0.6	Out & Back	✓							
10 Waihee Ridge	89	3	5.0	Out & Back	✓		✓				✓	
11 Waihee Valley	95	3	4.0	Out & Back	✓					✓		✓
12 Lahaina Pali	101	5	5.0	Point-to-Point	✓						✓	
2. Central & South Maui												
13 Iao Valley	119	1	0.6	Semiloop	✓					✓		
14 Kealia Pond	125	1	1.0	Out & Back	✓				✓	✓		
15 Kihei Coastal Trail	131	1	1.2	Out & Back	✓		✓			✓	✓	
16 Wailea Beach Walk	137	1	3.0	Out & Back	✓		✓		✓	✓	✓	
17 Hoapili Trail	143	3	4.0	Out & Back	✓							

USES & ACCESS
- Dayhiking
- Backpacking
- Running
- Biking
- Wheelchair Access
- Child Friendly
- Dogs Allowed
- Permit Required

TYPE
- Loop
- Out & Back
- Semiloop
- Point-to-Point

DIFFICULTY
-12345+
less more

TERRAIN
- Beach
- Forest
- Lava Flow
- Mountain
- Pond
- Summit
- Stream
- Waterfall

FLORA & FAUNA
- Birds
- Native Plants
- Tide Pools
- Wildlife

FEATURES
- Great Views
- Swimming
- Camping
- Geologic Interest
- Historic Interest
- Archaeological
- Secluded
- Shady
- Steep

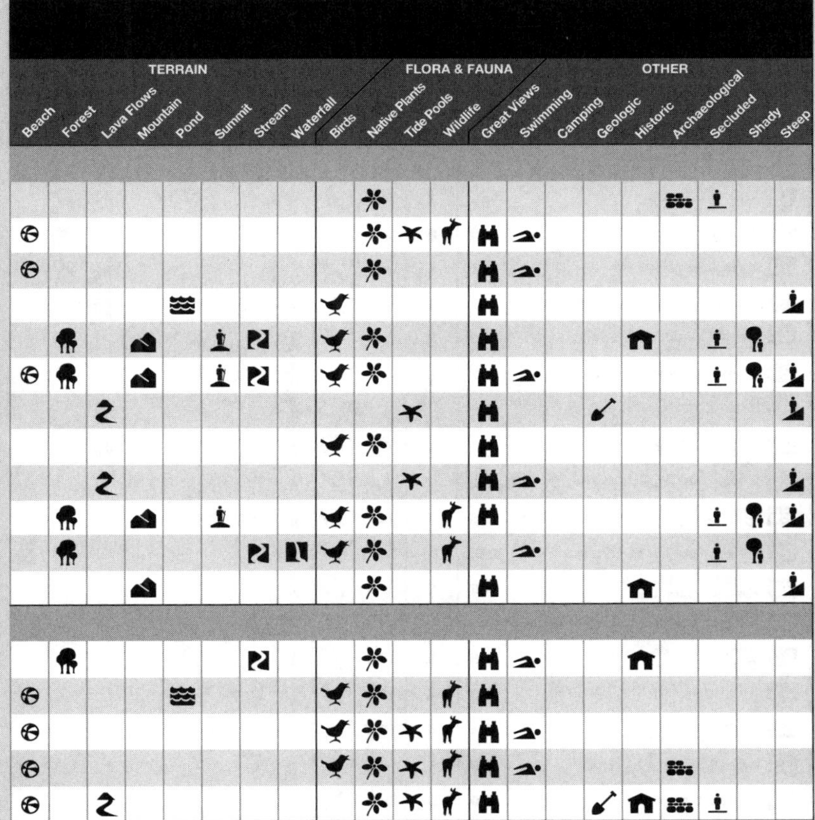
TERRAIN
FLORA & FAUNA
OTHER
Beach
Forest
Lava Flows
Mountain
Pond
Summit
Stream
Waterfall
Birds
Native Plants
Tide Pools
Wildlife
Great Views
Swimming
Camping
Geologic
Historic
Archaeological
Secluded
Shady
Steep

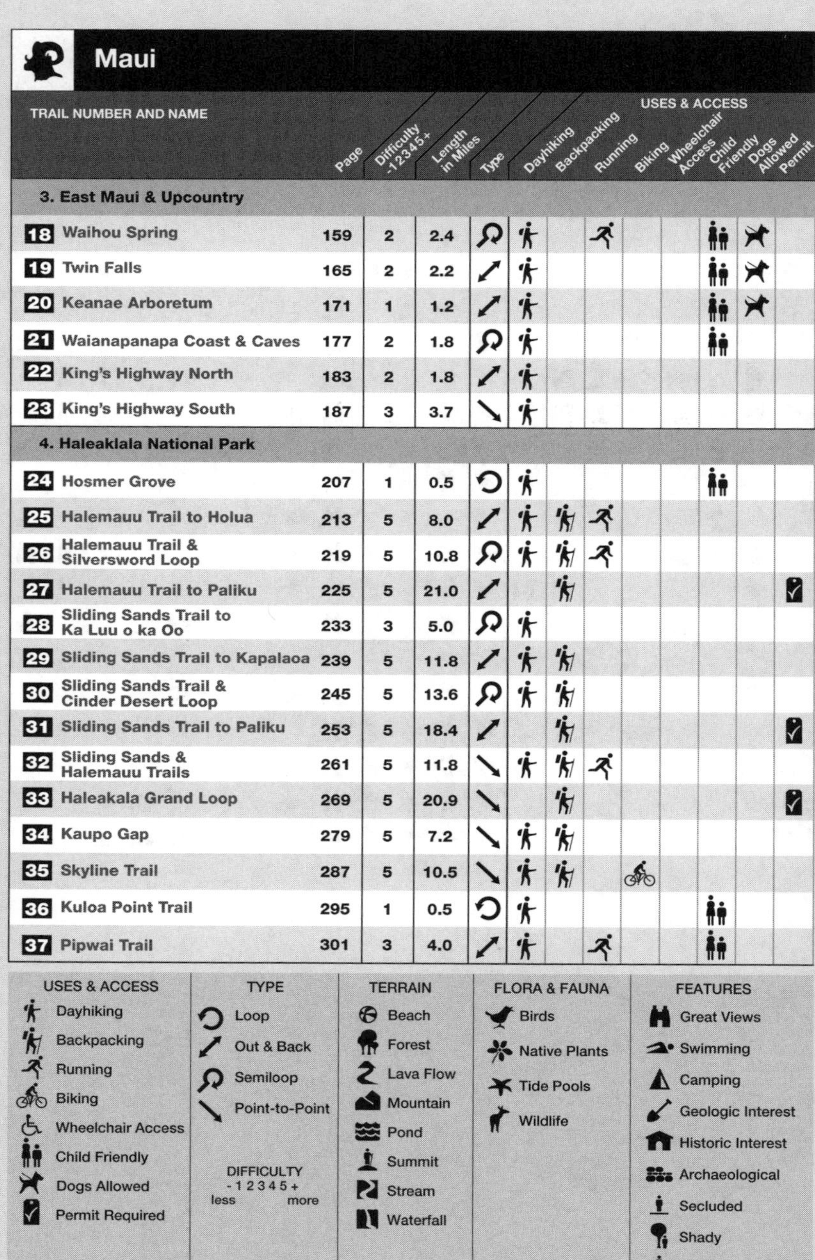

Maui

TRAIL NUMBER AND NAME	Page	Difficulty -12345+	Length in Miles	Type	Dayhiking	Backpacking	Running	Biking	Wheelchair Access	Child Friendly	Dogs Allowed	Permit
3. East Maui & Upcountry												
18 Waihou Spring	159	2	2.4	Semiloop	Dayhiking		Running			Child Friendly	Dogs Allowed	
19 Twin Falls	165	2	2.2	Out & Back	Dayhiking					Child Friendly	Dogs Allowed	
20 Keanae Arboretum	171	1	1.2	Out & Back	Dayhiking					Child Friendly	Dogs Allowed	
21 Waianapanapa Coast & Caves	177	2	1.8	Semiloop	Dayhiking					Child Friendly		
22 King's Highway North	183	2	1.8	Out & Back	Dayhiking							
23 King's Highway South	187	3	3.7	Point-to-Point	Dayhiking							
4. Haleaklala National Park												
24 Hosmer Grove	207	1	0.5	Loop	Dayhiking					Child Friendly		
25 Halemauu Trail to Holua	213	5	8.0	Out & Back	Dayhiking	Backpacking	Running					
26 Halemauu Trail & Silversword Loop	219	5	10.8	Semiloop	Dayhiking	Backpacking	Running					
27 Halemauu Trail to Paliku	225	5	21.0	Out & Back		Backpacking						Permit Required
28 Sliding Sands Trail to Ka Luu o ka Oo	233	3	5.0	Semiloop	Dayhiking							
29 Sliding Sands Trail to Kapalaoa	239	5	11.8	Out & Back	Dayhiking	Backpacking						
30 Sliding Sands Trail & Cinder Desert Loop	245	5	13.6	Semiloop	Dayhiking	Backpacking						
31 Sliding Sands Trail to Paliku	253	5	18.4	Out & Back		Backpacking						Permit Required
32 Sliding Sands & Halemauu Trails	261	5	11.8	Point-to-Point	Dayhiking	Backpacking	Running					
33 Haleakala Grand Loop	269	5	20.9	Point-to-Point		Backpacking						Permit Required
34 Kaupo Gap	279	5	7.2	Point-to-Point	Dayhiking	Backpacking						
35 Skyline Trail	287	5	10.5	Point-to-Point	Dayhiking	Backpacking		Biking				
36 Kuloa Point Trail	295	1	0.5	Loop	Dayhiking					Child Friendly		
37 Pipwai Trail	301	3	4.0	Out & Back	Dayhiking		Running			Child Friendly		

USES & ACCESS	TYPE	TERRAIN	FLORA & FAUNA	FEATURES
Dayhiking	Loop	Beach	Birds	Great Views
Backpacking	Out & Back	Forest	Native Plants	Swimming
Running	Semiloop	Lava Flow	Tide Pools	Camping
Biking	Point-to-Point	Mountain	Wildlife	Geologic Interest
Wheelchair Access		Pond		Historic Interest
Child Friendly	DIFFICULTY -12345+ (less … more)	Summit		Archaeological
Dogs Allowed		Stream		Secluded
Permit Required		Waterfall		Shady
				Steep

TERRAIN								FLORA & FAUNA				OTHER								
Beach	Forest	Lava Flows	Mountain	Pond	Summit	Stream	Waterfall	Birds	Native Plants	Tide Pools	Wildlife	Great Views	Swimming	Camping	Geologic	Historic	Archaeological	Secluded	Shady	Steep
	✓					✓		✓			✓	✓						✓	✓	✓
	✓					✓	✓	✓	✓				✓						✓	
	✓					✓		✓	✓									✓	✓	
✓		✓						✓	✓		✓	✓	✓	✓	✓	✓	✓			
✓		✓						✓	✓	✓	✓	✓				✓		✓		
✓		✓						✓	✓	✓	✓	✓				✓	✓	✓		
	✓		✓			✓		✓	✓		✓			✓					✓	
	✓	✓	✓					✓	✓		✓	✓		✓	✓	✓				✓
	✓	✓	✓					✓	✓		✓	✓		✓	✓	✓				✓
	✓	✓	✓					✓	✓		✓	✓		✓	✓	✓	✓	✓		✓
		✓	✓					✓	✓		✓	✓			✓					✓
		✓	✓					✓	✓		✓	✓			✓	✓				✓
		✓	✓					✓	✓		✓	✓			✓	✓	✓			✓
		✓	✓					✓	✓		✓	✓			✓	✓		✓		✓
	✓	✓	✓					✓	✓		✓	✓		✓	✓	✓				✓
	✓	✓	✓					✓	✓		✓	✓		✓	✓	✓	✓	✓		✓
	✓	✓	✓					✓	✓		✓	✓		✓	✓	✓	✓	✓		✓
	✓	✓	✓		✓			✓	✓		✓	✓		✓	✓			✓	✓	✓
						✓	✓	✓	✓		✓	✓	✓				✓			
	✓					✓	✓	✓	✓		✓	✓							✓	

Contents

CHAPTER 1

West Maui

CHAPTER 2

Central & South Maui

CHAPTER 3

East Maui & Upcountry

Using Top Trails™

Organization of Top Trails

Top Trails is designed so you can find the perfect trail and make every outing a success and a pleasure. With this guide it's a snap to find the right trail, whether you're planning a major hike or just a sociable stroll with friends.

The Region

At the front of this guide, the **Maui Map** (pages vi–vii) provides a geographic overview of the island, and shows the areas covered by each chapter.

The adjacent **Maui Trails Table** (pages viii–xi) lists every trail covered in the guide along with attributes for each trail. A quick reading of the regional map and the trails table gives you a quick overview of the entire region covered by this guide.

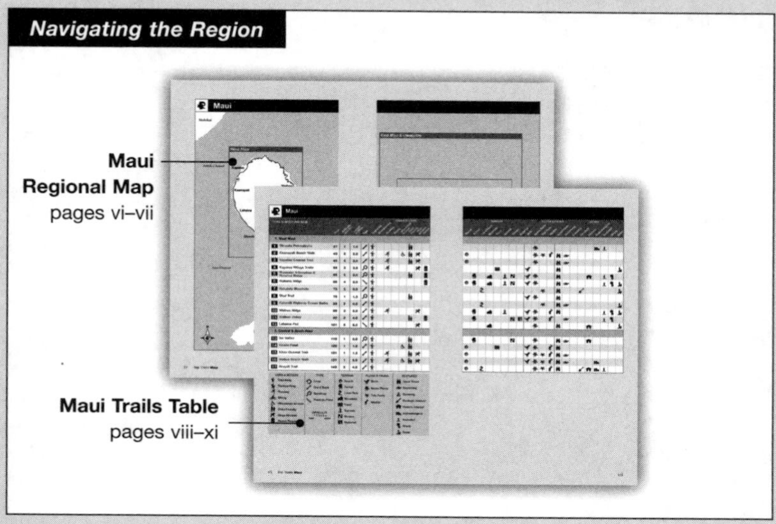

The Areas

The region covered in each book is divided into areas, with each chapter corresponding to one area in the region. Each area chapter introduction starts with information to help you choose and enjoy a trail every time out. Use the table of contents or the regional map to identify an area of interest, then turn to the area chapter to find the following:

- An overview of the area's parks and trails
- An area map showing all trail locations
- A trail features table providing trail-by-trail details
- Trail summaries highlighting each trail's unique experiences

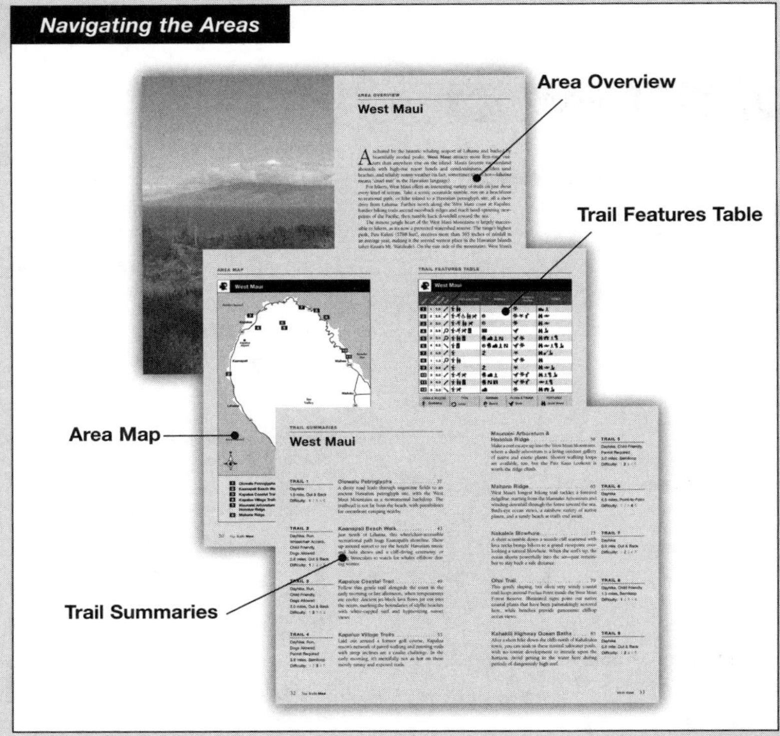

The Trails

The basic building block of the Top Trails guide is the trail entry. Each one is arranged to make finding and following the trail as simple as possible, with all pertinent information presented in this easy-to-follow format:

- A detailed trail map
- Trail descriptions covering difficulty, length, GPS coordinates (in decimal degrees) for start and end points, and other essential data
- A written trail description
- Trail milestones providing easy-to follow, turn-by-turn trail directions

Some trail descriptions offer additional information:

- An elevation profile
- Trail options
- Trail highlights
- GPS waypoints (in decimal degrees) for trail milestones

In the margins of the trail entries, keep your eyes open for graphic icons that signal features mentioned in the text.

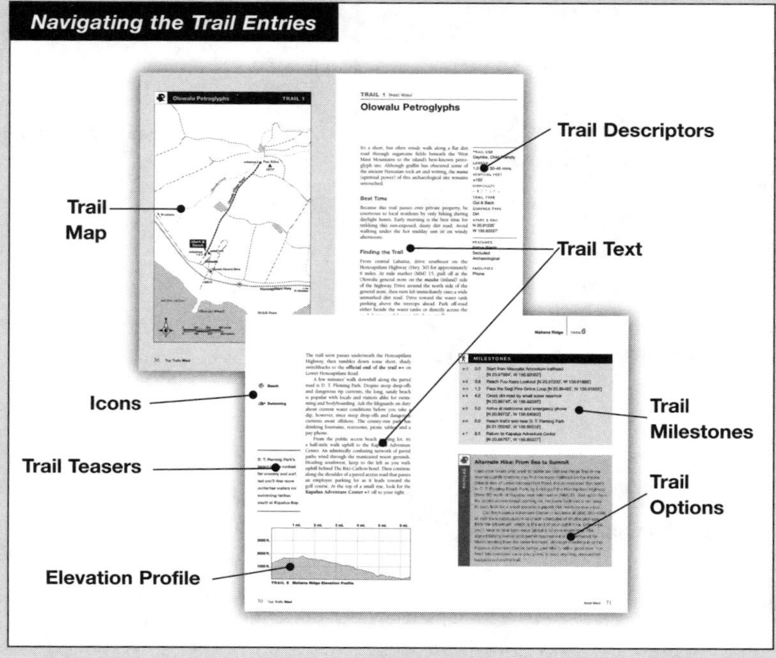

Choosing a Trail

Top Trails provides several different ways of choosing a trail, using easy-to-read tables and maps.

Location

If you know in general where you want to go, Top Trails makes it easy to find the right trail in the right place. Each chapter begins with a large-scale map showing the starting point of every trail in that area.

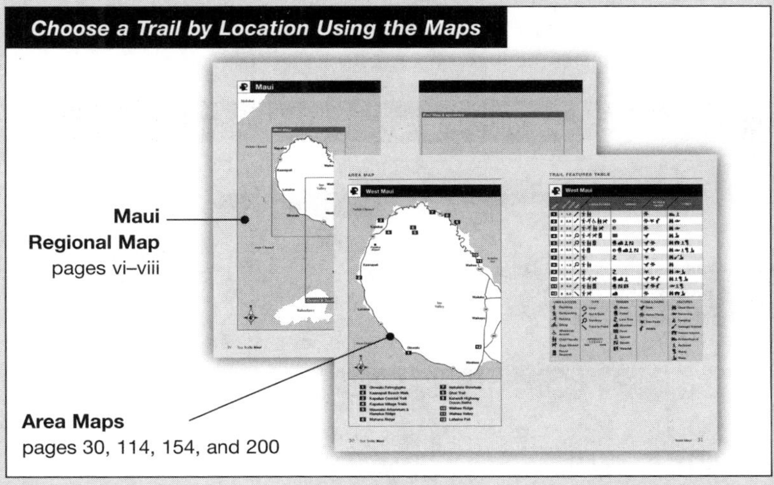

Features

This guide describes the Top Trails for the island of Maui. Each trail has been chosen because it offers one or more features that make it appealing. Using the trail descriptors, summaries, and tables, you can quickly examine all the trails to find out what features they offer, or seek a particular feature among the list of trails.

Season & Condition

Time of year and current conditions can be important factors in selecting the best trail. For example, an exposed low-elevation trail may be lush and cool (especially during winter) on the windward side of the island, but an oven-baked taste of hell come late summer or early fall on the leeward side.

Where relevant, Top Trails identifies the best and worst conditions for the trails you plan to hike.

Difficulty

Every trail has an overall difficulty rating on a scale of 1 to 5, which takes into consideration length, elevation change, exposure, trail quality, and more to create one (admittedly subjective) rating.

The ratings assume you are an able-bodied adult in reasonably good shape using the trail for hiking. The ratings also assume normal weather conditions—clear and dry.

Readers should make an honest assessment of their own abilities and adjust time estimates accordingly. Also, rain, snow, heat, wind, and poor visibility can all affect the pace on even the easiest of trails.

Choose a Trail by Length, Difficulty, or Features Using the Tables

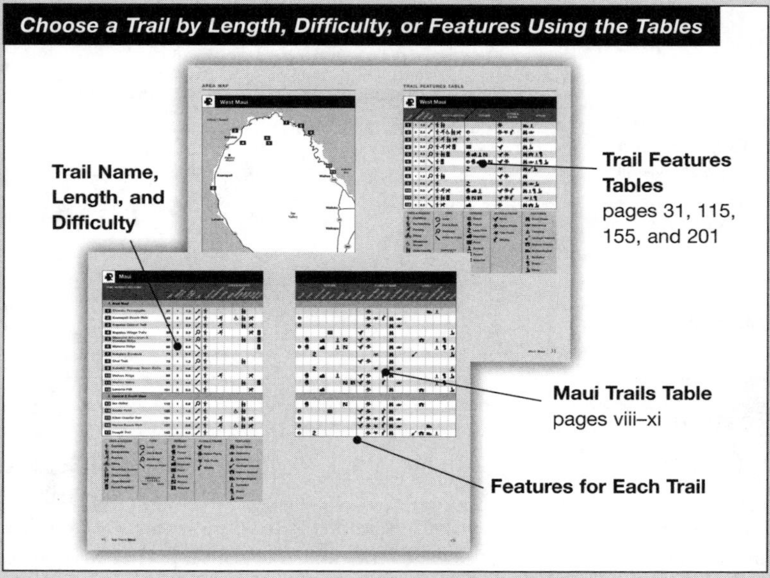

Vertical Feet

Every trail description contains the approximate trail length and the overall elevation gain and loss over the course of the trail. It's important to use both figures when considering a hike; on average plan one hour for every 2 miles, and add an hour for every 1000 feet you climb.

This important measurement is often underestimated by hikers when gauging the difficulty of a trail. The Top Trails measurement accounts for all elevation change, not simply the difference between the highest and lowest points, so that rolling terrain with lots of up and down is identifiable.

The calculation of vertical feet in the Top Trails guides is accomplished by a combination of trail measurement and computer-aided estimation. For routes that begin and end at the same spot—i.e., loop or out & back—the vertical gain exactly matches the vertical descent. With a point-to-point route, the vertical gain and loss will most likely differ, and both figures are provided in the text.

Finally, all Trail Entries with more than 1000 feet of elevation gain include an elevation profile, an easy means for visualizing the topography of the route. These profiles graphically depict the elevation throughout the length of the trail.

Surface Type

Each trail entry describes the surface of the trail. This information is useful in determining what type of footwear is appropriate. Surface type should also be considered when checking the weather—on a rainy day early or late in the hiking season a dirt surface can be a muddy slog; a boardwalk jaunt or a paved surface might be a better choice.

Top Trails Difficulty Ratings

1 A short trail, generally level, that can be completed in one hour or less.

2 A route of 1 to 3 miles, with some up and down, that can be completed in one to two hours.

3 A longer route, up to 5 miles, with uphill and/or downhill sections.

4 A long or steep route, perhaps more than 5 miles, or with climbs of more than 1000 vertical feet.

5 The most severe route, both long and steep, more than 5 miles long with climbs of more than 1000 vertical feet.

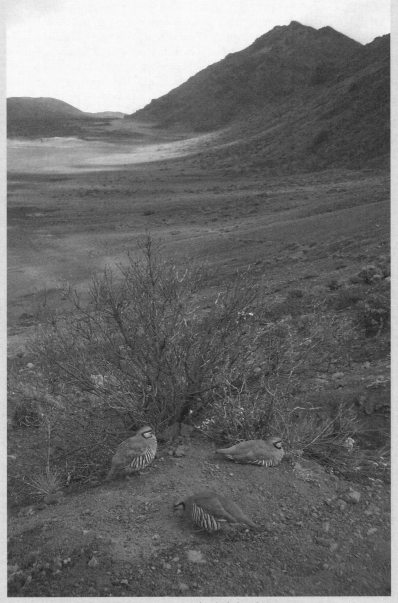

Bird life *thrives at the high-elevation summit of Haleakala volcano.*

Introduction to Maui

Hiking may not be what most people come to Hawaii to do. But don't let that stop you. Amazing trails crisscross the island, from meditative coastal beach walks to heady treks high atop a volcano. Hidden in cloud forest, more trails lead to tumbling waterfalls, hidden springs, and groves of bamboo that rustle musically in the Pacific trade winds. Back down on the coast, you can watch water spout through natural lava-rock blowholes and sea arches, take a dip or snorkel in ocean pools, and encounter deserted beaches to be savored in solitude. You can also wander across lava flows that feel primeval, examine ancient Hawaiian petroglyphs up close, or follow the King's Highway that Hawaiian royalty once trod. All this and more awaits on Maui's hiking trails, most of which are easily accessible day trips. No matter where you base yourself on the island, any of the dozens of trailheads pinpointed in this book is at most a couple hours' drive away, and often far closer than that. It's a hikers' paradise.

Geography

The Hawaiian Islands are the most geographically isolated landmass on earth, located about 2,400 miles from the nearest continent, North America. Hawaii sits at the apex of the Polynesian triangle, with the other two points positioned at Easter Island (Rapa Nui) and New Zealand (Aotearoa), both of the latter in the South Pacific. Maui is the second largest of the Hawaiian Islands (after the aptly nicknamed Big Island of Hawaii), with a total land area of 729 square miles and around 120 miles of coastline.

The island of Maui can be split roughly into two pieces. Smaller and shaped like a baseball, the northwestern section of the island is carved by the West Maui Mountains, which are cut by streams and valleys that are mostly inaccessible. Luckily, a few trails lead into the lush interior of the range, which tops out at Puu Kukui (elevation 5788 feet), the second wettest place in Hawaii, which receives more than 385 inches of rainfall annually. Only Kauai's Mt. Waialeale gets more precipitation each year. Lower elevation ridge climbs on Maui provide sweeping vistas of the Pacific and postcard panoramas of other Hawaiian Islands, while the island's drier west coast offers plenty of beach walks and strolls.

Shaped like an arrowhead, the larger southeastern section of the island of Maui is dominated by Haleakala volcano. With elevations ranging from sea level to 10,023 feet at the summit, this side of Maui offers hikers an enormous variety of terrain: tropical rain and cloud forests, *aa* (rough, jagged) and *pahoehoe* (smooth, unbroken) lava flows, rainbow-colored cinder deserts, and more. The windward east coast, especially around Hana, is famous for its pooling waterfalls, including at Kipahulu inside Haleakala National Park. Connecting the two sides of the island of Maui are coastal wetlands, where diverse native and migratory birds take refuge.

Geology

The Hawaiian archipelago measures 1,600 miles long and comprises more than 130 scattered points of land, including islands, islets, reefs, shoals, atolls, and underwater seamounts. Part of the Hawaiian Ridge–Emperor Seamount chain, as well as the much larger Pacific Ring of Fire, all of these islands are volcanic in origin. They slowly arise from columns of molten lava that build up on the ocean floor until eventually emerging above the ocean's surface, a process that takes eons. This process happens as the Pacific Plate moves northwest over a hot spot in the earth's mantle at the rate of just a few inches each year. Today, the Big Island of Hawaii straddles that hot spot, which accounts for its ongoing volcanic activity, notably at Kilauea Volcano inside Hawaii Volcanoes National Park. Having long since drifted away from the hot spot, Maui's volcanic activity has probably come to an end, although Haleakala—believed to have erupted most recently in the 1790s—is technically still an active volcano. Scientists continue to monitor Haleakala for signs of an eruption, which is possible even after hundreds of years of seeming inactivity.

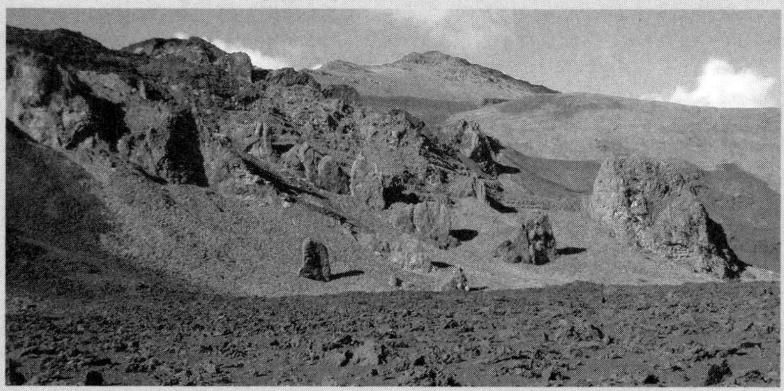

Ancient volcanic activity *is unearthed in Haleakala's eroded summit area.*

The island of Maui comprises two separate volcanoes joined together by ancient lava flows: the still-active Haleakala, which dominates East Maui's topography, and the now-extinct Puu Kukui that formed the West Maui Mountains. Both volcanoes were (and continue to be) shaped by the forces of erosion, namely wind, water, and time. In the case of Haleakala, precipitation at the volcano's summit, which traps moisture-laden trade winds, formed streams that cut channels down its slopes to the sea. What is left today at the volcano's summit is an erosional valley, popularly misnomered as Haleakala's "crater," even though it's *not* the product of a volcanic eruption. Another factor in the slow erosion of Hawaiian volcanoes, including those on Maui, is size: They slowly crush themselves under their own weight, eventually becoming underwater seamounts once again—just as they started out more than 70 million years ago.

For hikers, Maui's geological history provides a terrifically varied playground of terrain to explore. Keep in mind that the drama of plate tectonics can cause both earthquakes and tsunamis across the archipelago, although major events are rare. The majority of earthquakes in Hawaii take place on the Big Island, with minor shocks sometimes felt on Maui. The last locally generated tsunami occurred in 1975 following a magnitude 7.2 earthquake that jolted the Big Island. Seismic activity as far away as Australasia or Alaska can also cause tsunami events in the Hawaiian Islands.

Flora

Like Ecuador's Galapagos Islands in South America, the Hawaiian Islands spectacularly demonstrate Darwin's theory of adaptive radiation. All plant life that took root in this Polynesian archipelago originally arrived after drifting thousands of miles on the wind, the waves, or the wings of birds. Upon taking root, each type of plant had to adapt to its new environment, ultimately resulting in a rainbow of new species that are found only in this isolated island chain. In fact, botanists estimate that today there are at least 200 types of wild tree ferns alone growing here.

Starting around AD 500, the earliest human settlers arrived in long-distance seafaring canoes, bringing with them food and medicinal plants from elsewhere in Polynesia, including taro, coconuts, bananas, and sugarcane. Fast forward to the 19th century, when European, American, and Asian traders introduced exotic species into the fragile ecosystem of the Hawaiian Islands, while Hawaiians profitably harvested nearly all of the islands' sandalwood forests for export to China. Some of the newly introduced species of flora proved to be invasive, and today even more exotic plants arrive in Hawaii each year (e.g., in shipping containers or unwittingly stowed away in tourists' luggage). Other environmental threats include logging, grazing, agriculture, and tourist development. Today, Hawaii has the highest species extinction rate in the U.S. It is estimated that the islands have already lost almost half of their native forest cover.

But the news is not all bad. There is still an amazing diversity of flora for hikers to see on Maui, whether strolling on the beach or hiking deep in the rain forest, where wild orchids and ginger grow. Best of all, flowers bloom year-round in the Hawaiian Islands. The following are thumbnail descriptions of just a few of the most common plants seen along the island's hiking trails. For recommended field guides, turn to page 313.

The rarest plant of all is the threatened **silversword**. On Maui, silverswords only grow in the summit area of Haleakala volcano, where the plant's shiny silver leaves have adapted to reflect the intense solar radiation of high elevations from 7000 to 10,000 feet above sea level. Although a single plant can grow for up to 50 years, it blooms only once, at the end of its life cycle, when it shoots up a stalk of maroon blossoms before going to seed and dying. Another plant you'll find at high elevations in Haleakala's summit region is the **ohelo** shrub, which has serrated green leaves. A member of the cranberry family, its bright red berries are a favorite food of the nene (Hawaiian goose).

Also found colonizing ancient lava flows is **ohia lehua**, a versatile plant that can grow as a tree, shrub, or epiphytic vine, depending on the elevation of its immediate range, which can dip as low as 2000 feet. Ohia lehua, which happens to be the most common native forest tree in Hawaii, is easily recognized by its signature scarlet pom-pom flowers. Two other plants commonly seen on trails near the summit of Haleakala are **mamane**, which has oval green compound leaves and drooping clusters of star-shaped yellow flowers, and **pukiawe**, marked by five-pointed star-shaped white flowers and berries that vary in color from white to pink and red. Both of these alpine species can grow as either shrubs or trees, depending on environmental conditions.

Along Maui's beaches, you'll stumble across **naupaka**, a native shrub with thick, glossy green leaves and delicate white flowers streaked with purple that look as if they've been torn in half. **Pohuehue**, or beach morning glory, is another common coastal plant. Its tough vines, which help stabilize the sands, are twined with heart-shaped green leaves and delicate-looking pinkish or purplish flowers. Thorny **kiawe** (mesquite) and **ironwood** trees, the latter with drooping branches and shaggy needles, also help prevent beach erosion and may provide some welcome shade for beachgoers, but neither is native to the Hawaiian Islands.

Endemic coastal trees commonly seen include **coconut palms** and **hala** (screwpine, or pandanus). The latter has distinctive prop roots that support weak, brittle stems, which are often weighed down by green, pineapple-

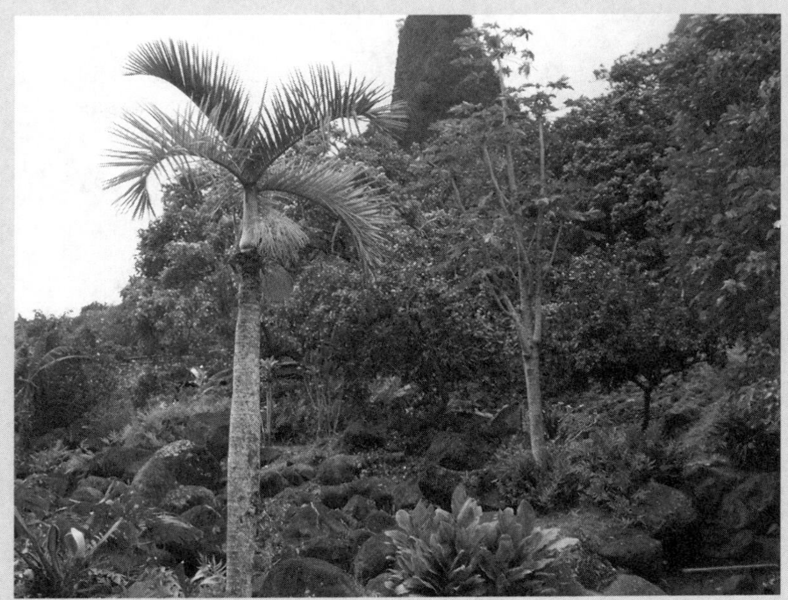

Hawaiian botanical gardens *flourish in Iao Valley.*

like female fruit that ripen into triangular orange seedpods. Traditionally in Hawaii, dried fiber strips from the plant's long, bladelike green leaves have been used for weaving (called *lauhala*). Not to be confused with hala, **hau** trees also have prop roots, but tend to grow together in dense, ankle-twisting thickets that pose a danger to hikers who don't watch their step. Hau trees can also be distinguished by their bright yellow flowers with dark red centers that open early in the morning, slowly change color over the course of a day to an orange or reddish hue, and then fall off in the evening.

Perhaps the most impressive native Hawaiian tree is **koa**, found at higher elevations up to 7500 feet. Starting off life looking like an oversized tree fern, these majestic beauties can grow up to a lofty 100 feet tall and are identified by their silver-green, sickle-shaped leaves and pale yellow pom-pom flowers. This hardwood has been traditionally harvested to make dugout canoes and surfboards, as well as for contemporary artistic carvings, furniture, and the tourist trade. Another native tree more commonly found in Maui's upland forests is the **kukui** (candlenut), which was brought to the islands by early Polynesian settlers. Its small, pale green leaves and tiny white flowers are less recognizable than its hard, dark brown nuts, which ancient Hawaiians used for candles and stringing lei. For hikers, fallen kukui nuts make trail surfaces slippery, especially when it rains.

Fauna

The story of Hawaii's fauna is similar to that of its flora (see the previous section), with adaptive radiation resulting in a spectacular array of species, especially among Maui's forest birds. Most species have evolved so far that they can't be traced to common ancestors elsewhere on earth.

Unfortunately, the modern introduction of both invasive and exotic species has taken a toll on the islands' endemic wildlife. Many native species have become extinct because of loss of habitat; predation by introduced species, especially feral pigs and grazing livestock; and exotic diseases, such as avian malaria (spread by mosquitoes), to which Hawaii's endemic birds have no natural immunity. Some native birds have evolved to lose some of their natural abilities, such as flight, making it even harder for them to escape from or defend themselves against predators.

Today, Hawaii has more fauna species that are either extinct or threatened than any other place in the U.S. Now, here's the good news: The islands also have just about the greatest diversity of native fauna of any state. Maui's immense variety of birds, as well as land and marine mammals, insects, and amphibians will not fail to impress even casual hikers. The following are brief descriptions of some of the most common wildlife seen while hiking on the island. For recommended field guides, turn to page 313.

The most diverse and colorful island bird family is the **honeycreepers**, which flit among Maui's upland forests, sipping nectar with their specially adapted bills. Although it is estimated that several dozen species of honeycreepers once existed in Hawaii, fewer than half are thought to still exist. Take heart that several colorful honeycreepers thrive on Maui. Often seen is the crimson-colored **apapane**, which has a black bill and white feathers under its tail. The **iiwi** also has bright red plumage, but sports an iconic curved orange bill. The yellow-green **amakihi**, identified by the brush-like black streak between its bill and each eye, is also common. The **Maui creeper** is similar in appearance to the amakihi, but it has a shorter, straight bill. A rarer honeycreeper is the **Maui parrotbill**, which uses its parrotlike beak to pry open plants to uncover the insects and grubs hidden within. The parrotbill can sometimes be spotted on guided hikes inside the Waikamoi Preserve, high on the slopes of Haleakala volcano (see the "Options" box on page 211).

On Maui, the bird that almost every hiker most wants to see is the **nene**, or **Hawaiian goose**. Hawaii's official state bird, this medium-sized goose has a black head, a buff-colored neck and cheek patches, and a grayish-brown body. On Maui, nene typically live in mountainous cloud forests and at higher elevations near the summit of Haleakala volcano, where they have evolved to walk on lava by losing some of the webbing on their feet. By the early 1950s, Hawaii's nene population was reduced to only about 30 birds, and so captive breeding programs were begun. Still an endangered species today, nene were first released back into the wild on Maui in Haleakala National Park in 1962. Now they can be spotted soaring across the volcano summit's cinder desert and rain forest, especially early in the morning and around sunset. The nene nesting season runs from October through March, when eggs are laid in shallow, bowl-shaped ground scrapes, usually hidden under vegetation. One of the biggest threats to nene is humans, sadly. Please do your part to help save these wild birds by driving slowly inside the park and by not feeding them or giving them water, as remaining untamed is critical to their survival.

Another endangered species that inhabits Haleakala National Park is the **uau**, or **Hawaiian petrel**. Averaging 16 inches long, these migratory seabirds are mostly black, with white foreheads and undersides. They nest from February through November inside underground burrows in the volcano's summit area and occasionally in the West Maui Mountains as well. These birds mainly feed on ocean squid, which requires making incredibly long flights from their homes at elevations of up to 10,000 feet down to sea level to feed. During these flights, petrels may become confused by the bright lights of developed areas and lose their way, becoming exhausted and eventually expiring on the ground, sometimes after fatally colliding with artificial objects.

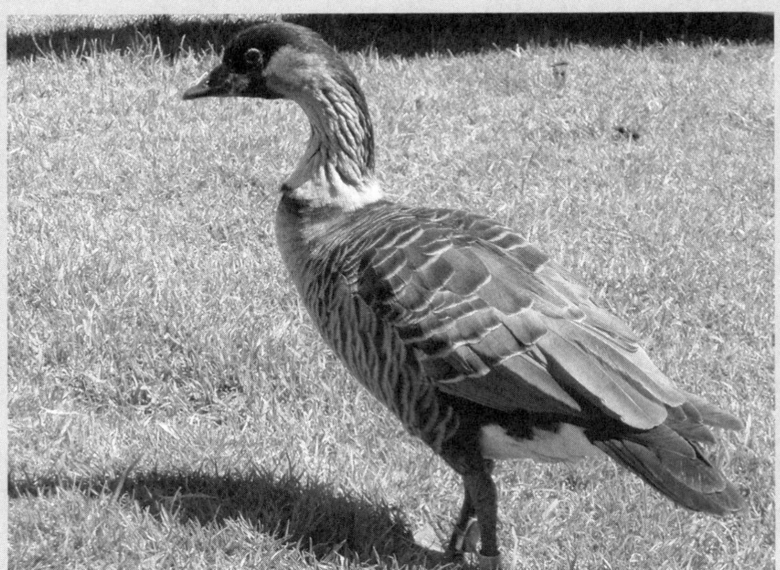

The endangered nene, *or Hawaiian goose, has made a comeback in Haleakala National Park.*

Another endangered resident of the national park—although its island-wide habitat extends all the way down to the coast—is the **opeapea**, or **Hawaiian hoary bat**, Hawaii's only native land mammal. Its name comes from the whitish tips of its body hair, which give it a "hoary" (aged) appearance. These bats usually roost in trees, although they have occasionally been known to inhabit lava tubes. They are most active in the early evening hours after dusk, when they fly and forage for insects. The endemic **pueo**, or **Hawaiian short-eared owl**, is most active during daylight hours, when it can be spotted flying over pastureland or in deep forests on the slopes of Haleakala. Like the Hawaiian petrel, these owls are particularly susceptible to light pollution.

Maui's coastal wetlands are excellent places to spot endemic and endangered waterbirds, as well as many migratory species. The plump-looking **alaekeokeo**, or **Hawaiian coot**, has a slate-gray body with a protruding frontal shield that can vary in color, but is often snow-white. The **aeo**, or **Hawaiian stilt**, is a noticeably skinnier bird, with black wings, back, and bill, a white forehead and underbelly, and long pink legs. The **koloa maoli**, or **Hawaiian duck**, are mottled brown and easy to recognize, though it's smaller than a mainland mallard. The **alea ula**, or **Hawaiian moorhen**, is seen more rarely, though its bright red frontal shield and bill really stand out against its black and dark-gray body with white feathers under its tail. Migratory birds include the **kolea**, or **Pacific golden plover**, spotted dark brown and gold. After flying south from their nesting grounds in Alaska, these plovers winter in Hawaii with their young between October and April. According to ancient Hawaiian legends, it was the kolea who guided the first Polynesians to this remote archipelago.

Naturally, Maui is home to an enormous variety of **fish** and other tropical coral-reef dwelling species, many of which can be seen while snorkeling at beaches near some of the island's hiking trails. Maui's most famous marine animal is the migratory **North Pacific humpback whale**, which can measure 45 feet long, weigh as much as 50 tons, and live for up to 50 years. Endangered after being hunted almost to extinction by the 1960s, populations of humpback whales are finally rebounding. Their recovery is thanks in part to protective legislation and the Hawaiian Islands Humpback Whale National Marine Sanctuary, which encompasses shallow ocean waters offshore from many Hawaiian Islands, including Maui, where humpback whales come to mate and give birth during the winter months. Whale-watching activity peaks between December and March, when you may spot these gigantic creatures breaching, blowing, and slapping the water off the West Maui and South Maui coasts.

Acrobatic **spinner dolphins** often come into Maui's protected bays to rest, including at the state's Ahihi-Kinau Natural Area Reserve in South

Maui. **Spotted dolphins** and **bottlenose dolphins** are two other common cetacean species seen in island waters. **Honu**, or **green sea turtles**, are the most abundant of Hawaii's three endemic species of sea turtles, which include the **leatherback** and **hawksbill**, all of which are endangered. Rarest of all are **Hawaiian monk seals**, likely so named for the cowl of skin at their necks, which resembles a Christian monk's clothing, as well as for their solitary habitats. These seals can live for 30 years, weigh up to 600 pounds, and measure almost 8 feet long. They mostly find shelter in the remote northwestern Hawaiian Islands, but recently have been hauling out on the beaches of the main islands, including Maui. If you are lucky enough to see any of these protected marine species, please help their chances of survival by not approaching or otherwise harassing them. Immediately report any monk seal sightings or marine mammal emergencies (e.g., injuries or entanglements) by calling (888) 256-9840.

Early Polynesian settlers were the first to import exotic species of wildlife to the Hawaiian Islands. They voyaged long distances from the South Pacific in their seafaring outrigger canoes packed with **pigs**, **dogs**, **rats**, **lizards**, **snails**, and **jungle fowl**. Beginning in the late 18th century, foreign explorers, traders, and settlers arrived in ships carrying **cattle**, **horses**, **sheep**, **goats**, **axis deer**, and various **game birds**. Many of these exotic grazing animals reproduced at unsustainably high rates, as they lacked any natural predators in Hawaii. This population explosion eventually decimated the island's natural ecosystems, wiping out an uncountable number of native plants and animals. Hunting is still a popular sport on Maui, mostly in forests where feral pigs, goats, axis deer, and game birds, such as **wild turkeys**, **quails**, **partridges**, **pheasants**, and **doves** survive.

In the early 19th century, whaling ships landing in Maui's busy port of Lahaina likely brought the first **mosquitoes** to the island, probably as sailors unloaded the ships' water casks. These mosquitoes carried malaria, which sickened Hawaii's human and animal populations, especially birds. Speaking of other pesky invaders, in the late 19th century, sugar plantation owners imported the **mongoose** to help control local rat populations in sugarcane fields. Unfortunately, the mongoose had no natural island predators, and has since adapted its diet to prey on the eggs of rare tropical birds, whose species extinction rate has been accelerated by these smart, ferocious hunters. Most hikers will rejoice that there are no snakes on Maui—at least, not yet.

When to Go

You can go hiking on Maui year-round. Average temperatures during midwinter (December to March) are less than 10°F lower than during the peak summer months (June to August). Year-round, ambient air temperatures range from the mid-60s into the high 80s. Winter brings Maui more frequent rain showers than other seasons, although most tropical storms don't last long. In summer, cooling trade winds make the island's hot, dry weather easier to bear. The hottest months are September and October, when island trade winds fade and ambient humidity can exceed 80 percent. April and May may be the most pleasant months for hiking—it's not too hot or humid, there are plenty of trade winds to cool things off, and it rains only occasionally. Peak tourist season runs from mid-December to mid-April and, to a lesser degree, from June through August. The autumn shoulder season (September to November) is the least busy time to visit Maui. Ocean waters are calmest then, too, before big winter storms arrive. Year-round, the island's tropical water temperatures average in the pleasantly warm mid-70s.

What determines the weather on Maui more than anything else is which side of the island you are on. The dry, leeward (western) side of the island experiences sunny weather year-round. The wet, windward (eastern) side of the island sees the most precipitation and cloudy conditions, thanks to Maui's high volcanic peaks, which prevent Pacific trade winds from passing overhead to the leeward side of the island. If it's raining in East Maui, you can probably still find a dry place to hike in South Maui or between Maalaea and Kapalua in West Maui. Otherwise, just wait out the inclement weather—chances are it will change in a few hours, or overnight. Consider carrying a lightweight waterproof jacket or poncho in your backpack at all times.

Elevation is also a major factor in the weather. In Maui's cloud-forest belt between 5000 and 7000 feet (e.g., at Polipoli Spring State Recreation Area and on the lower slopes of Haleakala volcano), it is often cold, rainy, and completely socked in. If you'll be hiking at elevations above 7000 feet in Haleakala National Park, beware that the weather in the park's summit area is more changeable than anywhere else on Maui. A day at high altitude that starts with sunshine and without a cloud in the sky can quickly turn rainy and cold. Overnight lows at the summit regularly dip below freezing, and daytime highs atop the volcano average just 50°F to 65°F year-round. Remember that you'll lose about 3°F for every 1000 feet of elevation gain, too. Expect it to be at least 30°F colder at the volcano summit than back down by the beach on the coast.

For island weather forecasts and current conditions, visit www.prh.noaa.gov/hnl online or call the National Weather Service recorded information line at (866) 944-5025.

Trail Selection

Only the premier dayhiking and overnight backpacking trips have been included in this book. Here you'll find trails suited to all levels of ability and interests. All of the trails selected for this guide offer scenic beauty and ease of access for hikers. Together, these trails represent the island's incredible diversity of ecological systems and environments, from lava flows and multi-colored cinder cones to cloud forests filled with native birdsong and hidden waterfalls. Some of the hiking trails described in this book are popular with both locals and visitors, while others are seldom trodden.

More than 80 percent of the hikes in this guide start and end in the same place. Of the remaining seven point-to-point hikes, one can be hiked as a long out-and-back trip simply by retracing your steps or walking along the highway back to the trailhead; one has a resort-sponsored shuttle to the trailhead; and two have an official hitchhiking zone from a hikers' parking lot to the trailhead. Only three hikes included in this guide are true point-to-point trails that require shuttling two vehicles (or alternatively, a friend to drop you off at the trailhead and pick you up at the other end). Of these three shuttle hikes, only one—the Skyline Trail from the summit area of Haleakala National Park down into Polipoli Spring State Recreation Area—might require a 4WD vehicle for access.

Other trails in Polipoli Spring State Recreation Area have not been included in this guide for a variety of reasons, including difficulty of access, shared use with hunters and mountain bikers, severe trail erosion, and the danger of falling trees in forests recently devastated by fire. Elsewhere, trails that enter private property without permission and violate posted NO TRESPASSING (KAPU) signs have not been included, out of respect for island residents.

Features & Facilities

Even on a relatively small tropical island like Maui, which has just 120 miles of shoreline and covers only 729 square miles of land, you'll find a surprising diversity of terrain. Island ecosystems start with coastal beach shrublands and range up through misty cloud forests and over knife-edged forest ridges to the summit of Haleakala volcano at 10,023 feet above sea level. See also the Using Top Trails section (page xvi) and overview table (page viii) near the front of this guide for a run-down of specific trail features and facilities, as well as what type of terrain you can expect from each.

On Maui, hikers will discover many treats that tourists who never leave the beach behind miss. To start with, there are plenty of coastal trails to pick from, ranging from peaceful boardwalks beloved by birders to beachfront recreational paths to adventurous hikes over lava flows. Today, a few coastal routes in South and East Maui still follow the historic King's Highway, which once laid unbroken around the entire island. In West Maui, you can also hike to ancient petroglyph sites, natural ocean baths, and lava-rock blowholes, and along forested ridgelines from misty mountain summits all the way down to the sea. If it's your first time visiting Maui, you won't want to miss Haleakala National Park. The park's volcanic summit region is a natural wonderland, comprising a kaleidoscopic cinder desert and lush rain forest. Meanwhile, beyond the end of East Maui's famously scenic Road to Hana, the park's coastal Kipahulu area is famous for its cascading waterfall pools and musical bamboo groves inside native rain forest.

Multiple Uses

All of the trails described in this book are suitable for hiking. Coastal hikes are mostly level, and appropriate for runners. Trail running is also a popular pursuit on a few mountain trails, from lowland forests right up to the summit of the Haleakala volcano. Only a few trails on Maui are open to mountain bikers, and the majority of these are in Polipoli Spring State Recreation Area; only one of these trails, the Skyline Trail, is also suitable for hiking, and so I've included it in this book. Guided horseback rides are available on the Sliding Sands Trail in the summit region of Haleakala National Park. At press time, the only company offering these trail rides was Pony Express Tours; make reservations in advance online at www.ponyexpresstours.com or by calling (808) 667-2200. Note that many hiking trails on Maui expressly prohibit mountain bikes, horses, and all motorized vehicles. Three of the coastal trails included in this book are suitable for wheelchair access, either via pavement or level boardwalks.

In Haleakala National Park, dogs are not allowed on any unpaved trails. Leashed dogs are allowed on the national park's paved paths and roadways, in parking lots, and at campgrounds. Working guide dogs are legally allowed inside all national park buildings. If you have a documented disability, ask a park ranger about hiking with your guide dog. In Maui's state parks, dogs are not allowed in campgrounds or cabins, at picnic pavilions, on beaches, or at any other swimming areas. With a maximum six-foot leash, dogs are allowed on Maui's state park trails, unless otherwise posted. For all other island trails, regulations regarding dogs varies. Details are given with individual hike descriptions later in this book.

Trail Safety

One of the biggest dangers for hikers on Maui is **flash floods**, which can be fatal. Several hikers have lost their lives to flash floods on Maui, including in the Kipahulu section of Haleakala National Park, as well as on waterfall and streamside trails on the island's windward (eastern) side. Always check the weather forecast before setting out on the trail, especially if you'll be crossing any streams or hiking through valleys prone to flash floods. If rain is predicted or dark clouds appear in the sky, do not start hiking (if you're already on the trail, turn back immediately or get to higher ground). When in doubt, pick a different hike—there are plenty to choose from on Maui, and it's usually not raining everywhere on the island at the same time. Be cautious walking around or swimming in waterfalls, because of the ever-present danger of **rockfall**, which also makes **climbing cliffs** on Maui's crumbly volcanic terrain a risky proposition. Keep in mind that some waterfalls, no matter how tempting they look, are simply too dangerous to swim in (e.g., waterfalls alongside the Pipiwai Trail in the Kipahulu section of Haleakala National Park). If you hear a **tsunami** warning siren while hiking on Maui's trails, evacuate from coastal areas immediately and seek higher ground. For tsunami updates, listen to almost any major island frequency on your vehicle's radio; call the Pacific Tsunami Warning Center at (808) 689-8207; or check online at www.prh.noaa.gov/ptwc.

Another serious danger for hikers on Maui is the trifecta of **dehydration**, **heat exhaustion**, and **heatstroke**, which can be fatal if not noticed in time and treated properly. Be prepared to start hiking early in the day, especially on the leeward side of the island and during the hottest months of the year (see the "When to Go" section, page 10). If you're going to be trekking across lava fields (e.g., South Maui's Hoapili Trail or in the summit area of Haleakala National Park) or up exposed mountain trails that lack shade (e.g., West Maui's Lahaina Pali Trail), plan to start hiking around dawn, stay properly hydrated (don't wait until you're already thirsty to drink), and carry plenty of extra water. Know the symptoms of heat exhaustion and heatstroke, and hike with a buddy if you can. Sunglasses, a wide-brimmed sun hat, and water-resistant sunscreen with a high SPF factor are all essential.

You must boil, filter, or otherwise treat all freshwater sources on Maui, as bacterial and parasitic microscopic organisms are omnipresent. **Giardia** and **leptospirosis** are the most common illnesses caused by drinking contaminated water. The latter can also result from swimming, wading or hiking in freshwater streams, ponds, or waterfall pools contaminated by animal urine and feces; infection is more likely if you have any open cuts. Wash your hands frequently and consider carrying a small bottle of hand sanitizer with you on the trail. **Dengue fever**, a viral illness transmitted by infected *Aedes* mosquitoes, is so far uncommon in Hawaii, with the last serious outbreak on Maui occurring from 2001 to 2002. Apply insect repellent to avoid mosquito bites, especially on the windward side of the island in East Maui, particularly around Hana town.

When hiking at **high elevations** (e.g., the summit area of Haleakala National Park), come prepared to experience any kind of weather, no matter what time of year it is and regardless of the weather forecast. Dress warmly and bring waterproof layers. Remember that **hypothermia** can occur in wet, windy conditions, even when the temperature stays above freezing. Wear plenty of sunscreen to protect yourself from the intense solar radiation. A few visitors experience **altitude sickness**, also known as acute mountain sickness (AMS), while atop the volcano, as the sudden change in elevation from sea level to summit can cause shortness of breath, hyperventilation, fatigue, weakness, dizziness, nausea, and difficulty sleeping. If symptoms do not resolve, the best treatment is to descend rapidly in elevation. Scuba divers must not travel to high elevations for at least 24 to 48 hours after their last dive. Pregnant women, young children, and anyone with heart, respiratory, or obesity medical issues should also consider avoiding the Haleakala summit region.

On some public lands on Maui, hunting is allowed. Usually, posted entry signs will warn you of the possible presence of **hunters** and let you know if it's currently open season or not. In popular hunting areas (e.g., Polipoli Spring State Recreation Area), hikers should keep their wits about them and consider wearing a safety vest or bright orange-colored clothing to warn hunters of their presence. Sticking to the trail is always a wise idea to minimize accidental interaction with hunters. In many of these hunting areas, you may also run into **wild boars** and **hunting dogs** off-leash. Give these animals a wide berth to avoid any ill-fated encounters. On a few hiking trails that skirt private property, you may also run into off-leash **guard dogs**, whose bite may indeed be as bad as their bark. When possible, politely ask the owners to leash the dogs until you pass by. Otherwise, consider turning back.

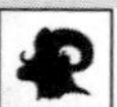

Warning

Unfortunately, vehicle break-ins are commonplace on Maui. Rental cars left at beach parking lots and trailheads are especially popular targets. Before leaving your vehicle parked anywhere on the island, make sure no valuable items are visible inside. Some locals advise leaving your vehicle completely unlocked with the windows rolled down, to show that there are no valuables hidden inside, which may deter any thieves from damaging the car to break into it. Thieves often hang out at popular tourist destinations, sizing up arriving vehicles for their potential value, so don't open your trunk in public places. If you decide to leave any of your belongings locked in the trunk, stow them there before arriving at the trailhead or parking area.

Don't rely on **cell phones** or **handheld GPS receivers** while hiking on Maui. The island's coastal trails typically enjoy decent cell phone reception and GPS coverage, but inland valleys, thick forests, and mountain peaks may have none whatsoever. Adverse weather, tall trees, and various topographical features can also prevent cell phones and GPS units from functioning.

Camping, Cabins & Permits

In Haleakala National Park, wilderness permits are only required for overnight trips into the summit area backcountry (for national park entry fees and passes, see page 198). You'll need a wilderness permit regardless of whether you are backpacking and carrying your own camping gear, or staying in the historic wilderness cabins at Holua, Kapalaoa, or Paliku. Each wilderness cabin has wood-burning and propane stoves, cookware and padded bunk beds, but no electricity; pit toilets are located nearby outside. Nonpotable water is usually available at the cabins, except occasionally during times of drought, when you must pack in all water. Reservations for cabins are accepted up to 90 days in advance online (https://fhnp.org/wcr), by calling (808) 572-4400 between 1 PM and 3 PM HST, or in person at the park headquarters' visitor center in the summit area. The standard nightly rate for wilderness cabin stays is $75, or $60 if you make your reservation less than 21 days in advance.

For overnight camping trips (i.e., not staying in the cabins), wilderness permits are free and not subject to daily trailhead quotas; no reservations are accepted. Backcountry camping is permitted only in designated areas at Holua and Paliku, where pit toilets and nonpotable water (except during occasional times of drought) are available. Backpackers may use the pit toilets and nonpotable water at Kapalaoa cabin, although camping there is prohibited. Whether you are staying in a cabin or camping, you must pick up your wilderness permit in person at the park headquarters' visitor center between 8 AM and 3 PM daily. Wilderness camping and cabin stays in the park are limited to 3 days in any 30-day period, with a 2-night maximum at any one backcountry site. The maximum group size is 12 people.

Haleakala National Park is also the best place for car camping on Maui, but don't expect well-equipped individual campsites like on the U.S. mainland. There are free drive-up dispersed camping areas at Hosmer Grove in the summit area of the national park and at Kipahulu in the park's coastal section. Both camping areas are little more than grassy meadows, outfitted with a few picnic tables, BBQ grills, and pit toilets. Dispersed camping is available on a first-come, first-served basis; reservations are not accepted for either camping area. Drinking water is available only at Hosmer Grove,

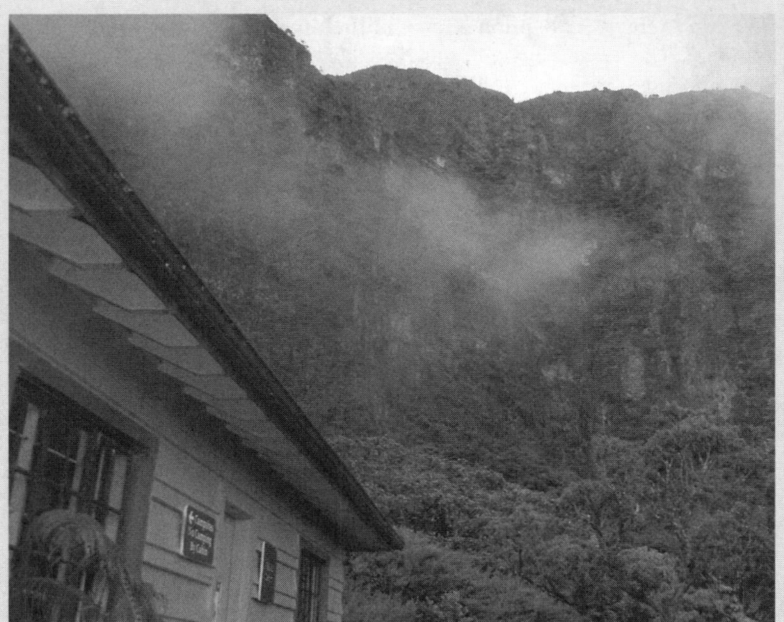

A historic 1930s-era wilderness cabin *beckons to backpackers atop Haleakala.*

located in the cloud forest on the volcano's slopes at an elevation of almost 7000 feet. The weather is often rainy and cold there, with overnight temperatures that can dip below freezing. The camping area at Kipahulu is situated on ocean bluffs, and can be either rainy or extremely sunny. Mosquitoes can be quite pesky there, so bring plenty of insect repellent, plus all the drinking water you'll need. Kipahulu is usually quieter than Hosmer Grove, which tends to be overcrowded and noisy, especially on weekends. Inside the park, car camping is limited to three nights per month at each campground with a maximum group size of 12 people. The Hosmer Grove campground, with a maximum capacity of 50 campers, may fill up, especially on weekends, so arrive early. Kipahulu (limit 100 campers) rarely fills.

Maui's state parks and recreation areas are less desirable places to camp or rent a cabin. In East Maui, coastal Waianapanapa State Park north of Hana is a popular place to camp, next to a black sand beach. The park also offers simple housekeeping cabins that have kitchens, bathrooms, cots, electricity, and hot showers; the maximum group size is six people. Located at an elevation above 6000 feet in dense cloud forest, Polipoli Spring State Recreation Area is very remote and usually only accessible by 4WD vehicle. It's lonely campground and housekeeping cabin (eight-person maximum) is typically frequented by hunters, not hikers. Camping at Maui's state parks costs $18 per night for up to six people, plus $3 for each additional person (children age 2 and under are free), with a maximum of $30 per night; Hawaii residents pay $12, plus $2 for each additional person, with a maximum of $20 per night. State park cabins cost from $90 per night for up to six people at Waianapanapa SP (eight people at Polipoli Spring SRA), or $60 for Hawaii residents. The maximum length of stay in any state park is five consecutive nights. For online reservations, visit https://camping.ehawaii.gov; otherwise, you must apply for a permit in person at a Hawaii State Parks district office, since mail-in applications are no longer accepted.

Maui's county parks are not always safe places to camp. Although located attractively near the beach, these roadside campgrounds tend to be popular places for late-night carousing and sometimes crime. Ask locals for advice first if you plan to camp at any county parks on Maui. At press time, camping was allowed at Papalaua Wayside Park, south of Lahaina in West Maui; and Kanaha Beach Park, near the airport in Central Maui. Papalaua is generally the safer of the two, although it has no drinking water and is currently closed on Mondays and Tuesdays for maintenance. Both campgrounds have picnic tables, BBQ grills, and swimming areas. Kanaha also has outdoors showers and potable water. To camp at Maui's county parks, you must reserve a permit. Fees range from $1 to $8 per person per night, depending on each camper's age, whether they live in Hawaii, and whether it's a weekday or weekend. There's a three-night camping limit at Maui County parks. Download mail-in camping permit applications in advance from the county parks website at www.co.maui.hi.us/parks.

Contact details for all national, state, and county parks and permit offices on Maui are provided in Appendix 2 (page 307).

Outside of Haleakala National Park, most hikes in this book do *not* require permits or entrance fees. To access a few trails in West Maui, hikers are currently required to self-register and sign a liability release; details about obtaining any necessary permits are given in the "Permits & Maps" section at the start of the "West Maui" chapter, page 28. West Maui is also currently home to the only private campground on Maui, Camp Olowalu. Located on the coast about 6 miles south of Lahaina, this private group retreat makes its 36 tent camping sites available on a first-come, first-served basis. Staff also rent camping equipment. Campground amenities include outdoor and enclosed cold showers, portable toilets, picnic tables, and drinking water. Rates are currently $10 per adult per night, plus $5 for each child ages 6 to 12 (children 5 and younger are free). The campground is about a half mile north of mile marker (MM) 14 on the *makai* (ocean) side of the Honoapiilani Highway (Hwy. 30). For more information, visit www.campolowalu.com online or call (808) 661-4303.

Note from the Author

In 2009 I rehiked every trail described in this guide. Many of the trails were old friends that I'd hiked several times before when I lived on Maui, as well as during frequent return visits to the island. Access to a few old favorites, like the Blue Pool off the Hana Highway, had sadly been closed, usually because of overcrowding or disrespectful use by nonresidents. Keep in mind that trail access on Maui can be fickle: A trail that was open to hikers when I researched this book may suddenly close if a private landowner decides to revoke thru-hiking privileges, so always have a back-up plan or another hike nearby that you're interested in doing that day. Future updates for this book will be posted online at www.toptrailsmaui.blogspot.com, where feedback and comments from enthusiastic hikers like you are always welcome.

While on Maui, please do your part to care for all of these wonderful trails, as well as the natural environment and Hawaii's cultural heritage, by showing plenty of *aloha aina* (literally, "love for the land" in the Hawaiian language). Practicing "Leave No Trace" principles is the best way to guarantee that these trails stay open. As a last word of advice, be careful out there. Although I've hiked and backpacked on six continents and have some wilderness medical training, while researching this book I suffered heat exhaustion that could easily have become life-threatening heatstroke. Emergencies can happen to anyone in the wilderness, even those who are well-prepared, experienced, and physically fit. Take care of yourself and the land, and have responsible fun out there. *Maui no ka oi* ("Maui is the best!").

On the Trail

Every outing should begin with proper preparation, which usually takes only a few minutes. Even the easiest trail can turn up unexpected surprises. People seldom think about getting lost or injured, but unexpected things can and do happen. Simple precautions can make the difference between a good story and a dangerous situation.

Use the Top Trails ratings and descriptions to determine if a particular trail is a good match with your fitness and energy level, given current conditions and the time of year.

Have a Plan

Choose Wisely The first step to enjoying any trail is to match the trail to your abilities. It's no use overestimating your experience or fitness—know your abilities and limitations, and use the Top Trails difficulty rating that accompanies each trail.

Leave Word About Your Plans The most basic of precautions is leaving word of your intentions with friends or family. Many people will hike the backcountry their entire lives without ever relying on this safety net, but establishing this simple habit is free insurance.

It's best to leave specific information—location, trail name, and intended time of travel—with a responsible person. However, if this is not possible or if plans change at the last minute, you should still leave word. If there is a registration process available, make use of it. If there is a ranger station, trail register, or visitor center, check in.

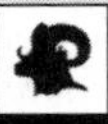

Prepare and Plan

- Know your abilities and your limitations.
- Leave word about your plans with family and friends.
- Know the area and the route.

Review the Route Before embarking on any hike, read the entire description and study the map. It isn't necessary to memorize every detail, but it is worthwhile to have a clear mental picture of the trail and the general area.

If the trail or terrain are complex, augment the trail guide with a topographic map. Maps and information about current weather and trail conditions are often available from local ranger and park stations—resources worth using.

Carry the Essentials

Proper preparation for any type of trail use includes gathering certain essential items to carry. Trip checklists will vary tremendously by trail and conditions.

Clothing When the weather is good, light, comfortable clothing is the obvious choice. It's easy to believe that very little spare clothing is needed, but a prepared hiker has something tucked away for any emergency, from a surprise shower to an unexpected overnight in a remote area.

Clothing includes proper footwear, essential for hiking and running trails. As a trail becomes more demanding, you will need footwear that performs. Running shoes are fine for many trails. If you will be carrying substantial weight or encountering sustained rugged terrain, step up to hiking boots.

In hot, sunny weather, proper clothing includes a hat, sunglasses, a long-sleeved shirt, and sunscreen. In cooler weather, particularly when it's wet, carry waterproof outer garments and quick-drying undergarments (avoid cotton). As a general rule, whatever the conditions, bring layers that can be combined or removed to provide comfort and protection from the elements in a wide variety of conditions.

Water Never embark on a trail without carrying water. At all times, particularly in warm weather, adequate water is of key importance. Experts recommend at least 2 quarts of water per day, and when hiking in heat a gallon or more may be more appropriate. At the extreme, dehydration can be life threatening. More commonly, inadequate water brings fatigue and muscle aches.

For most outings, unless the day is very hot or the trail very long, plan to carry sufficient water for the entire trail. Unfortunately, in Hawaii natural water sources are questionable, generally loaded with various risks, including bacteria, viruses, and fertilizers.

Water Treatment If it's necessary to make use of trailside water, you should filter or treat it. There are three methods for treating water: boiling, chemical treatment, and filtering. Boiling is best, but often impractical—it requires a heat source, a pot, and time. Chemical treatments, available in sporting goods stores, handle some problems, including the troublesome giardia parasite, but will not combat many artificial chemical pollutants. The preferred method is filtration, which removes giardia and other contaminants and doesn't leave an unpleasant aftertaste.

If this hasn't convinced you to carry all the water you need, one final admonishment: Be prepared for surprises. Water sources described in the text or on maps can change course or dry up completely. Never run your water bottle dry in expectation of the next source; fill up when water is available and always keep a little in reserve.

Food While not as critical as water, food is energy—don't underestimate its importance. Avoid foods that are hard to digest, such as candy bars and potato chips. Carry high energy, fast-digesting foods: nutrition bars, dehydrated fruit, gorp, and jerky. Bring a little extra food—it's good protection against an outing that turns unexpectedly long, perhaps because of weather or losing your way.

Useful but Less than Essential Items

Map & Compass (& the Know-How to Use Them) Many trails don't require much navigation, meaning a map and compass aren't always as essential as water or food—but it can be a close call. If the trail is remote or infrequently visited, a map and compass should be considered necessities. A handheld GPS unit is also a useful trail companion, but is no substitute for a map and compass; knowing your longitude and latitude is not much help without a map. (The GPS coordinates listed for key trail locations in this guide are in decimal degrees.)

Cell Phone Most populated areas of the main Hawaiian Islands, and even a few remote destinations, have some level of cellular coverage. In extreme circumstances, a cell phone can be a lifesaver. But don't depend on it; coverage is unpredictable and batteries fail. And be sure that the occasion warrants the phone call—a blister doesn't justify a call to search and rescue.

Gear Depending on the remoteness and rigor of the trail, there are many additional useful items to consider, such as a pocketknife, flashlight, fire source (waterproof matches, light, or flint), and first-aid kit.

Every member of your party should carry the appropriate essential items described above; groups often split up or get separated along the trail. Solo hikers should be even more disciplined about preparation, and carry more gear. Traveling solo is inherently more risky. This isn't meant to discourage solo travel, simply to emphasize the need for extra preparation.

Trail Etiquette

The overriding rule on the trail is "Leave No Trace." Interest in visiting natural areas continues to increase in Hawaii, even as the quantity of unspoiled natural areas continues to shrink. These pressures make it ever more critical that we leave no trace of our visits.

Never Litter If you carried it in, it's easy enough to carry it out. Leave the trail in the same, if not better, condition than you find it. Try picking up any litter you encounter and packing it out—it's a great feeling! Just one piece of garbage and you've made a difference.

Stay on the Trail Paths have been created, sometimes over many years, for many purposes: to protect the surrounding natural areas, to avoid dangers, and to provide the best route. Leaving the trail can cause damage that takes years to undo. Never cut switchbacks. Shortcutting rarely saves energy or time, and trampling plant life takes a terrible toll on the land and hastens erosion. Moreover, safety and consideration intersect on the trail. It's hard to get truly lost if you stay on the trail.

Share the Trail The best trails attract many visitors, and you should be prepared to share the trail with others. Do your part to minimize impact. Commonly accepted trail etiquette dictates that bike riders yield to both hikers and equestrians, hikers yield to horseback riders, downhill hikers yield to uphill hikers, and everyone stays to the right. Not everyone knows these rules of the road, so let common sense and good humor be the final guide.

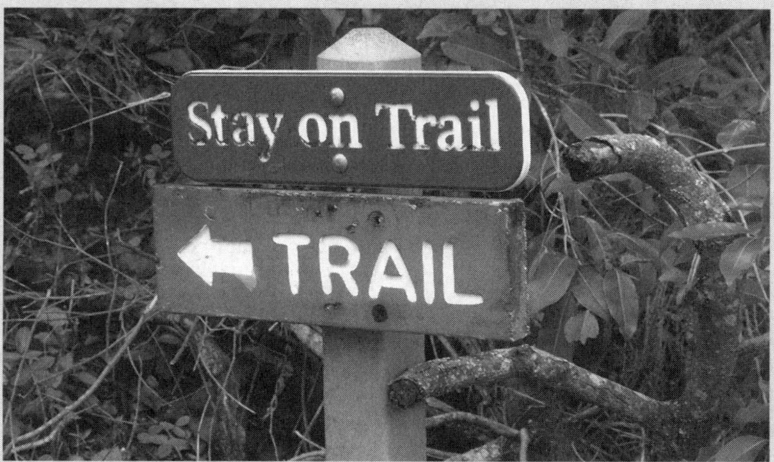

Rest assured *that helpful signs point the way.*

Trail Etiquette

- Leave no trace. Never litter.
- Stay on the trail. Never cut switchbacks.
- Share the trail. Use courtesy and common sense.
- Leave it there. Don't disturb wildlife.

Leave It There Destruction or removal of plants, animals, or historical, prehistoric, or geological items is certainly unethical and almost always illegal.

Getting Lost If you become lost on the trail, stay on the trail. Stop and take stock of the situation. In many cases, a few minutes of calm reflection will yield a solution. Consider all the clues available; use the sun to identify directions if you don't have a compass. If you determine that you are indeed lost, stay on the main trail and stay put. You are more likely to encounter other people if you stay in one place.

Map Legend

Trail
Other Trail
Freeway
Road
Railroad
Viewpoint
Feature
Picnic Area
Gate
Start/Finish — start & finish
River
Stream
Seasonal Stream
Body of Water
Marsh/Swamp
Dam
Peak
Park/Forest
North Arrow — N

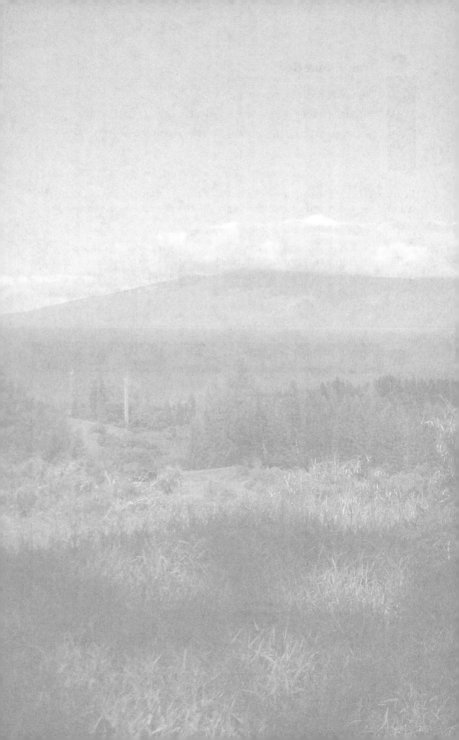

CHAPTER 1

West Maui

1. Olowalu Petroglyphs
2. Kaanapali Beach Walk
3. Kapalua Coastal Trail
4. Kapalua Village Trails
5. Maunalei Arboretum & Honolua Ridge
6. Mahana Ridge
7. Nakalele Blowhole
8. Ohai Trail
9. Kahekili Highway Ocean Baths
10. Waihee Ridge
11. Waihee Valley
12. Lahaina Pali

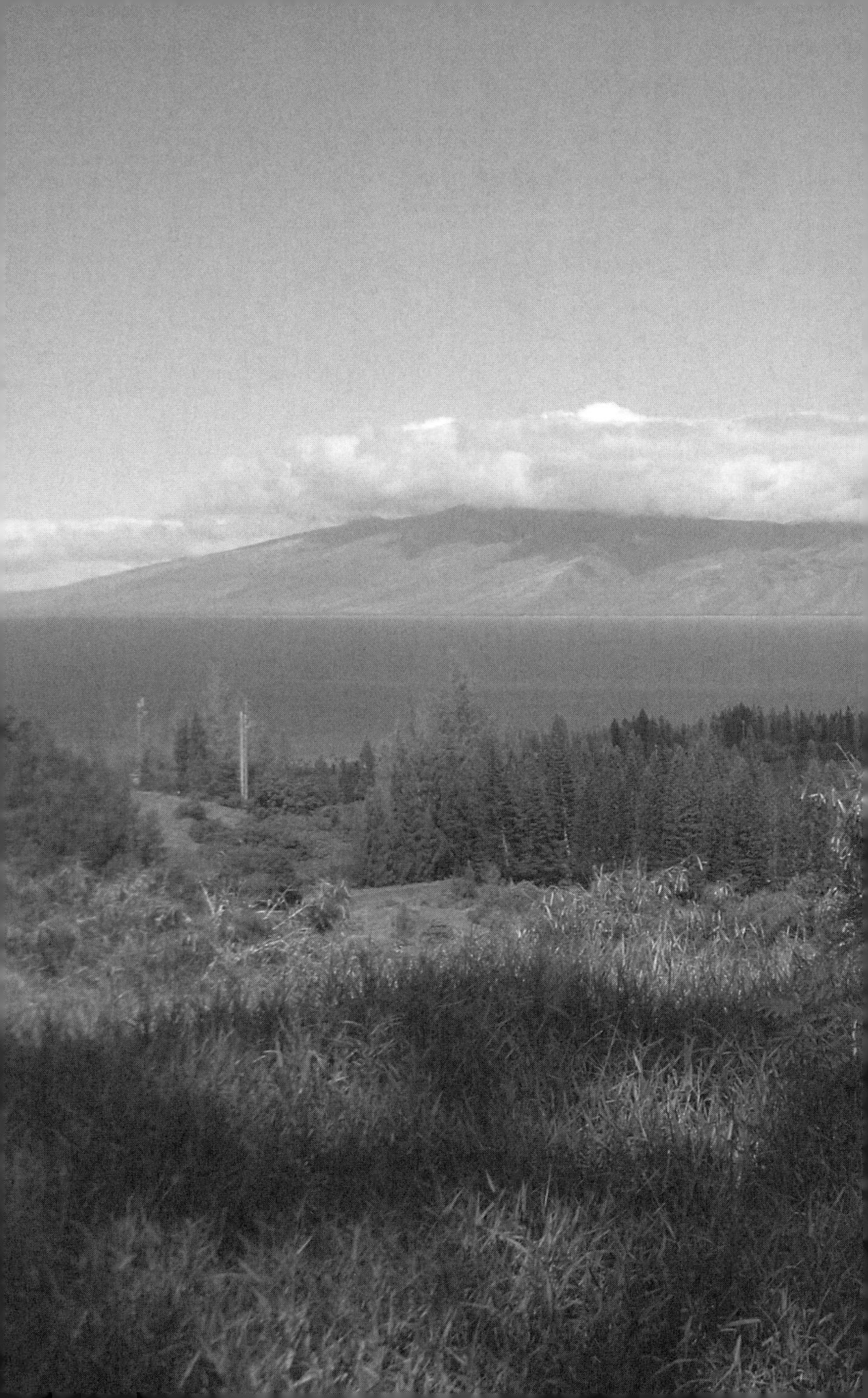

West Maui

Anchored by the historic whaling seaport of Lahaina and backed by enchantingly eroded peaks, **West Maui** attracts more first-time visitors than anywhere else on the island. Maui's favorite vacationland abounds with high-rise resort hotels and condominiums, golden sand beaches, and reliably sunny weather (in fact, sometimes it's too hot—*lahaina* means "cruel sun" in the Hawaiian language).

For hikers, West Maui offers an interesting variety of trails on just about every kind of terrain. Take a scenic oceanside ramble, run on a beachfront recreational path, or hike inland to a Hawaiian petroglyph site, all a short drive from Lahaina. Farther north along the West Maui coast at Kapalua, hardier hiking trails ascend razorback ridges and reach head-spinning viewpoints of the Pacific, then tumble back downhill toward the sea.

The remote jungle heart of the West Maui Mountains is largely inaccessible to hikers, as it's now a protected watershed reserve. The range's highest peak, Puu Kukui (5788 feet), receives more than 385 inches of rainfall in an average year, making it the second wettest place in the Hawaiian Islands (after Kauai's Mt. Waialeale). On the east side of the mountains, West Maui's windward coast is more lush, with fast-flowing streams, spritely waterfalls, spouting lava-rock blowholes, and natural ocean baths all accessible via trails off the Kahekili Highway, a favorite scenic drive for daytrippers.

Closer to Kahului and Wailuku, the Waihee Ridge Trail climbs to a viewpoint where you can gaze deep into the interior of the mountains. Nearby, the family-friendly Waihee Valley hike crosses swinging cable bridges to reach hidden waterfall pools. For a challenge, the sun-baked Lahaina Pali Trail follows a historic footpath and horseback route over the West Maui Mountains, granting panoramic views of Maalaea Bay.

Overleaf and opposite: *Panoramas of Molokai await on trails above West Maui's Kapalua resort.*

Permits & Maps

No permits or fees are required for hiking most trails described in this chapter, all of which are dayhikes. At Kapalua, hikers must sign a liability waiver inside the resort's Kapalua Adventure Center before hiking the resort's Kapalua Village, Maunalei Arboretum, and Honolua Ridge or Mahana Ridge trails (Trails 4, 5, and 6). Currently, no fees are charged to hike these trails, to park at the Kapalua Adventure Center, or to ride the resort's shuttle to the arboretum trailhead. The Waihee Valley Trail (Trail 11) passes over privately owned land; hikers must pay an entrance fee and sign a liability waiver. For more details, see the relevant hike descriptions later in this chapter.

Topographic maps are not necessary for any of the hikes in this chapter. At the Kaanapali and Kapalua resorts, coastal walking trails are clearly marked. Trails starting off the Kahekili Highway are usually not signposted, but distances are generally short and it's usually easy to follow the crowds, or even sight the trail's end from your starting point. The Lahaina Pali and Waihee Ridge trails have signposted trailheads and distance markers along their clearly laid-out routes. For the Olowalu Petroglyphs and Waihee Valley trails, the written directions and basic trail maps in this book should suffice. At the Kapalua Resort, the paved Kapalua Village Trails, the short Maunalei Arboretum nature trails, and the longer Honolua and Mahana Ridge trails are all marked and clearly signposted, often with laminated trail maps posted. Free hiking brochure booklets with basic trail descriptions and sketch maps are available from the resort's Kapalua Adventure Center. For more detailed topographic maps of West Maui, the USGS 7.5-minute (1:24,000) series does not show any of the trails described in this chapter except the coastal paths.

See Appendix 3 (page 312) for more recommended topographical and driving maps, both digital and printed, to help you navigate around Maui.

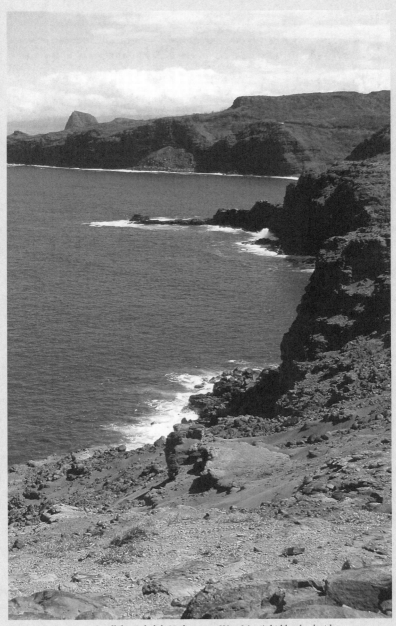

Ocean waves crash *off the Kahekili Highway on West Maui's hidden back side.*

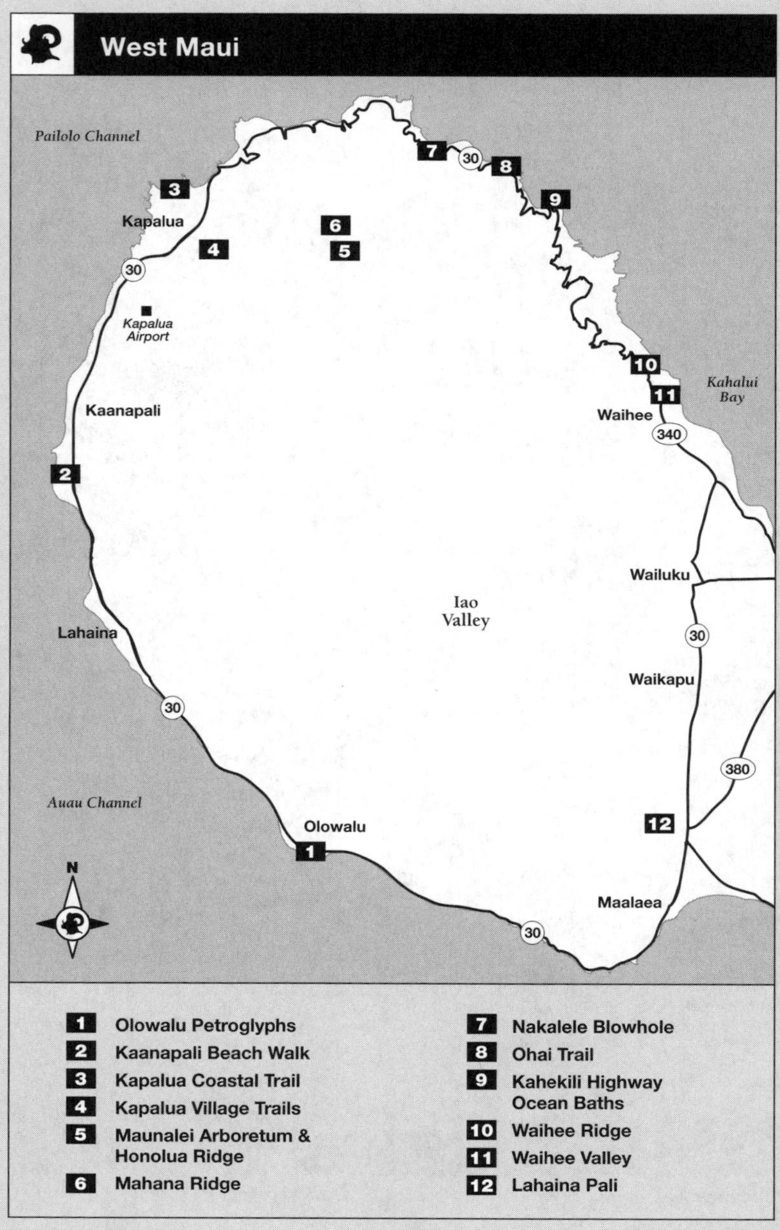
West Maui
Pailolo Channel
Kapalua
Kapalua Airport
Kaanapali
Lahaina
Auau Channel
Olowalu
Iao Valley
Kahalui Bay
Waihee
Wailuku
Waikapu
Maalaea
N
30
340
380
1 Olowalu Petroglyphs
2 Kaanapali Beach Walk
3 Kapalua Coastal Trail
4 Kapalua Village Trails
5 Maunalei Arboretum & Honolua Ridge
6 Mahana Ridge
7 Nakalele Blowhole
8 Ohai Trail
9 Kahekili Highway Ocean Baths
10 Waihee Ridge
11 Waihee Valley
12 Lahaina Pali

TRAIL FEATURES TABLE

West Maui

TRAIL	Difficulty	Length	Type	USES & ACCESS	TERRAIN	FLORA & FAUNA	OTHER
1	1	1.0	Out & Back	Dayhiking, Child Friendly		Native Plants	Archaeological, Secluded
2	2	2.8	Out & Back	Dayhiking, Running, Wheelchair Access, Child Friendly, Dogs Allowed	Beach	Native Plants, Tide Pools, Wildlife	Great Views, Swimming
3	2	3.0	Out & Back	Dayhiking, Running, Child Friendly, Dogs Allowed	Beach	Native Plants	Great Views, Swimming
4	3	3.9	Semiloop	Dayhiking, Running, Dogs Allowed, Permit Required	Pond	Birds	Great Views, Steep
5	2	3.0	Semiloop	Dayhiking, Child Friendly, Permit Required	Forest, Mountain, Summit, Stream	Birds, Native Plants	Great Views, Historic Interest, Secluded, Shady
6	4	6.5	Point-to-Point	Dayhiking, Permit Required	Beach, Forest, Mountain, Summit, Stream	Birds, Native Plants	Great Views, Swimming, Secluded, Shady, Steep
7	2	0.9	Out & Back	Dayhiking	Lava Flow	Tide Pools	Great Views, Geologic Interest, Steep
8	1	1.3	Semiloop	Dayhiking, Child Friendly		Birds, Native Plants	Great Views
9	2	0.6	Out & Back	Dayhiking	Lava Flow	Tide Pools	Great Views, Swimming, Steep
10	3	5.0	Out & Back	Dayhiking, Running, Dogs Allowed	Forest, Mountain, Summit	Birds, Native Plants, Wildlife	Great Views, Secluded, Shady, Steep
11	3	4.0	Out & Back	Dayhiking, Child Friendly, Permit Required	Forest, Stream, Waterfall	Birds, Native Plants, Wildlife	Swimming, Secluded, Shady
12	5	5.0	Point-to-Point	Dayhiking, Dogs Allowed	Mountain	Native Plants	Great Views, Historic Interest, Steep

USES & ACCESS
- Dayhiking
- Backpacking
- Running
- Biking
- Wheelchair Access
- Child Friendly
- Dogs Allowed
- Permit Required

TYPE
- Loop
- Out & Back
- Semiloop
- Point-to-Point

DIFFICULTY
-1 2 3 4 5+
less more

TERRAIN
- Beach
- Forest
- Lava Flow
- Mountain
- Pond
- Summit
- Stream
- Waterfall

FLORA & FAUNA
- Birds
- Native Plants
- Tide Pools
- Wildlife

FEATURES
- Great Views
- Swimming
- Camping
- Geologic Interest
- Historic Interest
- Archaeological
- Secluded
- Shady
- Steep

West Maui

TRAIL 1

Dayhike
1.0 mile, Out & Back
Difficulty: **1** 2 3 4 5

Olowalu Petroglyphs 37

A dusty road leads through sugarcane fields to an ancient Hawaiian petroglyph site, with the West Maui Mountains as a monumental backdrop. The trailhead is not far from the beach, with possibilities for oceanfront camping nearby.

TRAIL 2

Dayhike, Run,
Wheelchair Access,
Child Friendly,
Dogs Allowed
2.8 miles, Out & Back
Difficulty: 1 **2** 3 4 5

Kaanapali Beach Walk. 43

Just north of Lahaina, this wheelchair-accessible recreational path hugs Kaanapali's shoreline. Show up around sunset to see the hotels' Hawaiian music and hula shows and a cliff-diving ceremony, or bring binoculars to watch for whales offshore during winter.

TRAIL 3

Dayhike, Run,
Child Friendly,
Dogs Allowed
3.0 miles, Out & Back
Difficulty: 1 **2** 3 4 5

Kapalua Coastal Trail. 49

Follow this gentle trail alongside the coast in the early morning or late afternoon, when temperatures are cooler. Ancient jet-black lava flows jut out into the ocean, marking the boundaries of idyllic beaches with white-capped surf and hypnotizing sunset views.

TRAIL 4

Dayhike, Run,
Dogs Allowed,
Permit Required
3.9 miles, Semiloop
Difficulty: 1 2 **3** 4 5

Kapalua Village Trails. 55

Laid out around a former golf course, Kapalua resort's network of paved walking and running trails with steep inclines are a cardio challenge. In the early morning, it's mercifully not as hot on these mostly sunny and exposed trails.

Maunalei Arboretum & Honolua Ridge 59
Make a cool escape up into the West Maui Mountains, where a shady arboretum is a living outdoor gallery of native and exotic plants. Shorter walking loops are available, too, but the Puu Kaeo Lookout is worth the ridge climb.

TRAIL 5
Dayhike, Child Friendly, Permit Required
3.0 miles, Semiloop
Difficulty: 1 **2** 3 4 5

Mahana Ridge 65
West Maui's longest hiking trail tackles a forested ridgeline, starting from the Maunalei Arboretum and winding downhill through the forest toward the sea. Bird's-eye ocean views, a rainbow variety of native plants, and a sandy beach at trail's end await.

TRAIL 6
Dayhike, Permit Required
6.5 miles, Point-to-Point
Difficulty: 1 2 3 **4** 5

Nakalele Blowhole 73
A short scramble down a seaside cliff scattered with lava rocks brings hikers to a grand viewpoint overlooking a natural blowhole. When the surf's up, the ocean shoots powerfully into the air—just remember to stay back a safe distance.

TRAIL 7
Dayhike
0.9 mile, Out & Back
Difficulty: 1 **2** 3 4 5

Ohai Trail 79
This gently sloping, but often very windy coastal trail loops around Poelua Point inside the West Maui Forest Reserve. Illustrated signs point out native coastal plants that have been painstakingly restored, while benches provide panoramic clifftop ocean views.

TRAIL 8
Dayhike, Child Friendly
1.3 miles, Semiloop
Difficulty: **1** 2 3 4 5

Kahekili Highway Ocean Baths 83
After a short hike down the cliffs north of Kahakuloa town, you can soak in these natural saltwater pools, with no tourist development to intrude upon the horizon. Avoid getting in the water here during periods of dangerously high surf.

TRAIL 9
Dayhike
0.6 mile, Out & Back
Difficulty: 1 **2** 3 4 5

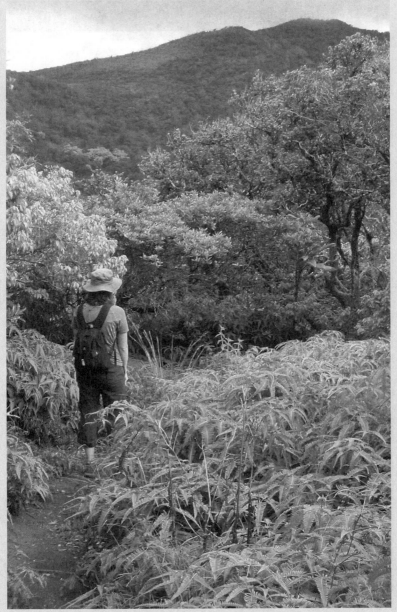

From Puu Kaeo Lookout, *hikers enjoy secret views of the rain-soaked West Maui Mountains.*

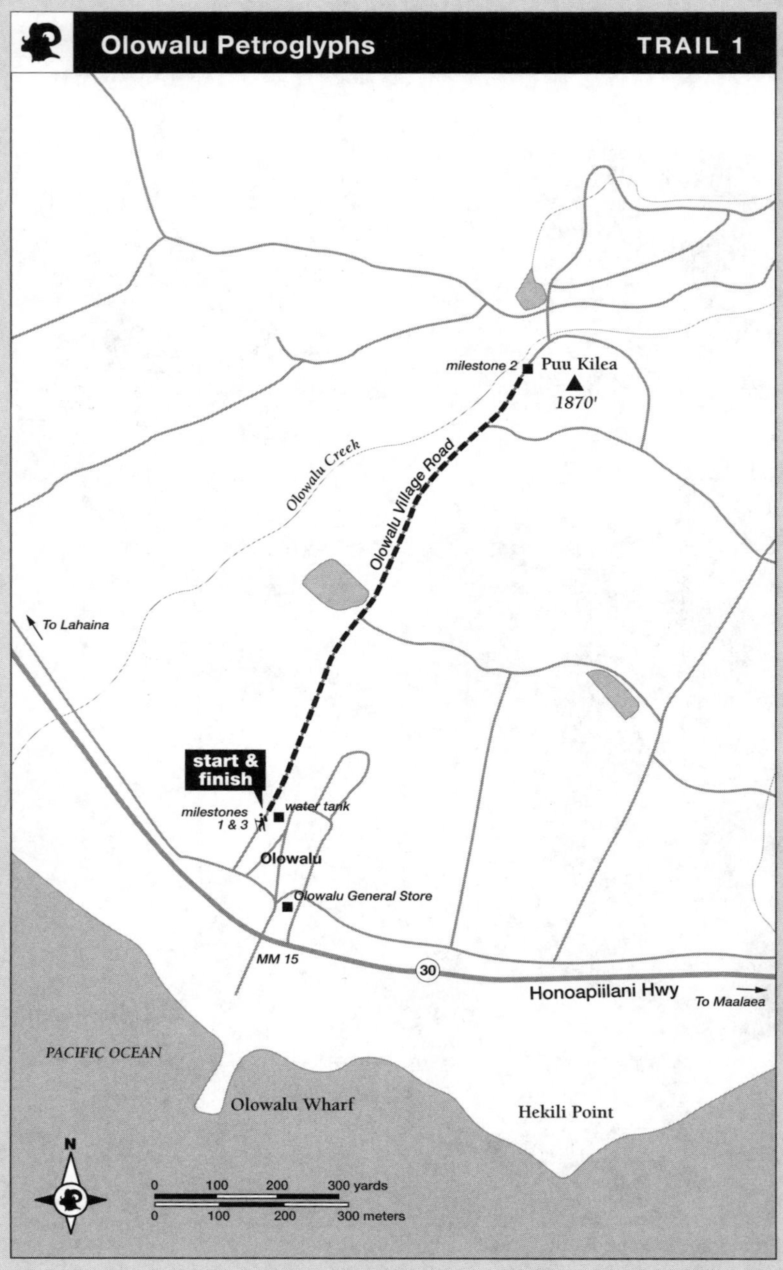
Olowalu Petroglyphs
TRAIL 1
milestone 2
Puu Kilea
1870'
Olowalu Creek
Olowalu Village Road
To Lahaina
start & finish
milestones 1 & 3
water tank
Olowalu
Olowalu General Store
MM 15
30
Honoapiilani Hwy
To Maalaea
PACIFIC OCEAN
Olowalu Wharf
Hekili Point
N
0 100 200 300 yards
0 100 200 300 meters

Olowalu Petroglyphs

It's a short, but often windy walk along a flat dirt road through sugarcane fields beneath the West Maui Mountains to the island's best-known petroglyph site. Although graffiti has obscured some of the ancient Hawaiian rock art and writing, the *mana* (spiritual power) of this archaeological site remains untouched.

TRAIL USE
Dayhike, Child Friendly

LENGTH
1.0 mile, 30–45 mins.

VERTICAL FEET
±150´

DIFFICULTY
– **1** 2 3 4 5 +

TRAIL TYPE
Out & Back

SURFACE TYPE
Dirt

START & END
N 20.81235°
W 156.62227°

FEATURES
Native Plants
Secluded
Archaeological

FACILITIES
Phone

Best Time

Because this trail passes over private property, be courteous to local residents by only hiking during daylight hours. Early morning is the best time for trekking this sun-exposed, dusty dirt road. Avoid walking under the hot midday sun or on windy afternoons.

Finding the Trail

From central Lahaina, drive southeast on the Honoapiilani Highway (Hwy. 30) for approximately 6 miles. At mile marker (MM) 15, pull off at the Olowalu general store on the *mauka* (inland) side of the highway. Drive around the north side of the general store, then turn left immediately onto a wide unmarked dirt road. Drive toward the water tank peeking above the treetops ahead. Park off-road either beside the water tanks or directly across the road, being careful not to block any traffic.

Trail Description

Although this is a relatively short hike, it can be surprisingly dehydrating because it follows an unshaded, dusty track heading inland across sugarcane fields. If you forgot to fill your water bottles before starting out, the Olowalu general store sells drinks.

Start walking along the dirt road next to the **water tank**, ▶1 making your way *mauka* (toward the mountains). The dirt road you're walking on passes over private property. There is no marked trailhead or any other helpful signposts for hikers along the way, but it's a straightforward walk. The foothills of the West Maui Mountains rise up and grow closer as you cross the commercial sugarcane fields. Especially in the afternoons, island winds tend to blow quite strongly here, so hang onto your hat!

About 0.2 mile from your starting point, the dirt road you're walking on reaches a Y-intersection. The side road leading off to the left into the cane fields is blocked by yellow posts usually with a heavy metal chain hanging between them. Stay to the right and keep walking inland on the main road, now roughly following a straight line of telephone poles with their wires hanging overhead.

During winter (from December to March), you can spot whales along the coast between Maalaea and Lahaina, including at Papawai Point, just south of mile marker 8 on the Honoapiilani Highway.

At the next major T-intersection, another dirt access road comes in from the right, off a paved road that heads back toward the highway. Ignore this side road as well. Instead continue walking straight ahead toward the prominent reddish volcanic cinder cone Kilea, keeping the few private homes along the road on your left. Beware that neighborhood guard dogs here are not always leashed, so exercise caution. As you continue walking inland along the narrowing road, a corrugated metal-roofed shed appears ahead. Now start paying close attention to the face of the lava rocks on the right-hand side of the trail. Parts of these rocks' surface are inscribed

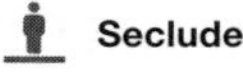

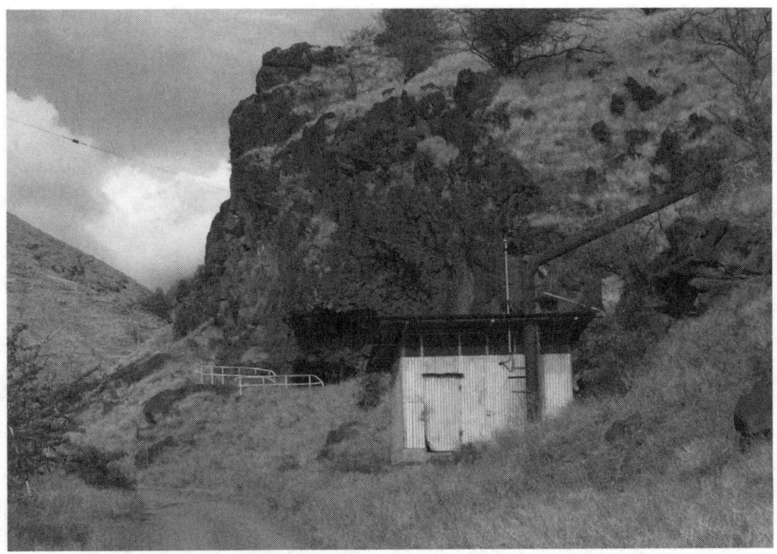

Images pecked by ancient Hawaiians *are hidden in the cliffs.*

with ancient Hawaiian petroglyphs, which you can inspect and photograph at eye level.

Just beyond the metal-roofed shed, you arrive at the **main petroglyph panels**. ▶2 Cautiously scramble up the dirt hillside beside the red railings (usually with peeling paint) and an old staircase that's probably still missing its rungs to reach the petroglyph panel's observation ledge. Although contemporary graffiti has obscured some of the lower petroglyphs, look up to discover others that are still well-preserved. Chiseled into the surface of the rocks using a stone hammer or sharp-edged rock, these chalk-white petroglyphs stand out strikingly against the rust-colored cliffs.

Archaeological

Look for triangle-shaped representations of humans and depictions of wildlife such as geckos, in addition to ancient ceremonial and abstract designs whose interpretation today cannot be definitive.

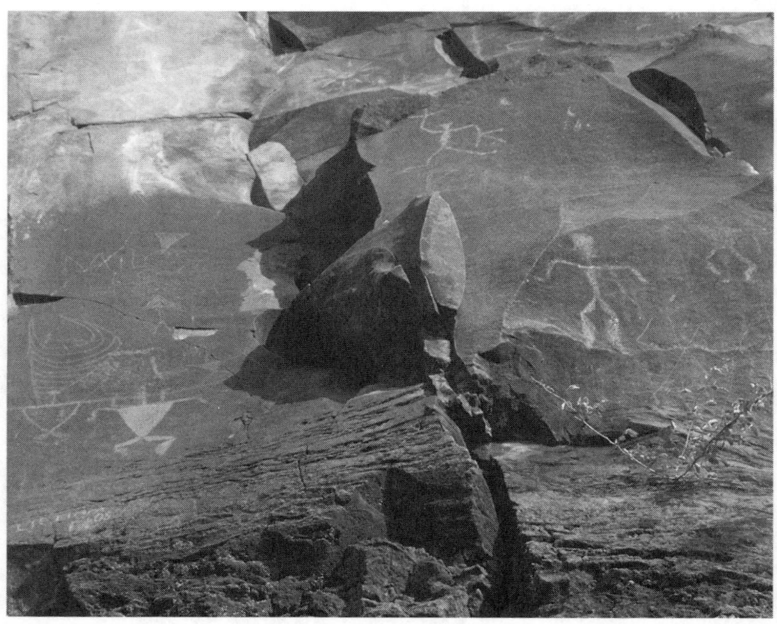

Human representations and abstract designs *tempt observers to guess at their meanings.*

Chiseled into the surface of the rocks using a stone hammer or sharp-edged rock, these chalk-white petroglyphs stand out strikingly against the rust-colored cliffs.

Although petroglyphs were once abundant on Maui, many are now hidden from public view on privately owned land or else were destroyed by developers in earlier centuries. Unusually, most petroglyphs on Maui are carved into the sides of sheer cliffs, which makes them more inaccessible—quite different from the petroglyph fields on the Big Island of Hawaii, which are often easily found in lava flows near the coast.

When you're ready, turn around and retrace your steps back along the dirt road and across the cane fields *makai* (toward the ocean) to the **water tank**, ►3 an easily spotted landmark en route. For details about nearby Camp Olowalu, Maui's only privately owned campground at press time, see page 17. Less inviting, there's also roadside camping at county-run Papalaua Wayside Park (see page 17).

Notice

The ancient Hawaiian village of Olowalu was the site of a historical massacre. In 1790, American sea captain Simon Metcalfe anchored offshore from Olowalu to trade and resupply his ship *Eleanora*. After one of his wooden skiffs was stolen during the night, the captain retaliated by opening fire on unsuspecting villagers that he had lured toward his ship under the pretense of trading. More than 100 Hawaiians—including men, women, and children—died that day, and another 200 were likely wounded. Most, if not all, were innocent of any crime.

MILESTONES

▶1	0.0	Start on road beside water tank [N 20.81235°, W 156.62227°]
▶2	0.5	Arrive at main petroglyph panels [N 20.81891°, W 156.61845°]
▶3	1.0	Return along road to water tank [N 20.81235°, W 156.62227°]

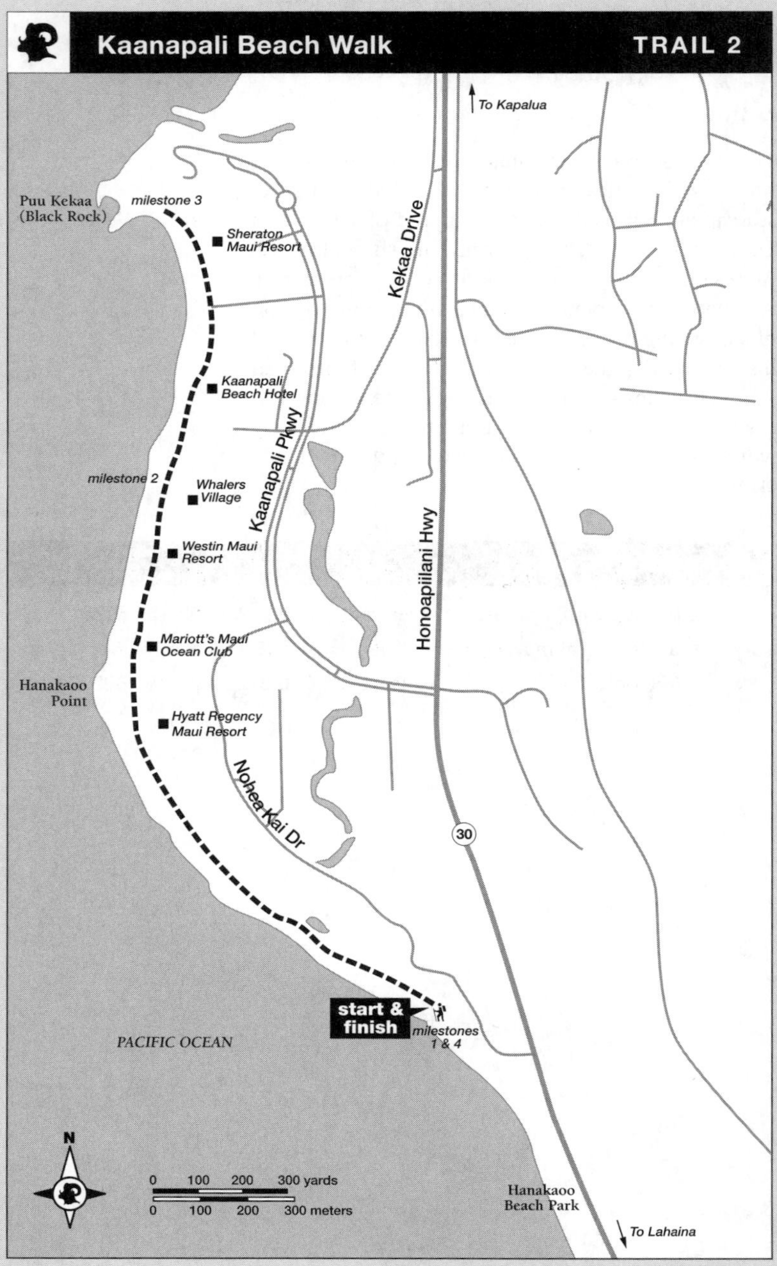
Kaanapali Beach Walk
TRAIL 2
To Kapalua
Puu Kekaa (Black Rock)
milestone 3
Sheraton Maui Resort
Kekaa Drive
Kaanapali Beach Hotel
Kaanapali Pkwy
milestone 2
Whalers Village
Westin Maui Resort
Honoapiilani Hwy
Mariott's Maui Ocean Club
Hanakaoo Point
Hyatt Regency Maui Resort
Nohea Kai Dr
30
start & finish
milestones 1 & 4
PACIFIC OCEAN
N
0 100 200 300 yards
0 100 200 300 meters
Hanakaoo Beach Park
To Lahaina

Kaanapali Beach Walk

Winding past Kaanapali's family-friendly resort hotels, just north of Lahaina, this recreational path is popular for early morning and late afternoon runs and strolls. Come around sunset to catch free live entertainment at hotels beside the beach, including a torch-lighting and cliff-diving ceremony near a popular snorkeling spot.

Best Time

You can walk this trail year-round. Pedestrians may access this coastal trail 24 hours a day, although walking along the beach itself after dark is not always safe because of crime. Avoid the midday heat by walking or running on this trail in the cool early morning (which is also when water conditions are best for snorkeling). Sunsets are also spectacular from this vantage point on the island's west coast.

Finding the Trail

From central Lahaina, drive north on the Honoapiilani Highway (Hwy. 30) for about 3 miles. Before mile marker (MM) 24, turn left onto Kaanapali Parkway at a stoplight intersection. Drive *makai* (toward the ocean) for 0.3 mile, then take the next major left onto Nohea Kai Dr. Follow this side road for 0.2 mile south past the Hyatt Regency Maui Resort to the most southern public access beach parking lot, signposted on your right. Parking spaces are limited here. Improve your chances of finding a spot by arriving either early or late in the day. (For alternative parking, see the "Options" box, page 47.)

TRAIL USE
Dayhike, Run, Wheelchair Access, Child Friendly, Dogs Allowed

LENGTH
2.8 miles, 1–1½ hours

VERTICAL FEET
±25′

DIFFICULTY
– 1 **2** 3 4 5 +

TRAIL TYPE
Out & Back

SURFACE TYPE
Paved, Sand

START & END
N 20.91121°
W 156.69022°

FEATURES
Beach
Native Plants
Tide Pools
Wildlife
Great Views
Swimming

FACILITIES
Restrooms
Phone
Water

Trail Description

From Kaanapali's southernmost public beach parking lot, walk *makai* to **the southern terminus of the coastal trail.** ►1 Farther south lies long, sandy Hanakaoo Beach, nicknamed "Canoe Beach" for its canoe house and the outrigger teams that practice here many afternoons. If you decide to detour south to the beach either before or after your hike, ask at the lifeguard station about current ocean conditions and water safety before taking a dip.

Otherwise, turn left onto the paved coastal recreational path and start heading north. You'll enjoy ocean views almost the entire way alongside Kaanapali Beach. The island of Lanai, formerly a pineapple plantation and now a luxury tourist resort, is visible directly across the Auau Channel. The channel's protected waters offer safe harbor for migratory North Pacific humpback whales, which travel down from Alaska to Hawaii's balmy waters each winter to give birth and mate. Your best chance of spotting whales offshore is between December and March—bring binoculars.

Great Views

Wildlife

The paved coastal trail winds north for 0.8 mile past the Hyatt Regency Maui Resort, which holds its Polynesian luau at sunset right next to the beach, and the grassy lawns of Marriott's Maui Ocean Club. At the south end of the Westin Maui Resort, the trail passes a statue of Buddha sitting atop a lotus blossom. The grounds of both the Hyatt and the Westin are known for their lush tropical gardens planted with native coastal species, as well as for their impressive public art collections. Fronting the resort hotels, Kaanapali Beach is popular for family-friendly water sports, including surfing, boogie boarding, and parasailing. Swimming conditions vary, depending on how strong the currents are. By the shoreline, beach-gear rental huts can give you the lowdown on current conditions and potential water hazards.

Swimming

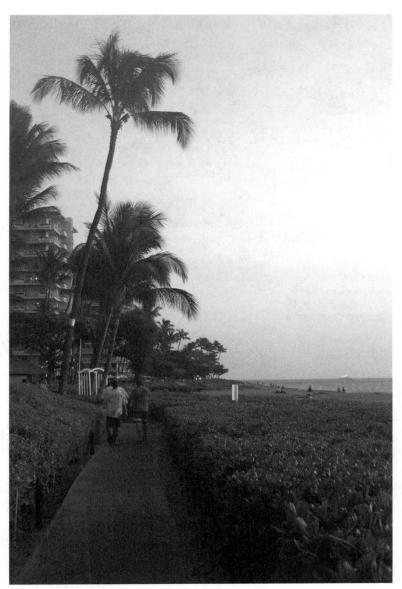

Take a sunrise or sunset stroll *along the beach resort's oceanfront path.*

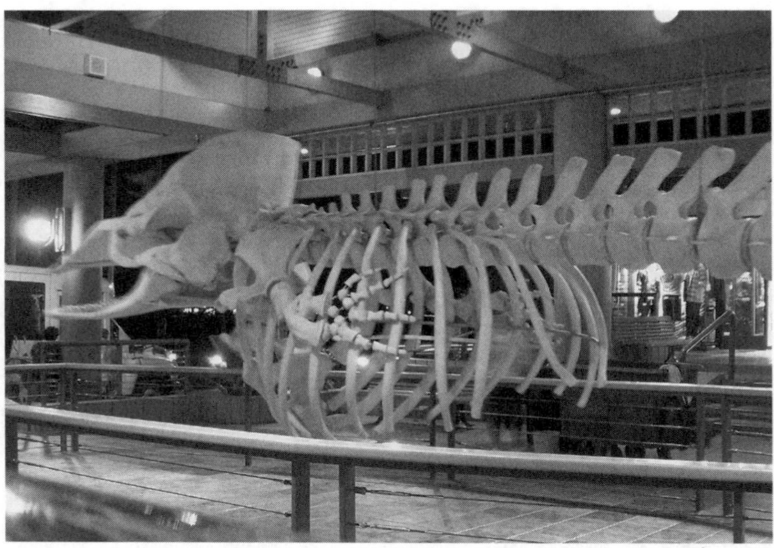

A whale of a skeleton *welcomes visitors in Kaanapali's Whalers Village.*

Inside the mall, the free Whalers Village Museum has a fascinating collection of whaling memorabilia and scrimshaw carvings from Maui's hurly-burly 19th-century whaling days. Visit www.whalersvillage.com or call (808) 661-5992 for details.

From the Westin, it's a short walk farther north to **Whalers Village** ▶2 shopping mall. Beachfront restaurants back onto the coastal path, their open-air patios blazing with tiki torches and often lively with the sounds of slack-key guitarists and ukulele players. The Kaanapali Beach Hotel—the next resort you encounter walking north along the path—holds its luau on the beach around sunset, too. As you're walking by, you might catch hotel staff unburying a slow-cooked kalua pig from a traditional Hawaiian underground pit, called an *imu*. Along this stretch of the Kaanapali Beach, you'll also find plenty of spots for lazily watching the sun sink into the sea.

The coastal path curves inland at the Sheraton Maui Resort, which hosts its own sunset luau with performances of Hawaiian music and hula. Walking another 0.2 mile northward brings you to the far edge of Kaanapali Beach, bordered by a prominent lava-rock outcropping, called **Puu Kekaa (Black**

Rock). ►3 Around sunset, listen for the sound of a conch shell being blown by a male performer dressed in traditional Hawaiian clothes, who will throw a lit torch into the waters below and then dive into the sea. (Posted signs prohibit you from doing likewise, however.)

When you're ready, turn around and retrace your steps for approximately 1.2 miles back to the **southern terminus of the coastal trail**, ►4 near the public beach-access parking lot.

When ocean waters are calm, experienced snorkelers can swim out to the small cove at the tip of Puu Kekaa, where coral thrives and sea turtles hang out.

MILESTONES

►1	0.0	Start from southern terminus of trail [N 20.91121°, W 156.69022°]
►2	0.8	Pass Whalers Village restaurants and shopping mall [N 20.92097°, W 156.69587°]
►3	1.4	Arrive at base of Puu Kekaa [N 20.92686°, W 156.69579°]
►4	2.8	Return to trail's southern terminus [N 20.91121°, W 156.69022°]

OPTIONS

Alternate Trailhead: Hanakaoo Beach Park

If Kaanapali's public beach access parking lots are full, drive back south along the Honoapiilani Highway and turn right into Hanakaoo Beach Park, which has more public parking. The county-run beach park also has restrooms, drinking water, outdoor showers, picnic tables, and pay phones. From its parking lot, head down to the beach, turn right and walk north across the sands to pick up the Kaanapali Beach Walk (that is, the official paved coastal trail) south of the Hyatt Regency Maui Resort, as described above. Starting from Hanakaoo Beach Park adds about a mile of total distance to your hike.

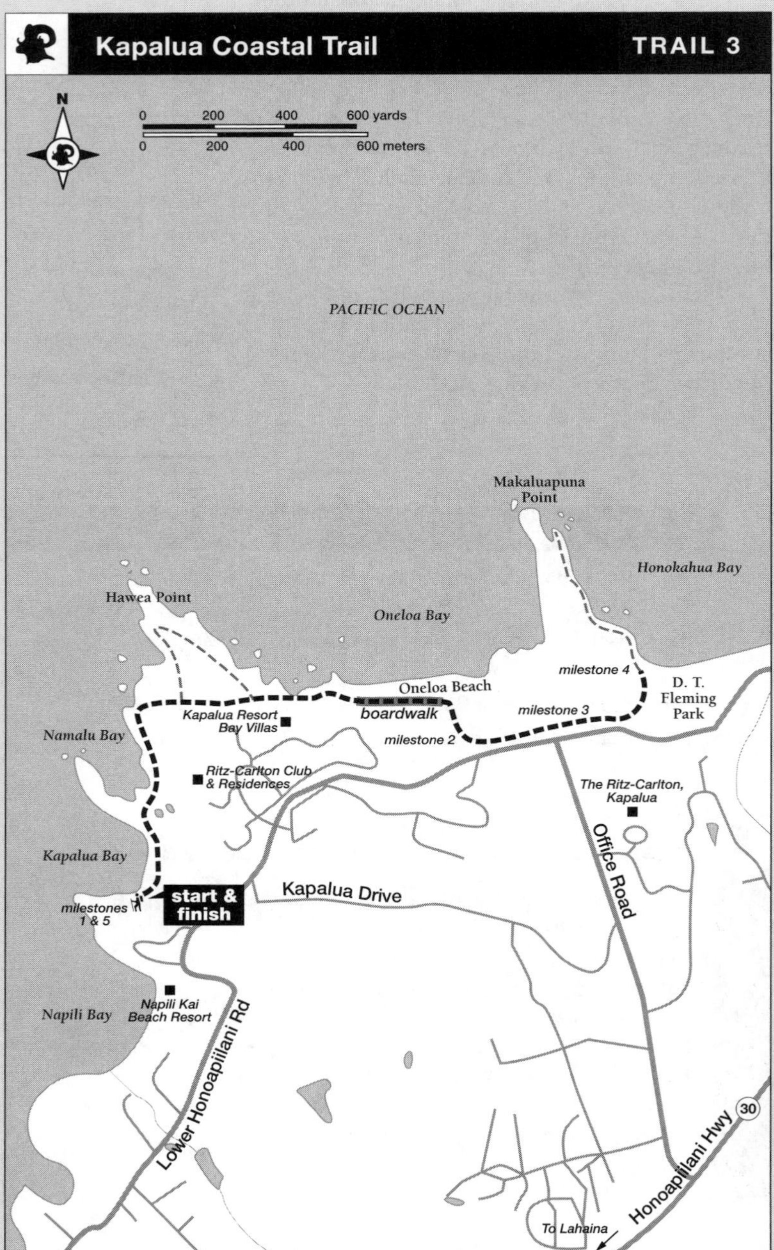

Kapalua Coastal Trail
TRAIL 3
N
0 200 400 600 yards
0 200 400 600 meters
PACIFIC OCEAN
Makaluapuna Point
Honokahua Bay
Hawea Point
Oneloa Bay
milestone 4
Oneloa Beach
D. T. Fleming Park
milestone 3
Kapalua Resort Bay Villas
boardwalk
Namalu Bay
milestone 2
Ritz-Carlton Club & Residences
The Ritz-Carlton, Kapalua
Office Road
Kapalua Bay
start & finish
Kapalua Drive
milestones 1 & 5
Napili Kai Beach Resort
Napili Bay
Lower Honoapiilani Rd
30
Honoapiilani Hwy
To Lahaina

Kapalua Coastal Trail

Stretch your legs along this resort's custom-built coastal path, passing white and golden strands of sand, scooting around small fields of crumbly lava, and wandering beside sand dunes anchored with native Hawaiian plants. Don't worry: Kapalua's low-rise resort buildings don't intrude on the gorgeous panoramic ocean views.

TRAIL USE
Dayhike, Run, Child Friendly, Dogs Allowed

LENGTH
3.0 miles, 1¼–1¾ hours

VERTICAL FEET
±300′

DIFFICULTY
– 1 **2** 3 4 5 +

TRAIL TYPE
Out & Back

SURFACE TYPE
Boardwalk, Dirt, Lava, Paved, Sand

START & END
N 20.99870°
W 156.66673°

FEATURES
Beach
Native Plants
Great Views
Swimming

FACILITIES
Restrooms
Picnic Tables
Phone
Water

Best Time

You can walk this trail year-round. Pedestrians may access this coastal path 24 hours a day, although walking along the beach itself after dark is not always safe because of crime. Avoid the midday heat by walking or running along this trail in the early morning or around sunset.

Finding the Trail

From central Lahaina, drive north along the Honoapiilani Highway (Hwy. 30) for about 8 miles, passing Kaanapali, Honokowai, and Kahana. Near mile marker (MM) 29, turn left at the stoplight with Hui Road, then right onto Lower Honoapiilani Dr., which winds slowly north past Napili's beach hotels and condos. Take the first left after the Napili Kai Beach Resort onto Kapalua Place, marked by a small public beach access sign. Park in the public beach lot here. Alternatively, if you'd rather walk this trail in reverse, drive north of Napili on the Honoapiilani Highway, turning left near MM 31 onto the short section of Lower Honoapiilani Road that abruptly dead-ends at D. T. Fleming Park.

Trail Description

Start from Kapalua Bay's **public beach parking lot**, ►1 which has restrooms, drinking water, and outdoor showers nearby. Head downhill toward the ocean and walk through a short concrete tunnel, then head north across the sands of the bay's crescent-shaped beach. Swimming and snorkeling are the most popular aquatic diversions here, with beautiful coral reefs protecting both ends of the beach. At the beach's north edge, you'll find a bench perfectly positioned for sitting while soaking up the views.

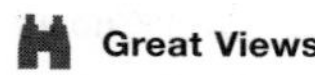

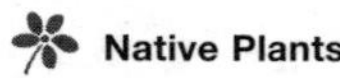

Most dunes are anchored by native plants such as naupaka, which has thick, glossy green leaves, or the twisted vines of pohuehue.

Heading north, you soon join the official coastal trail, which is signposted on the *makai* (ocean) side of the Ritz-Carlton Club and Residences. The trail skirts inland of Namalu Bay as you approach the Kapalua Resort Bay Villas. There you have an option to detour on a mixed sand-and-gravel path out to Hawea Point, a prominent black lava-rock outcropping off to your left. Otherwise, keep walking north along the signposted coastal trail, popular with everyone from families with young kids to locals out for an after-work run.

About 0.6 mile from where you started, step onto the coastal boardwalk that runs just inland from the sand dunes fronting Oneloa Bay. Most of these dunes are well anchored by vegetation, including native plants such as naupaka, which has thick, glossy green leaves, and the twisted vines of pohuehue (beach morning glory). Oneloa Beach often has high surf and strong currents, though, so don't expect to see many swimmers or snorkelers in the water here, unless conditions are unusually calm. This long stretch of sand is picturesque, backed by palm trees tossed by the wind.

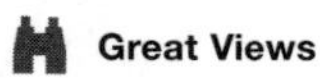

At the north end of the boardwalk, turn right and walk up the stairs to the public access parking lot for Oneloa Beach. Continue a short distance uphill on Ironwood Lane, then turn left at the main intersec-

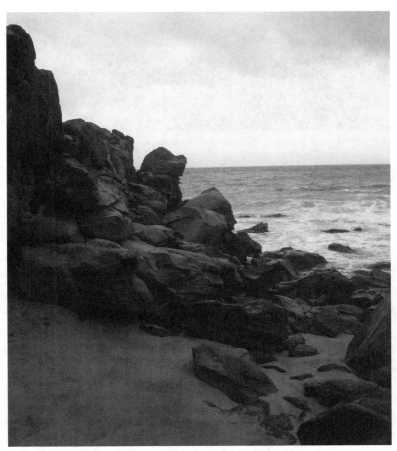

Detour out *to Kapalua's imaginatively named Dragon's Teeth formations.*

tion and **walk north along Lower Honoapiilani Road**. ▶2 After less than 0.2 mile, you pass the stop-sign intersection with Office Road and walk through another public access beach parking lot. Rejoin the paved coastal path at the back side of **The Ritz-Carlton, Kapalua**. ▶3 Keeping the golf course on your left, follow the winding path downhill through the resort all the way to Honokahua Bay.

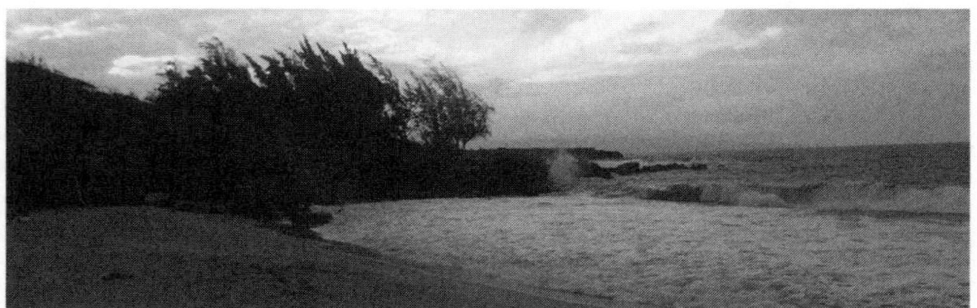

Surf crashes *at D. T. Fleming Park, one of West Maui's most popular beaches.*

After another half mile, the trail ends at **D. T. Fleming Park**. ▶4 Partly shaded by shaggy ironwood trees, this beach has consistently been voted among Maui's most beautiful, and also ranks among the best in Hawaii. Off to the left, you'll notice the sharply sculpted lava formations of Makaluapuna Point (for details, see the "Options" box, facing page). Broad and sandy, D. T. Fleming Beach is a favorite with local surfers and bodyboarders. If you want to swim, check in with park lifeguards about current water conditions. Steep drop-offs and dangerous rip currents await just offshore. On the north side of the beach, the county-run park offers restrooms, drinking fountains, picnic tables, and a payphone near the public parking lot, just off the Honoapiilani Highway.

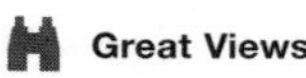

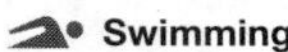

MILESTONES

▶1	0.0	Start from Kapalua Beach parking lot [N 20.99870°, W 156.66673°]
▶2	0.8	Walk north along Lower Honoapiilani Road [N 21.00300°, W 156.65854°]
▶3	1.0	Rejoin paved path at The Ritz-Carlton resort [N 21.00308°, W 156.65596°]
▶4	1.5	Turn around at D. T. Fleming Park [N 21.00463°, W 156.65393°]
▶5	3.0	Return to Kapalua Beach parking lot [N 20.99870°, W 156.66673°]

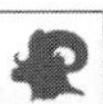

OPTIONS

Detour: The Dragon's Teeth

From D. T. Fleming Park, it's a 0.5-mile round-trip walk out to Makaluapuna Point, where you can inspect the lava-rock formations nicknamed the "Dragon's Teeth." True to their name, these volcanic rocks sculpted by the wind and waves are sharp and pointy. Although no official trail leads out here, it's not too difficult to find your way. Allow at least 30 minutes to get out to the tip of the point and back to the beach.

From the south side of the beach at Honokahua Bay, a faint use trail scrambles up the cliffs, then skirts north alongside the golf course and ancient Hawaiian burial grounds. Be careful not to walk on the grassy lawn inside the burial grounds, the boundaries of which are clearly marked by stone monuments. As soon as possible, drop back down into a field of surf-splashed boulders on your right and pick your way north toward the point. Exercise caution when taking this side trip, as high surf may make it dangerous.

When you're ready to leave D. T. Fleming Beach, retrace your steps for about 1.8 miles back south to Kapalua Bay's **public access beach parking lot**, ►5 where you started.

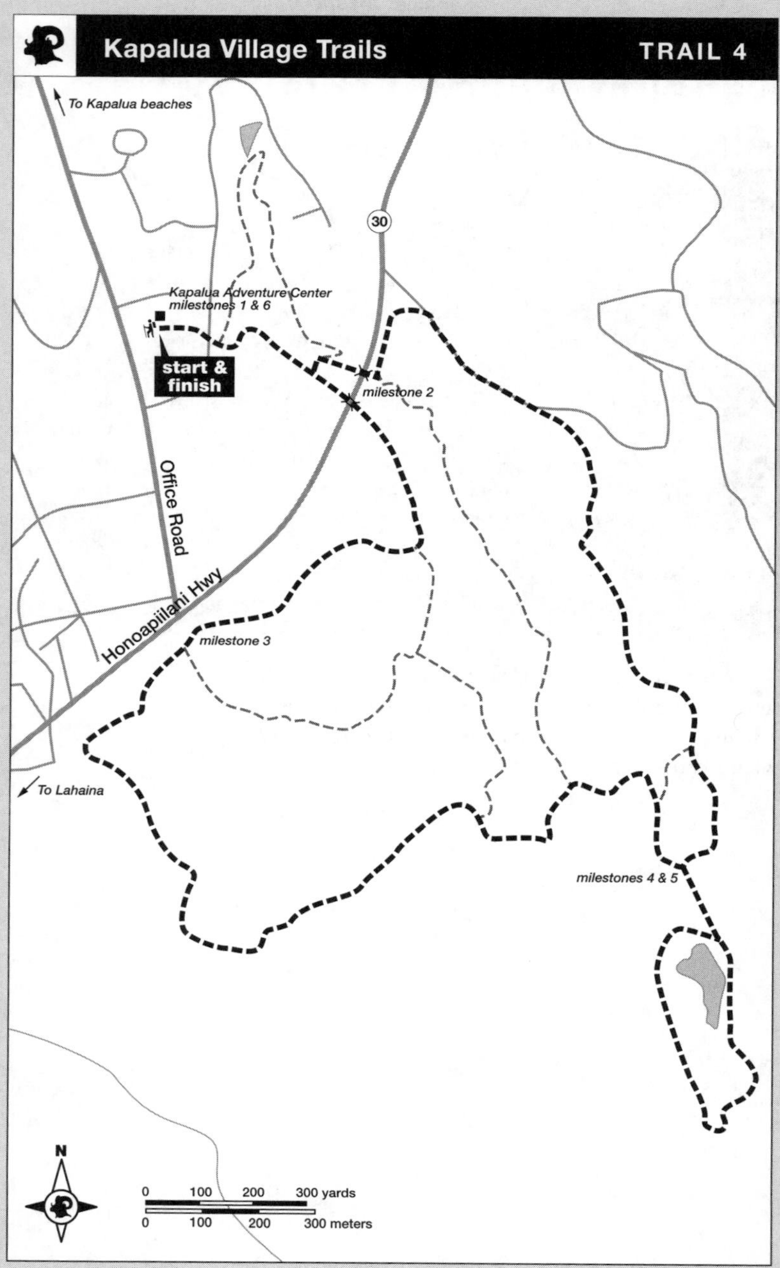
Kapalua Village Trails
TRAIL 4
To Kapalua beaches
30
Kapalua Adventure Center
milestones 1 & 6
start &
finish
milestone 2
Office Road
Honoapiilani Hwy
milestone 3
To Lahaina
milestones 4 & 5
N
0 100 200 300 yards
0 100 200 300 meters

Kapalua Village Trails

Home to West Maui's most exclusive luxury resort hotels, Kapalua also has some of the island's best-maintained paved recreational paths. Built atop a former golf course that's slowly being returned to its natural state, these walking and running loop trails climb the hillsides for uplifting ocean views.

TRAIL USE
Dayhike, Run, Dogs Allowed, Permit Required

LENGTH
3.9 miles, 1¾–2½ hours

VERTICAL FEET
±1900′

DIFFICULTY
– 1 2 **3** 4 5 +

TRAIL TYPE
Semiloop

SURFACE TYPE
Paved, Dirt

START & END
N 20.99767°
W 156.65327°

FEATURES
Pond
Birds
Great Views
Steep

FACILITIES
Visitor Center
Restrooms
Phone
Water

Best Time

The Kapalua Village Trails are open on an intermittent basis; they may be closed without notice at any time. To check if the trails are still accessible by the public, call the Kapalua Adventure Center at (808) 665-4386 or check www.kapalua.com. Normally, these trails are open year-round from 7 AM to sunset daily. Avoid the worst midday heat by hiking in the early morning. Visitors must check in first and sign a liability waiver inside the Kapalua Adventure Center (open 7 AM to 5 PM daily) on Office Road.

Finding the Trail

From central Lahaina, drive north along the Honoapiilani Highway (Hwy. 30) for approximately 9 miles, passing Kaanapali, Honokowai, and Kahana. North of mile marker (MM) 30, turn left at the main signs into the Kapalua Resort. Follow Office Road downhill for a short distance, keeping the driving range, putting green, and golf course on your right. Turn right into the signed Kapalua Adventure Center parking lot.

Trail Description

The resort's Kapalua Adventure Center offers scuba diving, snorkeling, and kayaking trips; zipline adventures; and guided tours of a pineapple plantation. All activities and tours are open to nonguests (fees vary); make reservations.

Inside the Kapalua Adventure Center, you'll find ice cold drinking fountains, restrooms, a cafe, and a small shop selling snacks and drinks. You must stop by the hikers' check-in desk to sign a liability waiver (retain the yellow copy as your permit). Also pick up a free copy of Kapalua's full-color hiking guide booklet, which contains sketch maps and descriptions of the resort's trails. Laminate signboards are posted at major junctions along the trails. Note that this hike follows the Master Loop, which is a little more than 3 miles long, adding a detour of less than a mile around the Lake Loop.

From the back porch of the **Kapalua Adventure Center,** ►1 which overlooks a busy golf course, walk downhill beside the driving range. The paved path, which is almost fully exposed to the sun, curves downhill around a disc golf course, and then passes through a pair of **concrete tunnels** ►2 about 0.2 mile from your starting point. On the far side of the tunnels, veer right and start following the red arrows pointing out the Master Loop. You'll begin climbing uphill, although not too steeply at first.

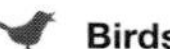 Birds

The trail's first views of the ocean and the island of Lanai, formerly a pineapple plantation owned by the Dole Food Company, appear about 0.5 mile from your starting point. Butterflies float by in the sunshine, while birdsong can be heard coming from the shady pine trees. Don't be surprised to find wildlife thriving here, since the Kapalua resort's golf courses are certified as Audubon Cooperative Sanctuaries.

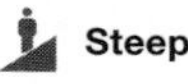 Steep

As the paved path steepens, continue following the red arrows and keep right at all major trail junctions to stay on the Master Loop. About 0.7 mile from your starting point, you **pass a mailbox and a locked gate** ►3 off the Honoapiilani Highway. The trail begins to ascend even more steeply, with only a little shade. The last stretch to the crest of the hill is a rather stiff climb. You may be glad to sit among the hilltop's shady trees and rest while making the ascent.

Detour right and start following the light blue arrows around the **Lake Loop**, ►4 about 0.7 mile long. This artificial pond, once a water hazard on the resort's former golf course, is now home to ducks. Once you've completed the lollipop loop around the pond, **rejoin the main trail** ►5 by veering right to stay on the Master Loop, marked with red arrows. As you head steeply downhill, pause every so often both to catch your breath and to soak up the panoramic ocean views, with Lanai again visible in the distance. Don't expect much shade on this final downhill stretch, however.

Near the bottom of the hill, turn right and walk back through the concrete tunnels. Then retrace your steps beside the golf course and driving range uphill along the curving paved path that leads back to the refreshingly air-conditioned **Kapalua Adventure Center**. ►6

Downhill from the Kapalua Adventure Center behind the Ritz-Carlton resort, D. T. Fleming Park is often voted one of Maui's most scenic beaches. But for calmer swimming conditions, head south to Kapalua Bay.

MILESTONES

►1	0.0	Start from Kapalua Adventure Center [N 20.99767°, W 156.65327°]
►2	0.2	Veer right after passing through concrete tunnels
►3	0.7	Continue past mailbox and off-highway gate [N 20.99238°, W 156.65280°]
►4	2.0	Detour right onto the Lake Loop
►5	2.6	Rejoin main trail and veer right to head downhill
►6	3.9	Return to Kapalua Adventure Center [N 20.99767°, W 156.65327°]

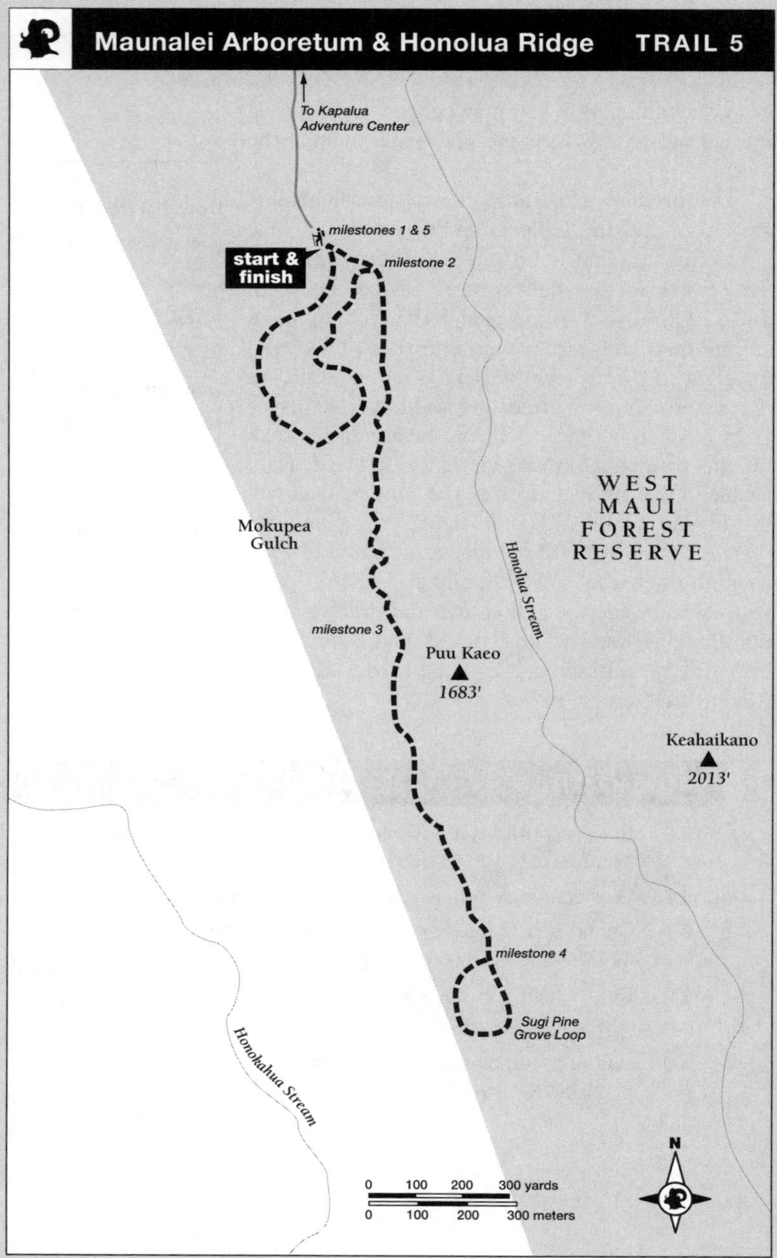
Maunalei Arboretum & Honolua Ridge
TRAIL 5
To Kapalua Adventure Center
milestones 1 & 5
start & finish
milestone 2
WEST MAUI FOREST RESERVE
Mokupea Gulch
Honolua Stream
milestone 3
Puu Kaeo
1683′
Keahaikano
2013′
milestone 4
Sugi Pine Grove Loop
Honokahua Stream
0 100 200 300 yards
0 100 200 300 meters
N

Maunalei Arboretum & Honolua Ridge

When the blisteringly hot sun is baking West Maui's coast, there's no better place for a cool, shady walk than this private arboretum with well-groomed intersecting hiking trails. If you're not up for the ridgeline climb to Puu Kaeo Lookout, the arboretum also offers easier half-mile and mile-long nature trail loops, which are family-friendly.

TRAIL USE
Dayhike, Child Friendly, Permit Required

LENGTH
3.0 miles, 1½–2 hours

VERTICAL FEET
±1300′

DIFFICULTY
– 1 **2** 3 4 5 +

TRAIL TYPE
Semiloop

SURFACE TYPE
Dirt, Grass

START & END
N 20.97984°
W 156.62062°

FEATURES
Forest
Mountain
Summit
Stream
Birds
Native Plants
Great Views
Secluded
Shady
Historic Interest

FACILITIES
Visitor Center
Restrooms
Picnic Tables
Phone
Water

Best Time

You can hike this trail year-round. Hikers must check in first and sign a liability waiver at the resort's Kapalua Adventure Center (open 7 AM to 5 PM daily) on Office Road (see "Finding the Trail" below), then catch a mandatory resort shuttle to the arboretum trailhead. At press time, those free shuttles were running four times daily, departing from the Kapalua Adventure Center between 8 AM and 2 PM, and picking up at the arboretum for the return trip between 9:50 AM and 5:20 PM. For more information and to check current shuttle schedules, visit www.kapalua.com or call (808) 665-4386.

Finding the Trail

From central Lahaina, drive north along the Honoapiilani Highway (Hwy. 30) for approximately 9 miles, passing Kaanapali, Honokowai, and Kahana. North of mile marker (MM) 30, turn left at the main signs into the Kapalua Resort. Follow Office Road downhill for a short distance, keeping the driving range, putting green, and golf course on your right.

Turn right into the signed Kapalua Adventure Center parking lot (see the map for Trail 4, page 54).

From the Kapalua Adventure Center's front entrance, catch a free resort shuttle to the arboretum trailhead (see the previous "Best Times" section for details). You can't drive your own vehicle to the trailhead because the arboretum lies inside a gated residential community.

Trail Description

The resort's Kapalua Adventure Center is equipped with restrooms, drinking fountains, pay phones, a small shop selling snacks and drinks, and a cafe. Visit the hikers' check-in desk to sign the liability waiver (retain the yellow copy as your permit). Also pick up a free copy of Kapalua's full-color hiking booklet, which includes sketch maps of the arboretum's loop trails. The resort's free shuttle drops you off at the arboretum entrance, where you'll find a portable toilet and a covered picnic table pavilion providing some shade, but no potable water. Check the posted shuttle schedule for pick-up times for the ride back downhill to Kapalua.

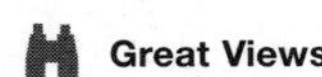

Start at the **arboretum entrance**, ►1 across the dirt road from the picnic pavilion. All three marked arboretum trails begin here: the Lower Arboretum Loop (0.5 mile), the Banyan Loop (1.0 mile), and the Honolua Ridge Trail (2.5 miles round-trip). The arboretum was originally an experimental garden planted in the early 20th century by D. T. Fleming, a ranch and pineapple plantation manager. The plants are a mix of native species and exotics imported from around the world, an attempt to make West Maui's arid landscape more profitable for agriculture and logging.

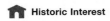

Historic Interest

Puu Kukui is the second wettest place in the Hawaiian Islands, after Mt. Waialeale on Kauai.

At first, you'll be walking along the same path shared by all three trails. At the first Y-junction split, stay to the right. Follow the combined Lower

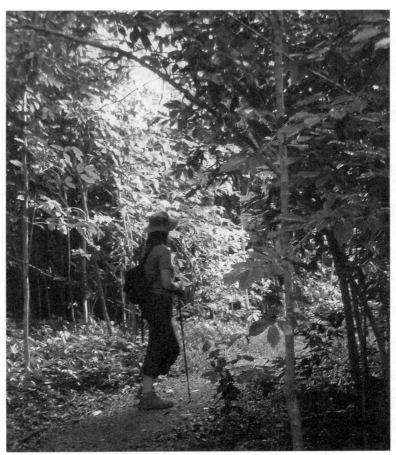

At Maunalei Arboretum *discover native and exotic flora on mountain trails.*

Arboretum and Banyan loops, which are color-coded red and green, respectively. At each fork in the trail that follows, take the right-hand path. The shady, forested footpath is bordered by plentiful native and exotic species, many of which are labeled, including Moreton Bay pines and Surinam cherry, bo, and tea trees.

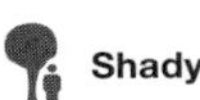

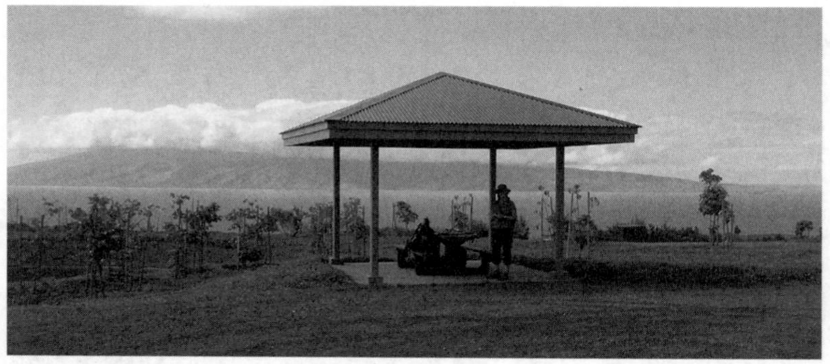

Take a break *and soak up the views of Molokai island.*

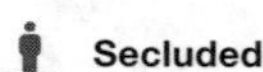

Where the Lower Arboretum and Banyan Loop trails finally split, stay to the right and follow the green-arrowed Banyan Loop. After about 0.3 mile, you pass through a gate into Puu Kukui Watershed Preserve. Receiving more than 385 inches of rainfall in an average year, Puu Kukui is the wettest place on the island. Deep inside the West Maui Mountains, the peak is remote and practically inaccessible on foot.

After meandering past tropical traveler's palms and a grove of giant banyan trees easily recognized by their sprawling, twisted root systems, **turn right onto the Honolua Ridge Trail**. ►2 Start ascending along the switchbacking dirt trail, fringed by native plants including maile, a fragrant vine with

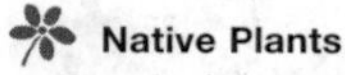

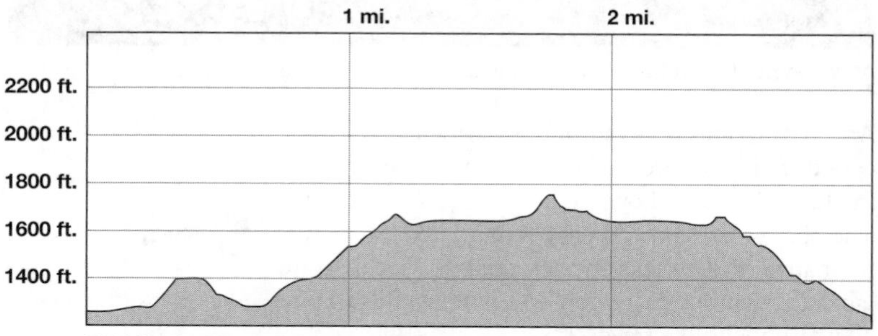

TRAIL 5 Maunalei Arboretum & Honolua Ridge Elevation Profile

yellow flowers and thick glossy leaves that's often used in making traditional Hawaiian lei. After a steady ascent, the trail pops out of the forest cover at **Puu Kaeo Lookout** ▶3 (elevation 1683 feet). The lookout grants panoramic views of the West Maui Mountains and the ocean, with the island of Lanai visible across the Auau Channel.

 Summit

 Great Views

The trail splits as it loops around the lookout, then reconnects and continues downhill, and hops across a seasonally dry stream gulch. Be aware that this section of the trail may be signposted as the Mahana Ridge Trail. About 0.5 mile from the lookout, detour right on the **Sugi Pine Grove Loop**. ▶4 Also called Japanese cedars, these stately evergreen trees are neither pines nor cedars, but instead belong to the cypress family.

After completing the short detour loop, rejoin the main trail and turn left to backtrack up to the Puu Kaeo Lookout, then downhill along the Honolua Ridge Trail back to the **arboretum trailhead**. ▶5 Ignore the Banyan Loop and Lower Arboretum side trips on your return hike, continuing straight ahead or staying to the right at every trail junction, following the orange-arrowed signs for the Honolua Ridge Trail.

Up for a longer hike? The Mahana Ridge Trail (see Trail 6, page 65) connects the arboretum's Honolua Ridge Trail with the beach at D. T. Fleming Park.

MILESTONES

▶1	0.0	Start from Maunalei Arboretum entrance [N 20.97984°, W 156.62062°]
▶2	0.7	Turn right onto the Honolua Ridge Trail
▶3	1.2	Arrive at Puu Kaeo Lookout [N 20.97200°, W 156.61888°]
▶4	1.7	Detour onto the Sugi Pine Grove Loop [N 20.96493°, W 156.61655°]
▶5	3.0	Return to Maunalei Arboretum entrance [N 20.97984°, W 156.62062°]

Mahana Ridge

TRAIL 6

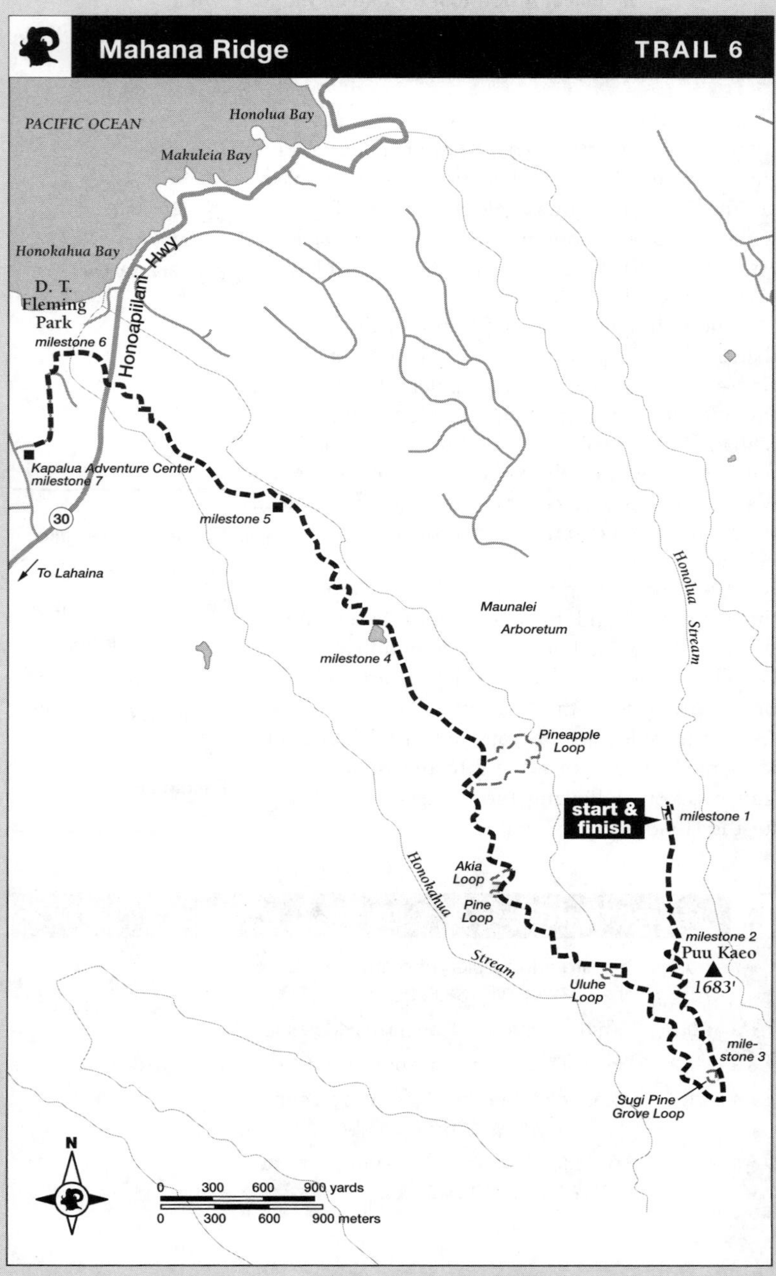

PACIFIC OCEAN
Honolua Bay
Makuleia Bay
Honokahua Bay
D. T. Fleming Park
Honoapiilani Hwy
milestone 6
Kapalua Adventure Center
milestone 7
30
milestone 5
To Lahaina
Maunalei
Arboretum
milestone 4
Honolua Stream
Pineapple Loop
start & finish
milestone 1
Honokahua Stream
Akia Loop
Pine Loop
milestone 2
Puu Kaeo
1683'
Uluhe Loop
mile-stone 3
Sugi Pine Grove Loop
N
0
300
600
900 yards
0
300
600
900 meters

Mahana Ridge

The Kapalua resort offers some of Maui's best groomed hiking trails, including this verdant forest trek that heads (mostly) downhill from a West Maui Mountain summit to the beach. A free resort shuttle drops you off at the trailhead inside a private arboretum planted with native and exotic flora.

TRAIL USE
Dayhike,
Permit Required

LENGTH
6.5 miles, 3–4 hours

VERTICAL FEET
±2750′

DIFFICULTY
– 1 2 3 **4** 5 +

TRAIL TYPE
Point-to-Point

SURFACE TYPE
Dirt, Grass

START
N 20.97984°
W 156.62062°

END
N 20.99767°
W 156.65327°

FEATURES
Beach, Forest
Mountain, Summit
Stream, Birds
Native Plants
Great Views
Swimming
Secluded
Shady, Steep

FACILITIES
Visitor Center
Restrooms
Picnic Tables
Phone
Water

Best Time

This trail is open year-round from sunrise to sunset daily. After it rains, expect some sections to be quite slick and muddy. Other parts are fully exposed to the sun, making a midday hike a hot, sweaty, and dehydrating endeavor. Hikers must check in first and sign a liability waiver inside the Kapalua Adventure Center (open 7 AM to 5 PM daily) on Office Road (see "Finding the Trail" below), then catch a mandatory resort shuttle to the arboretum trailhead. At press time, those free shuttles were running four times daily, departing from the Kapalua Adventure Center between 8 AM and 2 PM. For more information or to check current shuttle schedules, visit www.kapalua.com or call (808) 665-4386.

Finding the Trail

From central Lahaina, drive north along the Honoapiilani Highway (Hwy. 30) for approximately 9 miles, passing Kaanapali, Honokowai, and Kahana. North of mile marker (MM) 30, turn left at the main signs into the Kapalua Resort. Follow Office Road downhill for a short distance, keeping the driving range, putting green, and golf course on your right. Turn right into the signed Kapalua Adventure Center parking lot.

From the Kapalua Adventure Center's front entrance, catch a free resort shuttle to the arboretum trailhead (see the previous "Best Time" section for details). You can't drive your own vehicle to the trailhead, because the arboretum lies inside a gated residential community.

Trail Description

Just visible from the trail, although inaccessible on foot, remote Puu Kukui is the wettest place on Maui, averaging more than 385 inches of rain annually.

When you check in at the Kapalua Adventure Center and sign the liability waiver (the yellow copy is your hiking permit), pick up a free copy of Kapalua's full-color hiking booklet, which includes sketch maps of all of the resort's trails. A word of warning, though: The Mahana Ridge map shows the trail connecting directly back to the Kapalua Adventure Center, but at press time the trail finished near D. T. Fleming Park instead. The resort's Kapalua Adventure Center is equipped with restrooms, drinking fountains, pay phones, a small shop selling snacks and drinks, and a cafe. There is no drinking water available along this trail until near the end.

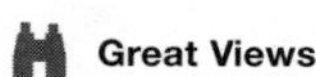

The resort's free shuttle drops you off outside the arboretum, next to a covered picnic table pavilion, which offers some shade and incredible ocean vistas. There's a portable toilet nearby. Start hiking from the **arboretum entrance ▸1** across the road. Follow the signs for the Honolua Ridge Trail, ignoring any paths leading off to the right onto the Lower Arboretum and Banyan loops. (For those side trips, see the previous hike, Trail 5, page 60.)

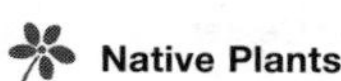

Beyond the last junction with the Banyan Loop Trail, the Honolua Ridge Trail starts ascending, eventually on gentle switchbacks. You'll notice a variety of native Hawaiian plants growing alongside the trail, including scented maile, a vine with glossy green leaves traditionally used for making Hawaiian

The Mahana Ridge Trail *makes its long, winding way down to the coast.*

lei. About 0.8 mile from the arboretum entrance, the trail emerges from the forest at **Puu Kaeo Lookout**. ►2 This modest summit (elevation 1683 feet) provides nearly 360-degree views of the West Maui Mountains and the ocean far below.

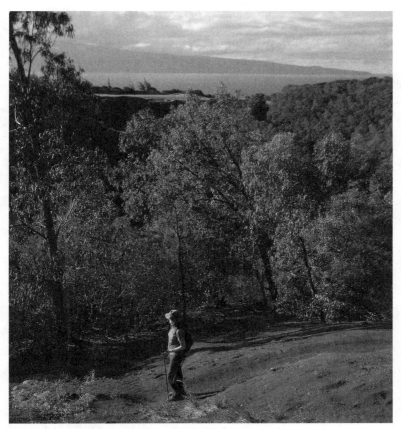
Summit

Great Views

As you continue beyond the lookout, you'll start following the officially signed Mahana Ridge Trail. The main trail splits as it circles around the lookout, reconnecting on the far side. Hike another 0.5 mile

Shady

Secluded

Native Plants

Birds

downhill, crossing a seasonally dry streambed, to reach the **Sugi Pine Grove Loop**. ►3 Here a short side trail ambles through a stand of *Crypotomeria japonica*, commonly called sugi pines or Japanese cedar, although these evergreens with spiral needles are actually a species of cypress.

Making a relatively easy downhill descent, the main Mahana Ridge Trail passes through a gate into the Puu Kukui Watershed Preserve, then contours uphill again. Soon you pass by the Uluhe Loop. This 0.3-mile side trail traipses through stands of uluhe (false staghorn ferns), which are endemic to Hawaii. Although they commonly grow only a few feet off the ground, when the ferns are able to brace themselves against taller trees, they can reach more dramatic heights. The main trail briefly grants peekaboo ocean views before passing into groves of nonnative eucalyptus trees.

Past the 0.1-mile Pine Loop detour, the trail enters a small clearing. Walk straight ahead to pick up the trail on the far side of the clearing, which is often sunny. The trail soon passes the 0.25-mile Akia Loop, named for the dark green shrubs with small yellow flowers and reddish berries that grow right alongside the main path, as well as on the side loop. About 0.3 mile past the clearing, you may want to skip the next detour along the 0.6-mile Pineapple Loop. Most of the fruit plants have gone to seed, so there's not much to see as you bushwhack through former pineapple plantation fields gone amok.

About 4 miles from the arboretum entrance, you'll see water tanks off to your left. Soon the trail runs onto a large jeep road with power lines strung overhead. Keep the **small water reservoir** ►4 on your left and follow the trail as it trudges through shoulder-high grasses, then reenters shady pine forest flush with the sounds of native birds. More sweeping ocean views open up to the northwest across the gulch as you continue downhill. Underfoot the trail

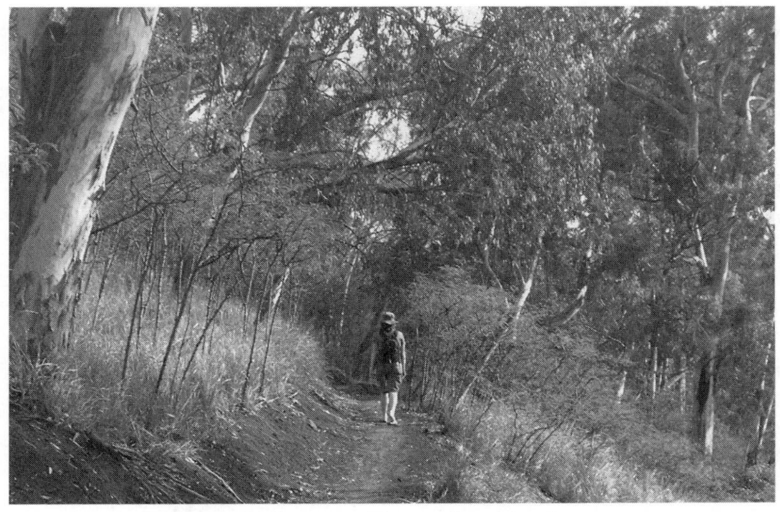

A gentle, shady forest path *drops you off at D.T. Fleming Beach.*

stops being a pine needle–carpeted path just before hitting a steeply eroded section of red dirt, subject to mudslides in rainy weather. Stone steps have been placed into the hillside here, beyond which the trail bottoms out onto a dirt 4WD jeep road. It's a short walk farther downhill to the **restrooms ►5** and emergency phone, placed here for the convenience of the resort's golfers, not hikers. The chilled drinking water dispenser may be working, but don't bet your life on it. Make sure you bring along enough water for the entire hike.

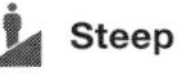 **Steep**

Don't follow the wide, paved golf-cart path leading downhill from the restrooms. Instead, look for a dirt footpath ascending a small hillside just south of the restrooms. At the top of a small hill, the trail jogs right along another dirt 4WD road for a short distance. Pick up the signposted Mahana Ridge Trail at the next major road intersection. With an industrial-looking maintenance yard visible below to your left, the sunny, exposed footpath ambles downhill.

The trail soon passes underneath the Honoapiilani Highway, then tumbles down some short, shady switchbacks to the **official end of the trail** ▶6 on Lower Honoapiilani Road.

Beach

A few minutes' walk downhill along the paved road is D. T. Fleming Park. Despite steep drop-offs and dangerous rip currents, the long, sandy beach is popular with locals and visitors alike for swimming and bodyboarding. Ask the lifeguards on duty about current water conditions before you take a dip, however, since steep drop-offs and dangerous currents await offshore. The county-run park has drinking fountains, restrooms, picnic tables, and a pay phone.

Swimming

D. T. Fleming Park's beach is top-ranked for scenery and surf, but you'll find more protected waters for swimming farther south at Kapalua Bay.

From the public access beach parking lot, it's a half-mile walk uphill to the Kapalua Adventure Center. An admittedly confusing network of paved paths wind through the manicured resort grounds. Heading southwest, keep to the left as you walk uphill behind The Ritz-Carlton hotel. Then continue along the shoulder of a paved access road that passes an employee parking lot as it leads toward the golf course. At the top of a small rise, look for the **Kapalua Adventure Center** ▶7 off to your right.

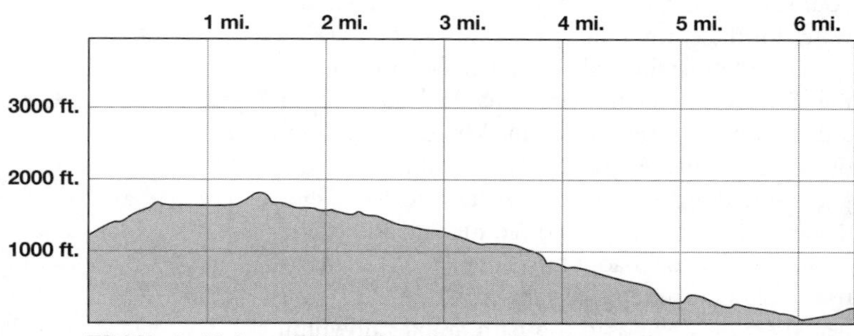

TRAIL 6 Mahana Ridge Elevation Profile

MILESTONES

▶1	0.0	Start from Maunalei Arboretum trailhead [N 20.97984°, W 156.62062°]
▶2	0.8	Reach Puu Kaeo Lookout [N 20.97200°, W 156.61888°]
▶3	1.3	Pass the Sugi Pine Grove Loop [N 20.96493°, W 156.61655°]
▶4	4.2	Cross dirt road by small water reservoir [N 20.98740°, W 156.63393°]
▶5	5.0	Arrive at restrooms and emergency phone [N 20.99702°, W 156.64020°]
▶6	6.0	Reach trail's end near D. T. Fleming Park [N 21.00243°, W 156.65019°]
▶7	6.5	Return to Kapalua Adventure Center [N 20.99767°, W 156.65327°]

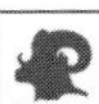

OPTIONS

Alternate Hike: From Sea to Summit

Hard-core hikers who want to tackle the Mahana Ridge Trail in the reverse (uphill) direction can find the lower trailhead on the *mauka* (inland) side of Lower Honoapiilani Road, the access road that leads to D. T. Fleming Beach Park, by turning off the Honoapiilani Highway (Hwy. 30) north of Kapalua near mile marker (MM) 31. Just uphill from the public access beach parking lot, the lower trailhead is not easy to spot; look for a small arrowed signpost that reads MAHANA RIDGE.

Call the Kapalua Adventure Center in advance at (808) 665-4386 or visit www.kapalua.com to check schedules of shuttle pick-ups from the arboretum, which is the end of your uphill hike. Otherwise, you'll have to hike both ways (about a 13-mile round-trip). The signed liability waiver and permit requirement is not enforced for hikers starting from the lower trailhead, although checking in at the Kapalua Adventure Center before your hike is still a good idea. It at least lets someone know your plans, in case anything unexpected happens out on the trail.

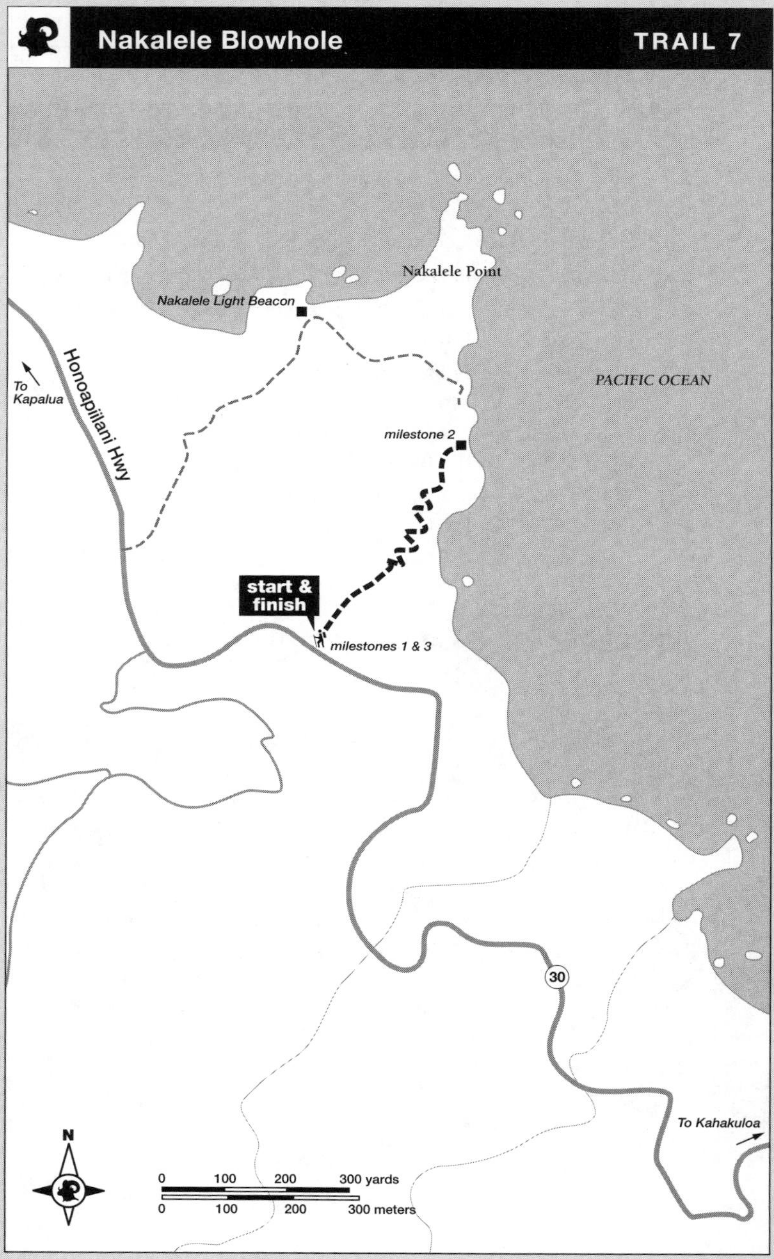
Nakalele Blowhole
TRAIL 7
Nakalele Point
Nakalele Light Beacon
PACIFIC OCEAN
To Kapalua
Honoapiilani Hwy
milestone 2
start & finish
milestones 1 & 3
30
To Kahakuloa
N
0 100 200 300 yards
0 100 200 300 meters

Nakalele Blowhole

The point of this short, but rugged coastal hike is to get as close as safely possible to the Nakalele Blowhole, a naturally occurring phenomenon. When the surf is high, the ocean spouts powerfully through lava rocks here, sometimes 50 feet or even higher into the air.

TRAIL USE
Dayhike
LENGTH
0.9 mile, 30–45 mins.
VERTICAL FEET
±250′
DIFFICULTY
– 1 **2** 3 4 5 +
TRAIL TYPE
Out & Back
SURFACE TYPE
Dirt, Lava, Sand
START & END
N 21.02461°
W 156.59038°

FEATURES
Lava Flows
Tide Pools
Great Views
Steep
Geologic Interest

FACILITIES
None

Best Time

You can hike this trail year-round from sunrise until sunset daily. You can't, however, predict exactly when the blowhole will sound off—it's a matter of luck as much as it is good timing. That said, try to visit on a windy day when the surf's up. After dark, the path can be dangerously tricky because of loose lava rocks and a lack of clear trail markings.

Finding the Trail

From Kapalua, drive northeast on the Honoapiilani Highway (Hwy. 30) for about 8 miles. A little more than 0.5 mile past mile marker (MM) 38, look for a dirt parking area pullout marked by boulders on the *makai* (ocean) side of the road.

Coming from Kahului in Central Maui, drive northwest on the Kahekili Highway (Hwy. 340), a winding cliffside route with blind curves and bridges that frequently narrows to one lane. After passing MM 17 on the Kahekili Highway, the mile markers reset for the Honoapiilani Highway at MM 41. Drive northwest almost 0.5 mile past MM 39 and look for the dirt parking area pullout on your right.

Trail Description

For daytrippers along the Kahekili Highway, West Maui's most twistingly narrow and remote scenic byway, the blowhole is a dramatic finish.

On the wilder windward side of the island, this short out-and-back hike is just a quick drive from the Kapalua resort area. For daytrippers along the Kahekili Highway, West Maui's most narrow and twisting scenic byway, the Nakalele Blowhole makes a dramatic finish. The trail itself is exposed and rocky, so bring along sunscreen and a hat that won't blow away in the strong winds that whip the coast here. Also wear shoes with good traction for the crumbly cliffside path that drops steeply to the coast.

Start hiking from the **parking area** ►1 off the Honoapiilani Highway. The trail starts off almost level, following a wide dirt road crisscrossed by hundreds of footprints. The road gently starts to drop as it heads *makai* (toward the ocean). A few minutes' walk from the highway, the blowhole already comes into view along the coast downhill to your left. Some people decide not to walk out any farther than this viewpoint: The panoramas of the black lava-rock coast, the ocean with its pounding white surf, and the spouting blowhole are impressive.

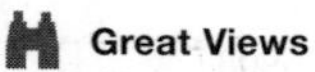

As you keep hiking downhill toward the blowhole, the road quickly narrows to a footpath that steeply descends the cliffs on switchbacks as the terrain changes from sand-colored dirt to jagged, jet-black lava. Multiple use trails crisscross this rocky area, so navigate your own way down as best you can using the *ahu* (stone cairns) left by other hikers. Just keep the blowhole in sight, generally heading in that direction.

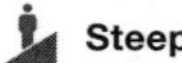

Steep

After less than 0.5 mile, the trail flattens out near sea level as you approach the *mauka* (inland) side of the **Nakalele Blowhole**, ►2 a natural geologic formation. When the ocean wears away the bottom of the lava shelf, an erosional hole is formed, through which the surf erupts much like a small geyser. Although you'll see some visitors walk right up to

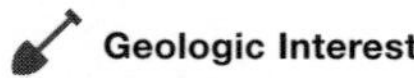

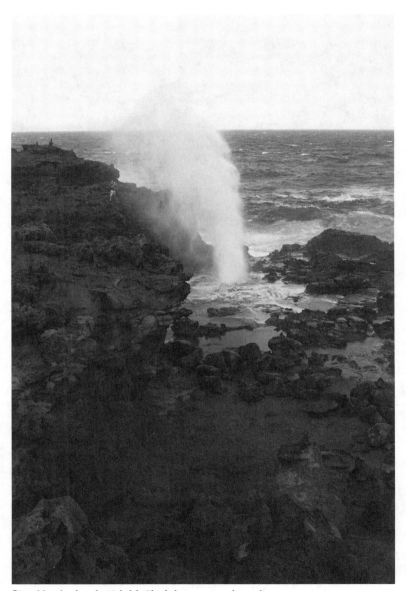

Stand back *when the Nakalele Blowhole is spouting skyward!*

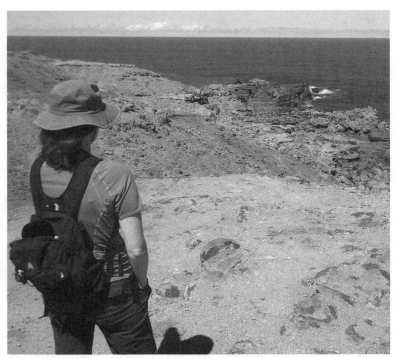

Pick your own way *down the lava-rock cliffs to the coast.*

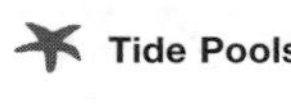

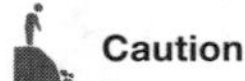

the mouth of the blowhole, that can be dangerous. It's smarter to stand back and observe the blowhole from a safe distance. There are also tide pools along the lava-rock coast that you can explore carefully here. The waves are unpredictable, so remember to never turn your back on the sea.

MILESTONES

►1	0.0	Start from roadside parking area [N 21.02461°, W 156.59038°]
►2	0.4	Approach *mauka* (inland) side of the blowhole
►3	0.9	Arrive back at roadside parking area [N 21.02461°, W 156.59038°]

When you've snapped enough photos or video, turn around and make your way back up the cliffs, following the cairns or whatever use trail looks easiest. From the top of the cliffs, it's a short walk back along the dirt 4WD road to the **parking area ▶3** beside the highway.

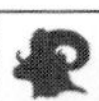

OPTIONS

Alternate Hikes off the Kahekili Highway

Another route for hikers approaches the Nakalele Blowhole from the north. To find the alternate trailhead, park on the *makai* (ocean) side of the Honoapiilani Highway at mile marker (MM) 38. Walk down a dirt 4WD road that descends steeply toward the modern Nakalele Light Beacon, near the tip of Nakalele Point. From there, pick your way carefully over to the rocky, windblown coast east toward the blowhole—there is no actual trail. During periods of high surf, avoid this risky walk near the coast.

Want more coastal scenery? It's easy to combine a hike to the Nakalele Blowhole with the nearby Ohai Trail (see Trail 8, page 79), which loops through native plant restoration areas and around a clifftop with ocean views. On calm days when the blowhole isn't sounding off, the natural ocean baths farther south along the Kahekili Highway are a good alternative hike (see Trail 9, page 83).

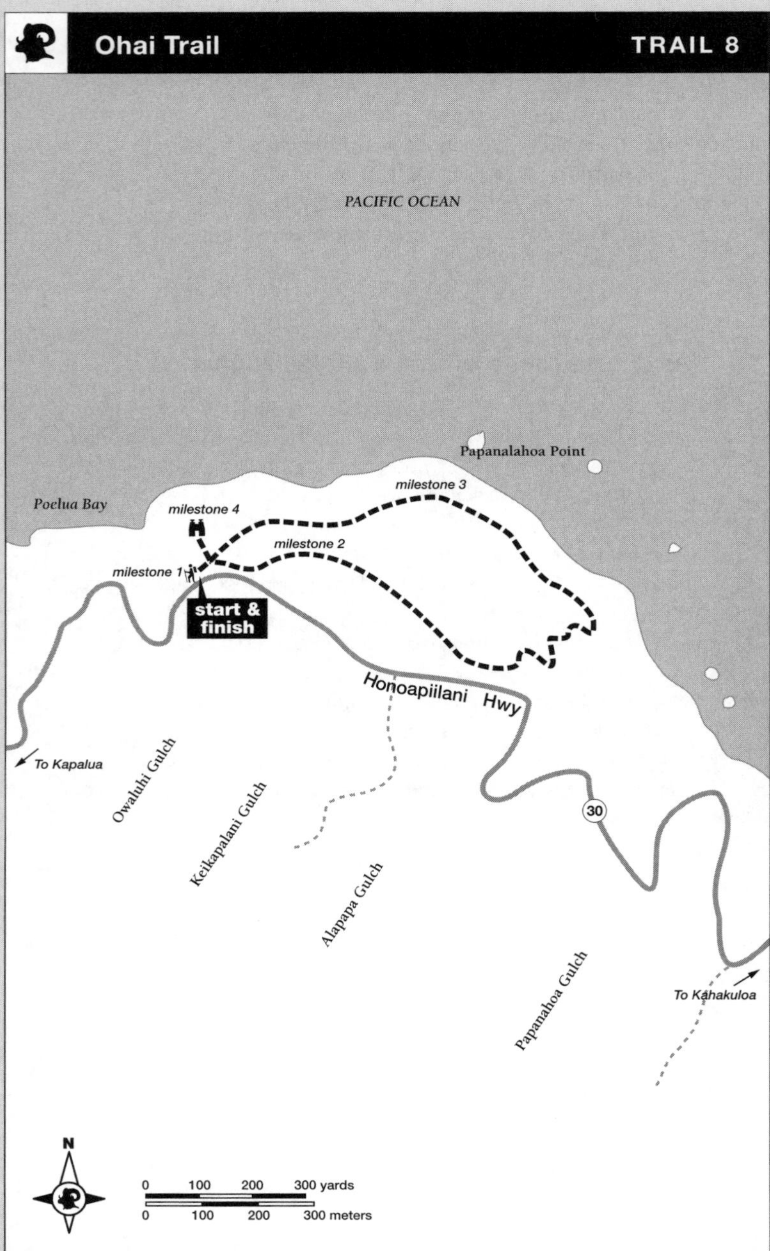
Ohai Trail
TRAIL 8
PACIFIC OCEAN
Papanalahoa Point
milestone 3
Poelua Bay
milestone 4
milestone 2
milestone 1
start & finish
Honoapiilani Hwy
To Kapalua
Owaluhi Gulch
Keikapalani Gulch
30
Alapapa Gulch
Papanahoa Gulch
To Kahakuloa
N
0 100 200 300 yards
0 100 200 300 meters

Ohai Trail

Often overlooked by drivers on the Kahekili Highway, this clifftop trail winds past beautifully restored native vegetation at the coastal edge of the West Maui Forest Reserve. It's a quick leg-stretching hike, either before or after visiting the Nakalele Blowhole (see Trail 7, page 73).

TRAIL USE
Dayhike, Child Friendly

LENGTH
1.3 miles, 30–45 mins.

VERTICAL FEET
±850′

DIFFICULTY
– **1** 2 3 4 5 +

TRAIL TYPE
Semiloop

SURFACE TYPE
Dirt, Grass, Paved

START & END
N 21.01586°
W 156.57675°

FEATURES
Birds
Native Plants
Great Views

FACILITIES
None

Best Time

You can hike this trail year-round. Avoid hiking midday, when the sun is strongest. Late afternoon tends to be windier than early in the morning. Sunrise is a pretty time to hike, as many of the trail's panoramic views face eastward.

Finding the Trail

From Kapalua, drive northeast on the Honoapiilani Highway (Hwy. 30) for almost 11 miles. Around 0.8 mile past mile marker (MM) 40, look for a parking area pullout on the *makai* (ocean) side of the road.

Coming from Kahului in Central Maui, drive northwest on the Kahekili Highway (Hwy. 340), a winding cliffside route with blind curves and bridges that frequently narrows to one lane. After passing MM 17 on the Kahekili Highway, the mile markers reset for the Honoapiilani Highway at MM 41. Drive 0.2 mile farther along the Honoapiilani Highway and look for a parking area pullout on your right.

Trail Description

Many people stop here for the viewpoint, but few take advantage of the trail that loops around the windswept cliffs.

Just northwest of Kahakuloa village, the parking lot for the untrammeled Ohai Trail is often full. Many people stop here just for the viewpoint, but few take advantage of the hiking trail that loops around the windswept cliffs of Poelua Point. The trail is exposed and often sunny, so bring sunscreen and a hat that won't blow away in the wind. Thanks to recent habitat restoration and volunteer trail maintenance, including by the Sierra Club (see Appendix 2, page 307), this mostly level trail is usually in very good condition. You won't need hiking boots.

Start walking toward the ocean from the **roadside parking area.** ►1 Ignore the paved path leading left toward the viewpoint. Instead, look for a signposted trailhead and a dirt path heading off to your right. About 0.1 mile from the parking area, veer right at the **first trail junction** ►2 to begin walking counterclockwise around the main loop of this lollipop-shaped trail. When you arrive at a relatively flat, large dirt area crisscrossed by many use trails, stick to the main trail, which is bordered by large rocks placed here to guide hikers.

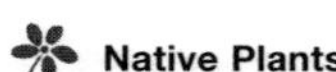

On the far side of the flatlands, the trail gently ascends the oceanfront cliffs. As you gaze out across the hillsides thick with vegetation, it's easy to spy where the trail goes next, as it snakes around and curves up and down around Poelua Point. Take time to look around at the immense variety of native plants that have been restored here. Shrubby naupaka is easily recognized by its thick glossy green leaves and white flowers that look as if they've been torn in half. Pauohiiaka is another low-growing vine, but with smaller pale blue and white flowers and leathery leaves covered in fine silver hairs. The trail's namesake, the rare ohia plant, is an endangered member of the pea family. It has stems of oval green leaves and floppy, bright pinkish-orange flowers that stand out brightly against the hillside.

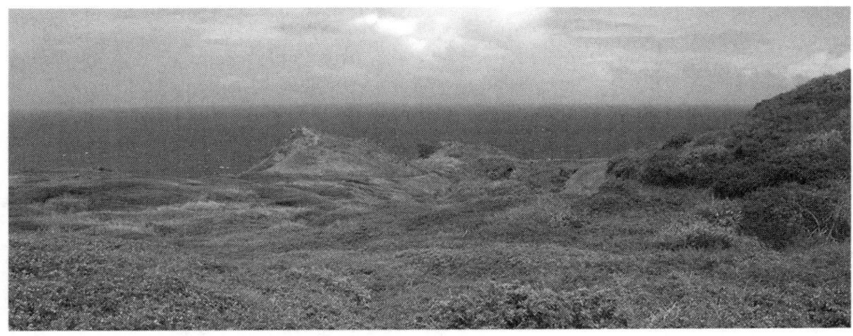

Stretch your legs *atop West Maui's highest sea cliffs.*

Less than a mile from the parking lot, you reach a **hikers' bench**. ►3 From here you can sit and peer down into the azure waters hundreds of feet below or observe seabirds soaring just offshore. When you're ready to press on, stand up and rejoin the main trail, which heads gradually uphill back toward the trailhead. Close the loop at the main trail junction, staying to the right and walking straight ahead toward the parking area by the highway.

Just before reaching the highway, veer right along a paved path that briefly leads out to the main **coastal viewpoint**. ►4 Looking south, you can see stony Kahakuloa Head jutting up above the coast, while to the north the spouting Nakalele Blowhole is often barely visible with the naked eye. When you're ready, retrace your steps for a few minutes along the paved path back to the **roadside parking area**. ►5

For guided hikes and volunteer clean-up days on the Ohai Trail, check the group outings calendar of the Maui group of the Hawaii chapter of the Sierra Club, at www.hi.sierraclub.org/maui.

 **Great Views**

MILESTONES

►1	0.0	Start from roadside parking area [N 21.01586°, W 156.57675°]
►2	0.1	Veer right at first trail junction [N 21.01622°, W 156.57619°]
►3	0.8	Arrive at hikers' bench [N 21.01729°, W 156.57233°]
►4	1.2	Detour to viewpoint
►5	1.3	Return to roadside parking area [N 21.01586°, W 156.57675°]

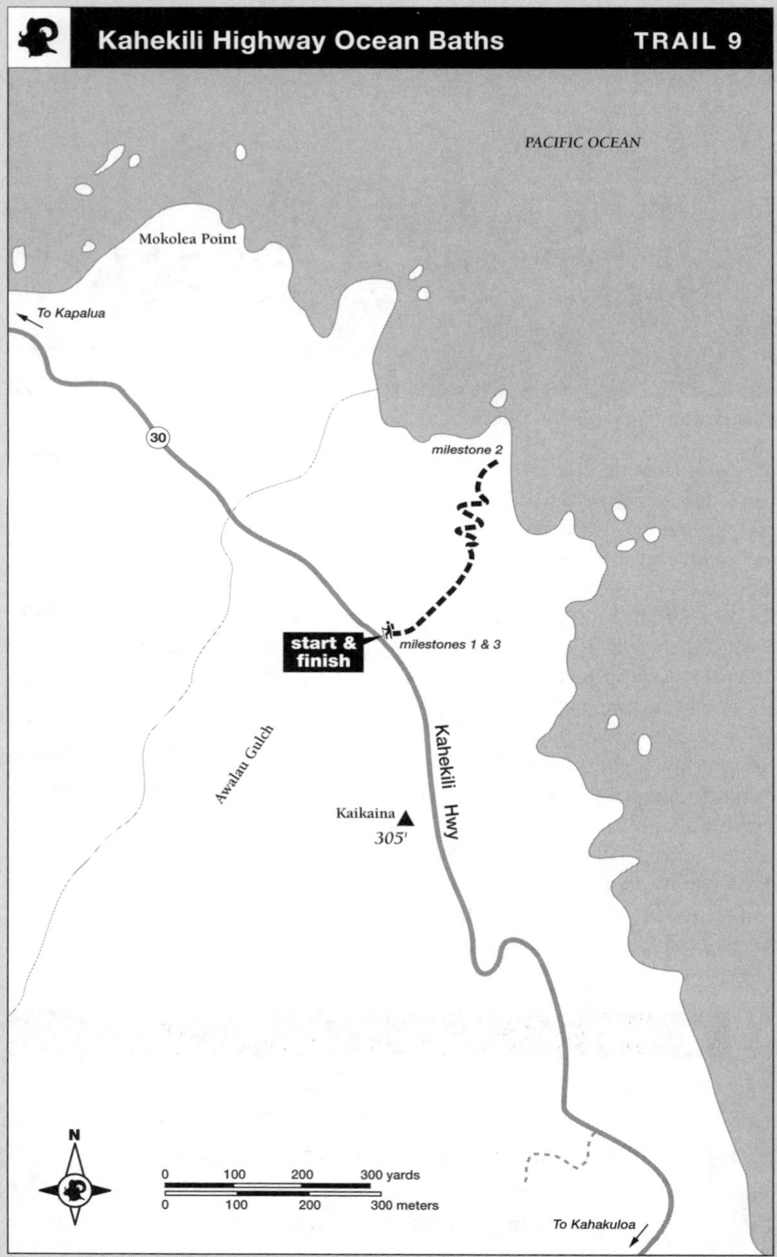
Kahekili Highway Ocean Baths
TRAIL 9
PACIFIC OCEAN
Mokolea Point
To Kapalua
30
milestone 2
start & finish
milestones 1 & 3
Awalau Gulch
Kahekili Hwy
Kaikaina
305'
N
0 100 200 300 yards
0 100 200 300 meters
To Kahakuloa

Kahekili Highway Ocean Baths

A quick scramble down the cliffs off the Kahekili Highway, these natural pools encircled by lava-rock walls will entice swimmers and snorkelers. Don't take a dip if strong winds are blowing or the surf is crashing high upon the rocks, as drownings have unfortunately occurred here.

TRAIL USE
Dayhike
LENGTH
0.6 mile, 30–45 mins.
VERTICAL FEET
±225′
DIFFICULTY
– 1 **2** 3 4 5 +
TRAIL TYPE
Out & Back
SURFACE TYPE
Dirt, Grass, Lava
START & END
N 21.00757°
W 156.55748°

FEATURES
Lava Flows
Tide Pools
Great Views
Swimming
Steep

FACILITIES
None

Best Time

The best time to visit the pools is during summer, when ocean waves are generally calmer and fewer rainstorms happen. If you see dark clouds overhead, big waves approaching, or the sea level starting to rise, get out of the water immediately. At low tide, there may not be enough water to fill the pools; then again, high tide can be a risky time to take a dip. There are no lifeguards, so use your own best judgment (see also the warning on page 87).

Finding the Trail

From Kahului in Central Maui, drive northwest on the Kahekili Highway (Hwy. 340), a winding cliffside route with blind curves and bridges that frequently narrows to one lane. Past the village of Kahakuloa, look for a dirt parking pullout area on the *makai* (ocean) side of the road just before mile marker (MM) 16.

Coming from Kapalua, drive northeast on the Honoapiilani Highway (Hwy. 30) for about 11 miles. After MM 41 on the Honoapiilani Highway, the mile markers reset for the Kahekili Highway at MM 17. Drive another mile farther along the

Kahekili Highway and look for a dirt parking pull-out area on your right, just past MM 16.

Trail Description

Olivine is the same mineral found on the Big Island of Hawaii's famous green sand beach near Ka Lae (South Point).

There are no facilities at the trailhead, although Kahakuloa village farther south along the highway has fruit stands and a few roadside vendors selling snacks, shave ice, and island-style plate lunches. Because this trail is fully exposed to the sun, bring sunscreen and a hat that won't blow away in the strong coastal winds. Shoes with good traction will help on the initial descent, as parts of the cliffside trail can be crumbly. Most visitors wear swimsuits underneath their shorts and T-shirts, as nudity is frowned upon at the pools.

From the **roadside parking area**, ►1 face the ocean and start walking straight ahead past the yellow sign warning you about ocean hazards. The wide dirt area here is crisscrossed by several confusing use trails. Generally speaking, if you stay to the right, you can make a more gentle descent toward the coast. If you head to the left, there are steeper, but also more direct routes down to the shore. Taking the right-hand path on the way down and the left-hand route on the way back up is probably your best bet for gradients that aren't too steep for basic running shoes to handle.

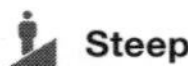
Steep

Inland along the highway just south of the trailhead, look for a large boulder known as Pohaku Kani, or simply the bellstone, for the way it can resonate when struck.

Pick your way carefully down for about 0.3 mile to the coast, where you'll spy the **natural ocean baths**. ►2 (If you don't see them, that means that the sea level is so high that the pools have been completely overrun, in which case you should stay out.) Nicknamed by some tourist guidebooks as the "Queen's Baths," these lava rock–encircled pools of varying sizes are spread out along the rocky shoreline. The views are incredible, with frothy surf and aquamarine water crashing against jet-black lava rocks. Some of the lava sparkles in the sun because

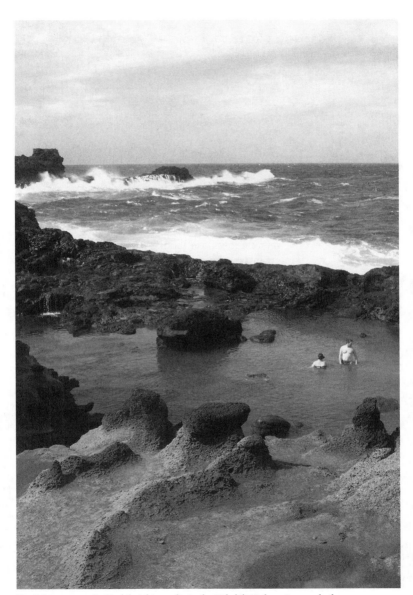

Daytrippers cool off *while taking a dip in the Kahekili Highway's ocean baths.*

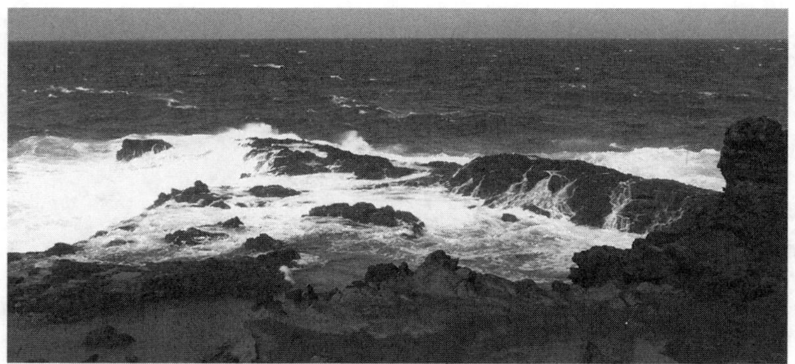

Remember *to never turn your back on the sea.*

of its green olivine content. Olivine is the same mineral found on the Big Island of Hawaii's famous green sand beach near Ka Lae (South Point).

Swimming

Caution

Tide Pools

Although it's always too rough for open-ocean swimming along this coast, you can take a dip in the pools when the waves are not too rough here. Most people enter the pools using the lava-shelf ledges or natural stepping stones. Bring a snorkel mask to peek into the pools' submarine life, too. There are also smaller tide pools that you can explore along the coast nearby. Just remember that you should never turn your back on the sea, for safety's sake.

After you've had a good soak, turn around and retrace your steps back up the rocky cliffs and along the dirt trail back to the **roadside parking area**.›3

Notice

Warning! Drownings have occurred in the Kahekili Highway ocean baths, mostly when people have been knocked over and pinned underwater or else swept out to sea by rogue waves. Do not attempt to enter the pools during rainstorms or periods of high surf. When in doubt, stay out. On days when the surf's up, you're better off watching the Nakalele Blowhole instead (see Trail 7, page 73).

MILESTONES

▶1	0.0	Start from roadside parking area [N 21.00757°, W 156.55748°]
▶2	0.3	Arrive at natural ocean baths [N 21.00949°, W 156.55604°]
▶3	0.6	Return to roadside parking area [N 21.00757°, W 156.55748°]

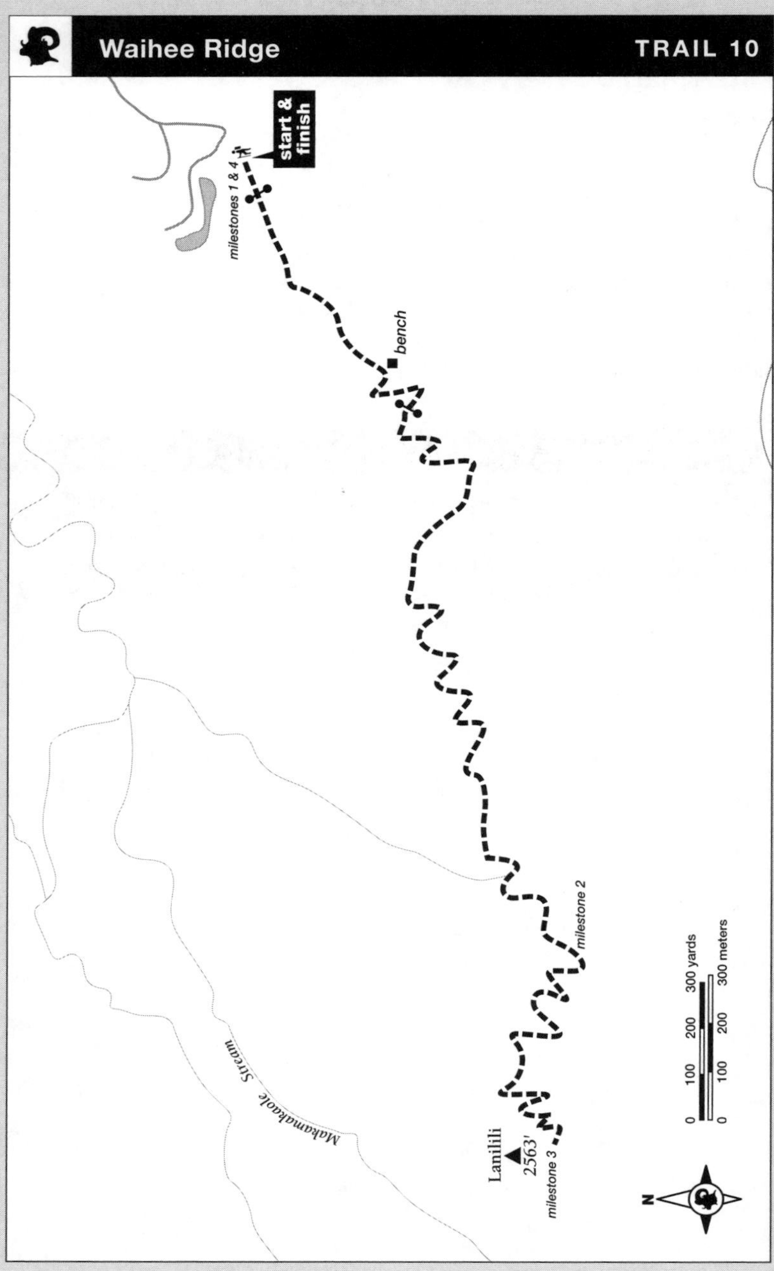
start & finish
milestones 1 & 4
bench
milestone 2
milestone 3
Lanilili
2563'
Makamakaole Stream
300 yards
0 100 200
300 meters
0 100 200
N

Waihee Ridge

On the lush windward side of the West Maui Mountains, this trail ascends to a head-spinning viewpoint that looks deep into the range—when the summit isn't completely veiled by clouds and mist, that is. Native plants and birds are both bonuses along this classic forest trail.

TRAIL USE
Dayhike, Run, Dogs Allowed

LENGTH
5.0 miles, 2½–3 hours

VERTICAL FEET
±1750

DIFFICULTY
– 1 2 **3** 4 5 +

TRAIL TYPE
Out & Back

SURFACE TYPE
Dirt, Grass, Paved

START & END
N 20.95294°
W 156.53230°

FEATURES
Forest
Mountain
Summit
Birds
Native Plants
Wildlife
Great Views
Secluded
Shady
Steep

FACILITIES
Picnic Tables

Best Time

You can hike this trail year-round. The gated trailhead access road is open from 7 AM to 6 PM daily. Take this partly shady hike on sunny days when there are no rain clouds in the sky to obscure the promised views. Getting an early start may also help you avoid disappointingly overcast conditions. Locals go running and walk their dogs here every day, but weekends tend to be more crowded.

Finding the Trail

From Central Maui, take Highway 340 (Kahului Beach Road, which turns into Waiehu Beach Road) northwest of Kahului or follow Highway 330 northeast of Wailuku. From the intersection of Highways 340 and 330, keep driving north on Highway 340 (now called the Kahekili Highway) for a little more than 4 miles. Past the Mendes Ranch near the END OF STATE HIGHWAY sign at a hairpin turn, turn left onto a paved access road signposted for the Boy Scouts of America's Camp Maluhia. (If you reach mile marker 7 on the Kahekili Highway, you've gone too far.) Drive 0.9 mile uphill along the winding paved road to the trailhead, then another 0.1 mile farther to the designated dirt parking area. Do not park at the gated trailhead or alongside the access road.

Trail Description

Seldom crowded, it's a tranquil forest escape from Maui's crowds of beachgoers and sun worshippers down on the coast.

Seldom crowded, the Waihee Ridge Trail makes for a tranquil forest escape from Maui's crowds of beachgoers and sun worshippers down on the coast. Over on the rainy side of the West Maui Mountains, this trail ascends to a summit where you can peek into the lush interior of this ancient volcanic range. There is no water available anywhere along the route, so bring all you'll need. Sunscreen and a hat will shield you from the most exposed sections at the beginning and near the end of the trail. Because hunters also use this forest reserve land, it's smart to wear bright-colored clothing. Leashed dogs are allowed.

From the designated dirt parking area, backtrack 0.1 mile along the paved access road to the **trailhead gate**, ▶1, marked by a brown-and-yellow NA ALA HELE sign. Step through the hikers' pass-through on the left side of the gate. The trail climbs stiffly uphill through pastureland along broken pavement partly overgrown with grasses. Straight ahead, you can see the trail continuing to rise on the hillside before passing into shady lowland forest. Don't forget to turn around for sweeping ocean views.

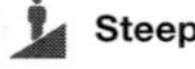

A little more than 0.1 mile from the trailhead, you pass a water tank on the left. The trail continues on the other side of a smaller hikers' pass-through, where it becomes a dirt (or muddy, if it has been raining recently) trail. You pass through another small pedestrian gate as the trail climbs on long, lazy switchbacks, which alternate with less strenuous ridgeline contours. The footpath is often shaded by tall Norfolk pines, tropical ash, and eucalyptus trees, as well as guava and thimbleberry plants whose fragrant smashed fruit often falls right onto the path itself.

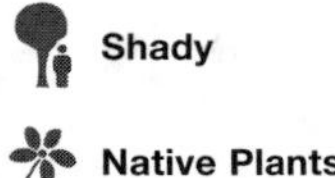

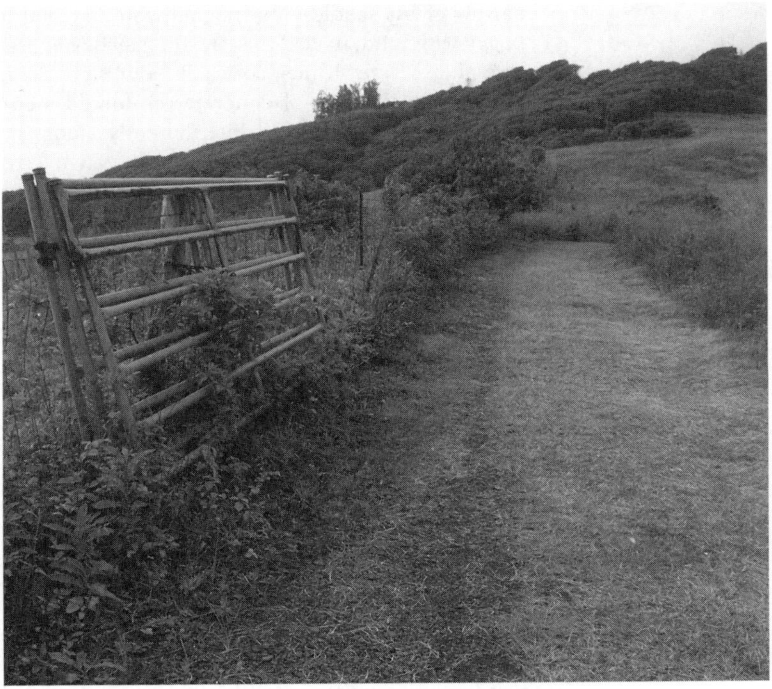

Sunny days *are your best bet for heart-stopping views from the summit.*

A little more than 0.5 mile from the trailhead, a bench appears beside the trail. There you can sit and admire the vistas of the Waihee and Makamakaole valleys carpeted with native foliage and waterfalls visible on the cliffside. Around the next bend in the trail you glimpse even broader ocean panoramas, followed by another hikers' pass-through. As the trail keeps switchbacking upward through the forest, alternating with ridgeline contours that make only modest elevation gains, look for more memorable glimpses of the mountainous interior valleys, lacy waterfalls, and the ocean.

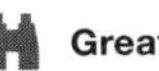

Great Views

Less than 1.5 miles from the trailhead, the trail breaks out of the forest cover and emerges onto a narrow grassy saddle. After rainfall, you may find it boggy with mud; in fact, this section may be impassable after severe storms, so watch your step. Soon you'll reach the start of **concrete-reinforced steps** ▶2 that have been placed intermittently along the trail, which suddenly gets steeper. Lush native ferns and ohia lehua trees grow alongside the path as you doggedly huff and puff ever upward. Those flashes of crimson seen in the trees are likely apapane, a common species of Hawaiian honeycreeper. After ascending a twisted knob, the trail reaches a flat tableland. If you're running on this trail, take it easy on the final ridgeline ascent to the summit, especially whenever the trail is muddy and slick, because there are steep drop-offs all around. Depending on the weather, this can be ankle-twisting territory.

Steep

Birds

About 2.5 miles from your starting point, the trail unceremoniously ends at a picnic table at the **summit** ▶3 of Lanilili (elevation 2563 feet).From this small peak, lucky hikers get sweeping views of the West Maui Mountains and the Pacific Ocean. But perhaps more often than not, the peak is shrouded in clouds and mist. That's not too surprising, given that it gets an average of 40 to 80 inches of rainfall each year. Thankfully, the winds that often blow at this elevation can push the clouds away within a matter of minutes, so stick around for a while if at

Summit

Great Views

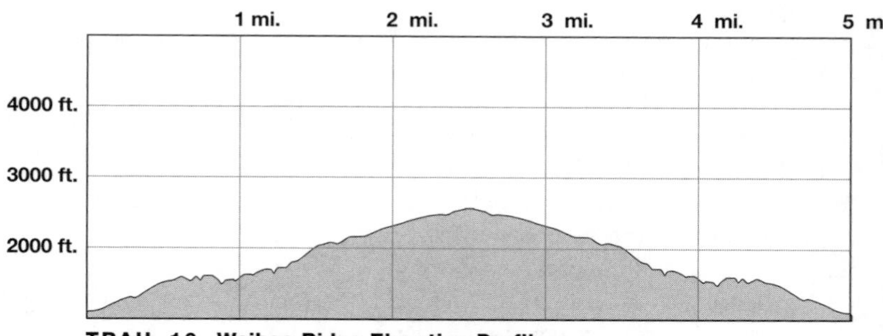

TRAIL 10 Waihee Ridge Elevation Profile

first your views are hemmed in. You never know whether or not the skies might quickly clear. Hiking beyond the end of the trail is illegal and not smart, given the perilously steep terrain.

Once you've captured that perfect photo from the summit, or perhaps you've finally gotten tired of waiting for the skies to clear, turn around and retrace your steps back downhill to the gated trailhead. On the other side of the gate, turn left and walk back along the paved road to the **designated dirt parking area** ►4 where you started.

Near the trailhead access road, the Mendes Ranch offers *paniolo* (cowboy) horseback rides in the West Maui Mountains, costing from $110 per person. Call (808) 871-5222 or visit www.mendesranch.com for reservations.

MILESTONES

►1	0.0	Start from gated trailhead [N 20.95294°, W 156.53230°]
►2	1.5	Climb concrete-reinforced steps [N 20.94799°, W 156.54558°]
►3	2.5	Reach summit of Lanilili (end of trail) [N 20.94678°, W 156.55171°]
►4	5.0	Return to gated trailhead [N 20.95294°, W 156.53230°]

Waihee Valley TRAIL 11

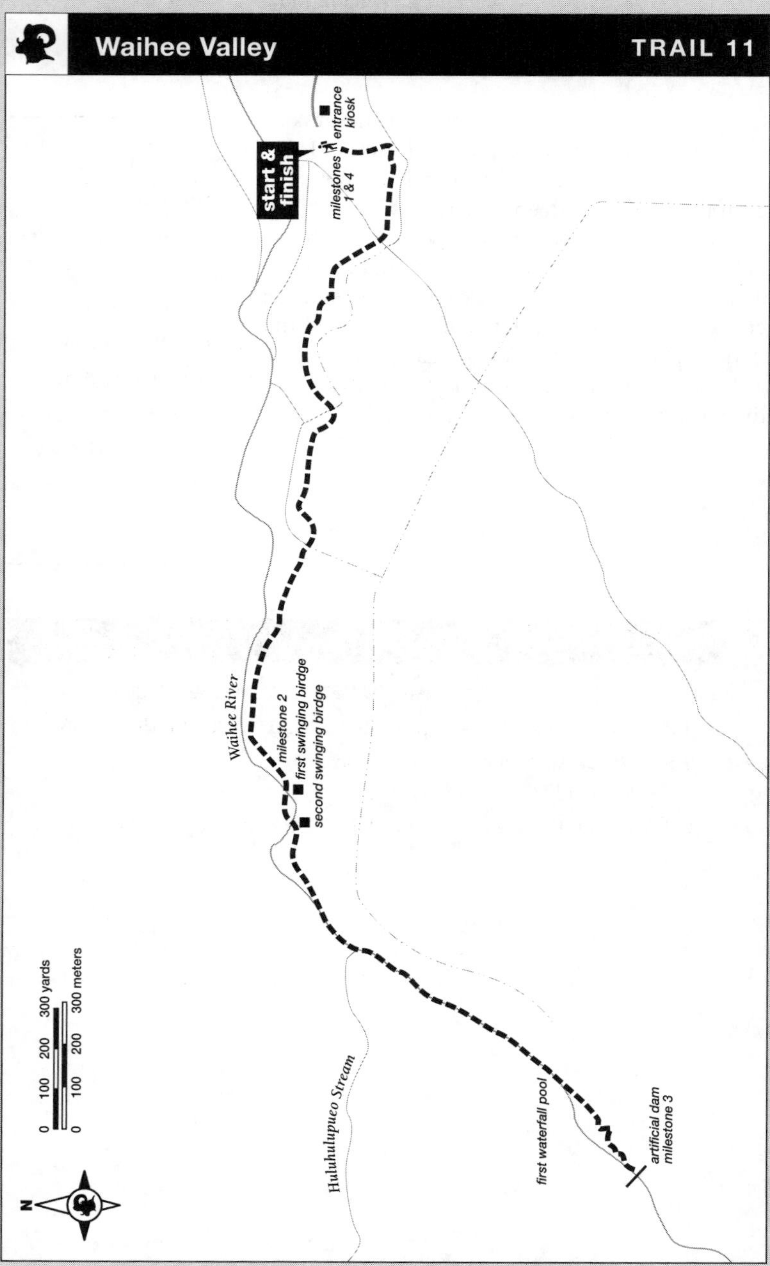
start & finish
entrance kiosk
milestones 1 & 4
Waihee River
milestone 2
first swinging birdge
second swinging birdge
Huluhulupueo Stream
first waterfall pool
artificial dam
milestone 3
0 100 200 300 yards
0 100 200 300 meters
N

Waihee Valley

Famous for its swinging cable bridges, this trail passes over private property that has been reopened to hikers for a fee. Bring plenty of insect repellent to ward off the mosquitoes along this streamside path, which ends at hidden waterfall pools and an artificial dam. Watch out for flash floods!

TRAIL USE
Dayhike, Child Friendly, Permit Required

LENGTH
4.0 miles, 1½–2½ hours

VERTICAL FEET
±800′

DIFFICULTY
– 1 2 **3** 4 5 +

TRAIL TYPE
Out & Back

SURFACE TYPE
Dirt, Grass

START & END
N 20.94143°
W 156.52464°

FEATURES
Forest
Stream
Waterfall
Birds
Native Plants
Wildlife
Swimming
Secluded
Shady

FACILITIES
Visitor Center
Restrooms

Best Time

The gated entrance kiosk is open from 9 AM to 5 PM daily. You can hike this trail year-round, although flash floods are more likely to occur during winter and spring. Beware if stream levels suddenly start to rise, as some hikers have drowned in Waihee Valley. Don't start hiking if any rain is forecast or if there are dark clouds in the sky. Weekday mornings tend to be quietest, while weekend afternoons can get quite busy.

Finding the Trail

From Central Maui, take Highway 340 (Kahului Beach Road, which becomes Waiehu Beach Road) northwest of Kahului or Highway 330 northeast of Wailuku. From the intersection of Highways 340 and 330, keep heading north on Highway 340 (now called the Kahekili Highway) for around 2.2 miles. Just before mile marker (MM) 5, turn left onto Waihee Valley Road, which winds through a residential subdivision for about 0.5 mile to the entrance gate. Turn right and drive another 0.2 mile to the staffed kiosk.

Trail Description

Stick to the main dirt 4WD road, lined by sweet-smelling guava trees, ti and thimbleberry plants, and wild ginger blooming.

At the small entrance kiosk, adult hikers are each charged $6 (Hawaii residents with ID $3), plus $2 for each child aged 5 to 10. You must also sign a liability waiver before hiking. The kiosk sells drinks and snacks for the trail, and staff can advise you about current trail conditions and the weather forecast. Just beyond the kiosk stand a few portable toilets. Farther down the road is the **trailhead parking area**. ►1 Most hikers layer their swimsuits under their shorts and T-shirt, and you should do likewise if you plan to take a dip.

From the parking area, walk toward the metal chain strung across a dirt 4WD road. Walk straight along this often muddy road, strewn with rocks and potholes, which leads gently uphill toward the first stone bridge. Stay to the right, ignoring a side road that heads off to the left. By now, you should be able to hear the stream running downhill to the right. Past the next stone bridge, continue walking ahead while keeping the irrigation ditch on your left. Stick to the main dirt 4WD road, which is lined by sweet-smelling guava trees, ti and thimbleberry plants, and wild ginger blooming in a variety of hues. Ignore any side roads or false trails leading off to the right. About 0.6 mile from your starting point, the irrigation ditch passes through a tunnel. You can hear the stream crashing loudly off to your right, but it's not visible yet from the trail.

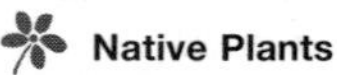

About 1 mile from your starting point, the irrigation ditch briefly rejoins the trail and runs alongside it for a while. A rocky, often dry streambed soon comes into view off to your left. It's only a few minutes' walk now to the **first swinging bridge**, ►2 the feature that famously makes this trail so fun. Climb up the stone piling steps, then walk across the wooden planks laid atop cables, which bounce up and down with every footstep. It's best if one hiker crosses the cables at a time. Once you are safely on

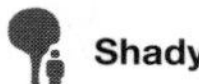

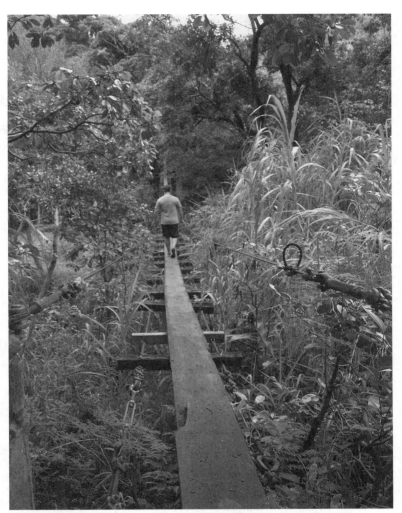

The Waihee Valley Trail *is better known by its nickname, Swinging Bridges.*

the other side, the trail continues across a short section of muddy banyan tree roots before reaching the second (and longer) swinging bridge, beyond which you pass among tall stands of bamboo plants.

Waterfall

A pretty, lacy cascade drops over the lip of the rocks into a mossy, fern-filled forest grotto.

Swimming

About 1.5 miles from your starting point, you reach the first waterfall pool. A pretty, lacy cascade drops over the lip of the rocks to form a mossy, fern-filled grotto deep in the forest. Local families and groups of teenagers often splash and swim in the usually calm waters here. But the trail doesn't end here. Ford the stream (if water levels are low enough to do so safely), then continue along the dirt path to the second stream crossing. On the other side, follow an even narrower dirt trail that's partly overgrown, heading upstream for about 10 minutes. At first it may feel like bushwhacking, but halfway along the trail becomes easier to follow.

Before you know it, the trail emerges beside an **artificial dam**. ▶3 Although not as naturally scenic as the first waterfall pool, the swimming hole here beneath the dam is larger and deeper. The dam also has rungs set into the side of the pool nearest the trail, making it easy to get into and out of the water. Continuing upstream beyond the dam is forbidden, as this is a protected watershed area. There is no real trail to follow anyway, and walking in the stream itself can be unsafe because of the danger of flash floods and strong currents.

Once you've taken a cool dip and devoured your picnic lunch, turn around and retrace your steps—fording the stream two more times and crossing both swinging bridges again—to arrive back at the **trailhead parking area**. ▶4

MILESTONES

▶1	0.0	Start from trailhead parking area [N 20.94143°, W 156.52464°]
▶2	1.1	Cross first swinging bridge [N 20.94242°, W 156.53825°]
▶3	2.0	Trail ends at artificial dam [N 20.93481°, W 156.54765°]
▶4	4.0	Return to trailhead parking area [N 20.94143°, W 156.52464°]

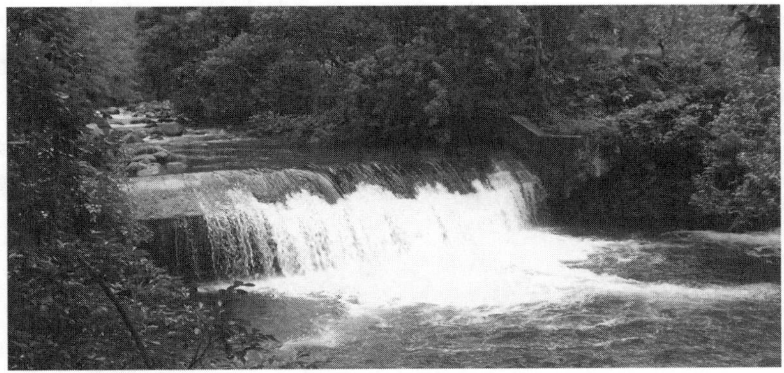

An artificial dam *has created a popular swimming hole at trail's end.*

Notice

Warning! Many flash floods have occurred in Waihee Valley. Some hikers have drowned while swimming in the stream or alongside irrigation ditches. If dark clouds appear in the sky overhead or farther up the valley, or if it starts raining and stream levels suddenly rise, get out of the water immediately and head to higher ground for safety.

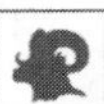

OPTIONS

Detour: Ancient Hawaiian Temples

Off Highway 340 (Waiehu Beach Road), south of its intersection with Highway 330, **Halekii-Pihana Heiau State Monument** (open 7 AM to 7 PM daily) is an off-the-beaten path archaeological site with ocean views. Along the easy 0.5-mile out-and-back trail, you can visit the platform ruins of two ancient Hawaiian temples. Admission is free.

To find the site, turn left onto Kuhio Place, just south of mile marker (MM) 2 on Highway 340, then turn left again onto Hea Place. If the monument gates are locked, park downhill on the street in the residential area, then walk uphill to the site. Don't leave anything valuable behind in your car, as vehicle break-ins are always possible. For more information about the monument, visit www.hawaiistateparks.org/parks/maui.

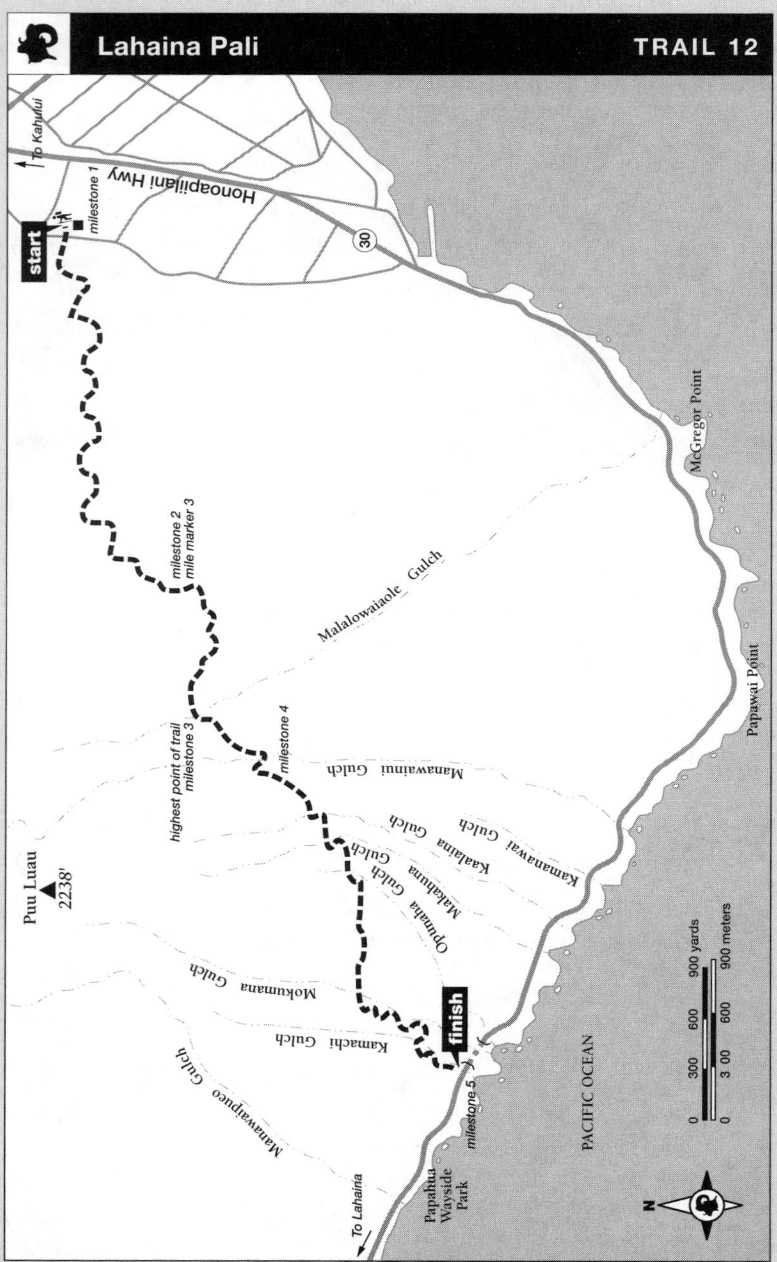

Lahaina Pali
TRAIL 12
To Kahului
Honoapiilani Hwy
milestone 1
start
30
McGregor Point
milestone 2
mile marker 3
Malalowaiaole Gulch
Papawai Point
highest point of trail
milestone 3
milestone 4
Manawainui Gulch
Kaalaina Gulch
Kamanawai Gulch
Makahuna Gulch
Opunaha Gulch
Puu Luau
2238'
Mokumana Gulch
Kamachi Gulch
finish
milestone 5
Manawaipueo Gulch
PACIFIC OCEAN
0 300 600 900 yards
0 300 600 900 meters
To Lahaina
Papahua Wayside Park
N

Lahaina Pali

This trail ranks as the most difficult on West Maui, not just for its rocky terrain and long distance, but also its full exposure to the blazing hot sun. This ancient footpath and 19th-century horseback trail across the West Maui Mountains boasts spectacular ocean panoramas en route.

Best Time

This trail is best attempted during the cooler winter months. Start hiking soon after sunrise and avoid strenuous exertion during the hottest midday hours. Dehydration, heat exhaustion, and heatstroke are all serious risks on this trail (see "Notice," page 107).

Finding the Trail

This is a point-to-point shuttle hike. To find the eastern trailhead, drive north from Maalaea on the Honoapiilani Highway (Hwy. 30) past the intersection with North Kihei Road. At the intersection with the Kuihelani Highway (Hwy. 380), make a U-turn and turn right almost immediately onto a paved road, then left onto a rutted dirt side road that passes over a small bridge. Look for the brown-and-yellow NA ALA HELE trail marker sign. You can park near the bridge, but if road conditions and your vehicle allow, keep driving inland and turn left onto a dirt road (normally barely passable by 2WD vehicles) for 0.6 mile until you reach the dirt trailhead parking lot, marked by a fence and more NA ALA HELE signs.

TRAIL USE
Dayhike, Dogs Allowed

LENGTH
5.0 miles, 3–4 hours

VERTICAL FEET
+1650′/-1550′

DIFFICULTY
- 1 2 3 4 **5** +

TRAIL TYPE
Point-to-Point

SURFACE TYPE
Dirt, Grass, Lava

START
N 20.80842°
W 156.51207°

END
N 20.78869°
W 156.55709°

FEATURES
Mountain
Native Plants
Great Views
Steep
Historic Interest

FACILITIES
None

To find the western trailhead, drive northwest from Maalaea along the Honoapiilani Highway (Hwy. 30) past mile marker (MM) 10. Almost immediately after driving through the highway tunnel, pull off into a wide dirt parking area on your right, where you'll find NA ALA HELE signs and an interpretive marker by the Lahaina Pali Trailhead. If you reach Papalaua Wayside Park on the *makai* (ocean side) of the road, you've gone too far.

Trail Description

The Lahaina Pali is a rugged hike, so make sure you're well-prepared before starting. There are no facilities or water anywhere along the route. If you find yourself getting a late start (say, after 6 AM), consider not hiking here at all, because the sun exposure can be brutal. Plan on hydrating more than you normally would for a hike of this distance at such a relatively low elevation. All of that aside, for adventurous hikers who like a challenge, or for anyone interested in Maui history, this historic trail is worth trying. It follows a 19th-century shortcut that once took travelers and traders on horseback over the West Maui Mountains. Archaeologists speculate it was built atop an ancient Hawaiian footpath that once circled the entire island.

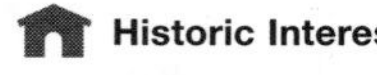

If you can't set up a shuttle, consider hiking the latter half of this point-to-point trail in reverse, from the western trailhead to the trail's highest point and back.

You can start hiking from either end of the Lahaina Pali Trail. Because the eastern trailhead is more difficult to find, it's recommended that you start there instead (that way, your friends can pick you up afterward at the more easily located western trailhead). In addition, hiking from east to west helps keep the sun out of your eyes, assuming you start early in the morning. Sometimes the dirt access road to the eastern trailhead can be impassable after heavy rains, though. If that's the case, you can walk inland to the eastern trailhead from the Honoapiiliani Highway, adding a little more

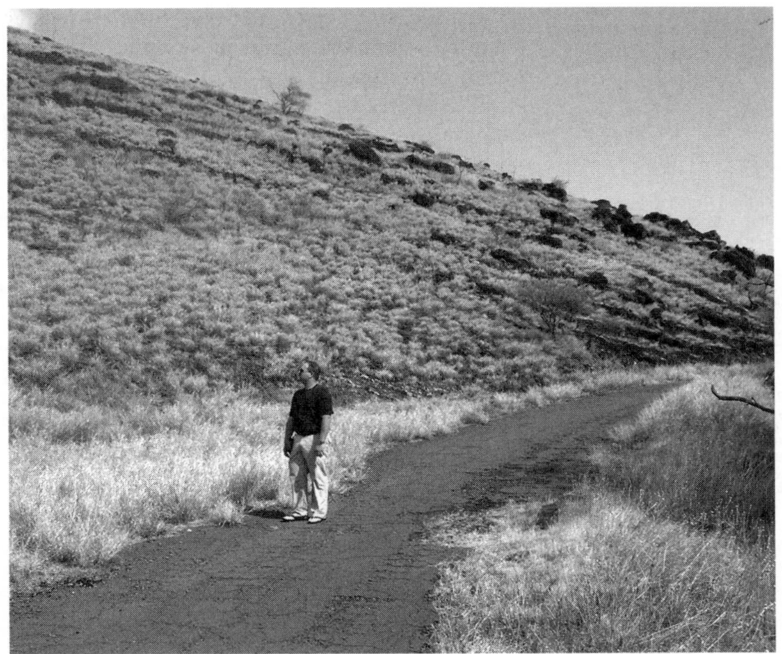

Don't forget *to stop along the way to enjoy the views—and catch your breath!*

than 0.5 mile of total distance to your hike. Note that there are no facilities (e.g., restrooms, drinking fountains, or pay phones) at either trailhead.

At the **eastern trailhead**, ▶1 interpretive plaques explain the trail's history and give hikers a brief overview of what lies ahead. The often dusty trail heads uphill, but there are few views from this point in the hike, except of central Maui's industrial sugarcane fields and passing highway traffic. You soon pass Na Ala Hele's trailpost mile marker (MM) 4.5 on your right, beyond which the trail switchbacks slowly, then more steeply uphill. There are only a few kiawe trees growing alongside the trail, but none large enough to provide sufficient shade for hikers to take a rest.

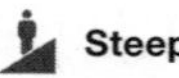

Past the MM 4 post, the trail becomes rockier and ever more steep as grueling switchbacks trudge ever upward. Around the MM 3.5 post, you pass a small kiawe tree overhanging the trail, a lone landmark on this sunburnt landscape. If you're lucky, **where the trail passes the MM 3 post**, ►2 a larger kiawe tree will still be growing beside the trail. It provides a decent amount of shade for taking a much-needed break and cooling off, but don't bet your life on its being there.

Once you've rested for a bit and rehydrated, keep climbing for another 0.5 mile, gaining about 200 feet in elevation. If you're curious, those white wind turbines now visible on the hillsides above are the property of Maui's first clean-energy wind farm. Expect things to get a little more breezy as you approach **the trail's highest point**. ►3 Although this isn't a true mountain summit (but rather the top of a ridge), you can't help but feel a sense of accomplishment in making it this far. With the hardest part of the trail now behind you, pause to gaze back at Haleakala volcano or look over the ocean toward the island of Kahoolawe.

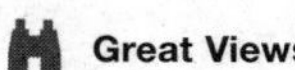

Near the western trailhead, Papalaua Wayside Park has a sandy beach for watching sunsets, longboard surfing, morning snorkeling, and camping.

Most hikers won't want to linger long at the top of the trail, because the exposed ridgetop is mercilessly unshaded. Continuing downhill, the trail quickly descends into **Manawainui Gulch**, ►4 the first and deepest gulch you'll hike through on the west side of the mountains. Alternating between a wide dirt road and a rocky footpath, the trail traverses several more gulches, with individual descents varying from gradual to steep. The views on the western side of the trail are much more interesting than where you started on the east side, thanks to the ocean lying right in front of you for much of the way.

Less than a mile from the western trailhead, you climb out of the trail's last gulch and soon encounter some sparse kiawe trees that provide a little shade over boulders conveniently placed for taking a

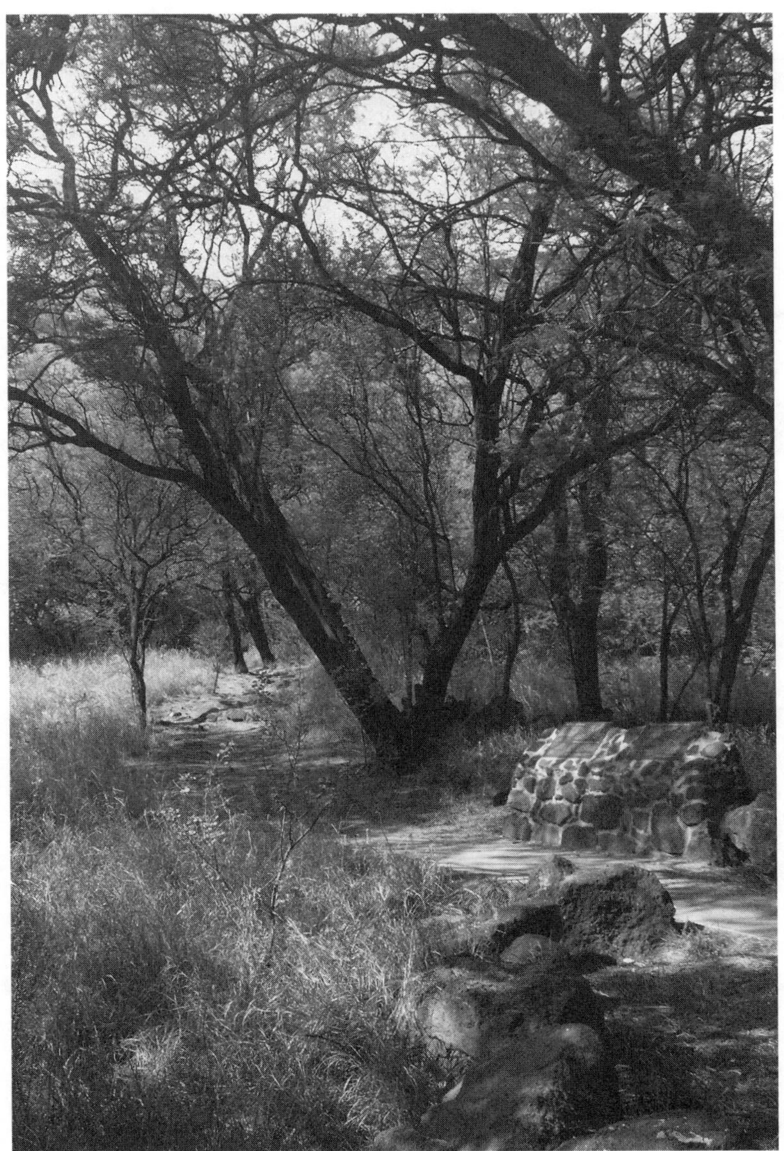

Shade is sparse *along this historic route, except at the western trailhead.*

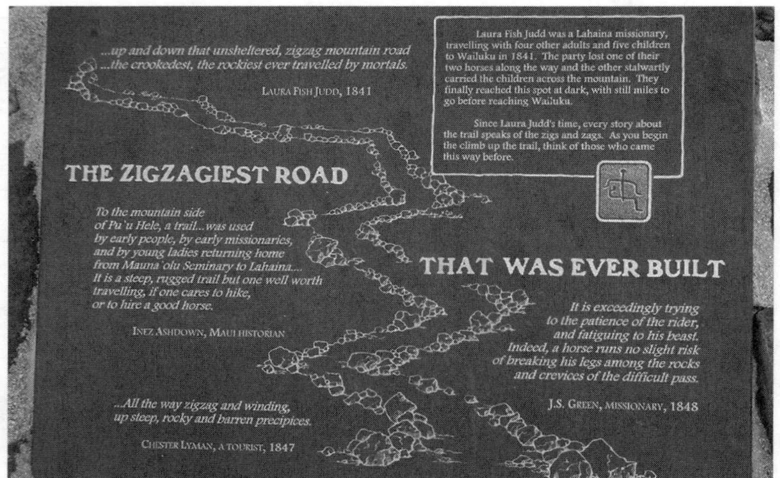

...up and down that unsheltered, zigzag mountain road
...the crookedest, the rockiest ever travelled by mortals.
LAURA FISH JUDD, 1841
Laura Fish Judd was a Lahaina missionary, travelling with four other adults and five children to Wailuku in 1841. The party lost one of their two horses along the way and the other stalwartly carried the children across the mountain. They finally reached this spot at dark, with still miles to go before reaching Wailuku.
Since Laura Judd's time, every story about the trail speaks of the zigs and zags. As you begin the climb up the trail, think of those who came this way before.
THE ZIGZAGIEST ROAD
THAT WAS EVER BUILT
To the mountain side of Pu'u Hele, a trail...was used by early people, by early missionaries, and by young ladies returning home from Mauna'olu Seminary to Lahaina... It is a steep, rugged trail but one well worth travelling, if one cares to hike, or to hire a good horse.
INEZ ASHDOWN, MAUI HISTORIAN
It is exceedingly trying to the patience of the rider, and fatiguing to his beast. Indeed, a horse runs no slight risk of breaking his legs among the rocks and crevices of the difficult pass.
J.S. GREEN, MISSIONARY, 1848
...All the way zigzag and winding, up steep, rocky and barren precipices.
CHESTER LYMAN, A TOURIST, 1847

Interpretive signs *explain this challenging route's layered history.*

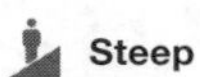
Steep

breather. The trail keeps pushing onward downhill, eventually joining a dirt 4WD road that descends more steeply. Once you veer left to enter a shady corridor of kiawe trees, it's only another few minutes' walk downhill to the **western trailhead**, ▶5 marked by Na Ala Hele markers and an interpretive sign. The dirt parking area here has room for only a few cars in scant shade.

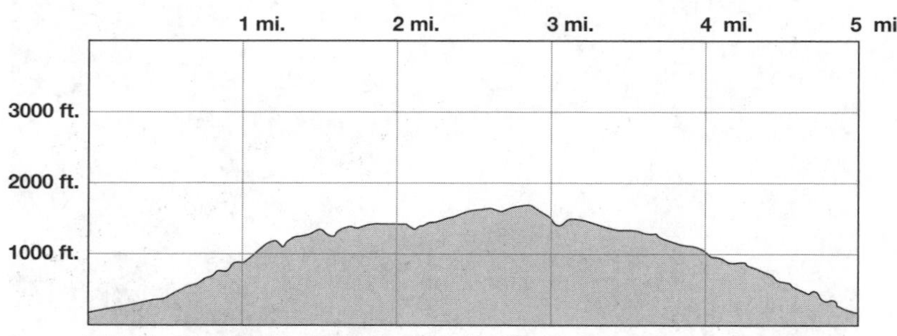

TRAIL 12 Lahaina Pali Elevation Profile

To find portable toilets and basic campsites (but no drinking water or pay phones), either drive or cautiously walk north alongside the Honoapiilani Highway (keeping the ocean on your left) for about 0.5 mile to reach the beach at Papalaua Wayside Park.

Notice

Don't underestimate the difficulty of this trail, which even Maui County firefighters find challenging on sunny days. Dehydration can quickly lead to heat exhaustion and life-threatening heatstroke, even for experienced hikers who are in good shape. Carry plenty of water and wear sunscreen, a hat, and sun-protective clothing. Hiking with a buddy is also smart. If you get into trouble, cell phone coverage is spotty along this trail—you can try climbing to the top of the nearest ridge to improve reception.

MILESTONES

▶1	0.0	Start at eastern trailhead [N 20.80842°, W 156.51207°]
▶2	2.0	Pass trailside mile marker 3 [N 20.80223°, W 156.53171°]
▶3	2.5	Reach the trail's highest point [N 20.80164°, W 156.53854°]
▶4	3.0	Descend through Manawainui Gulch
▶5	5.0	Finish at western trailhead [N 20.78869°, W 156.55709°]

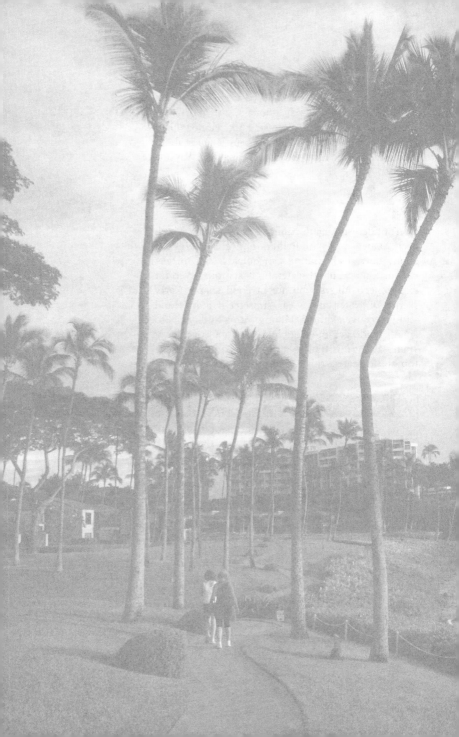

CHAPTER 2

Central & South Maui

13. Iao Valley
14. Kealia Pond
15. Kihei Coastal Trail
16. Wailea Beach Walk
17. Hoapili Trail

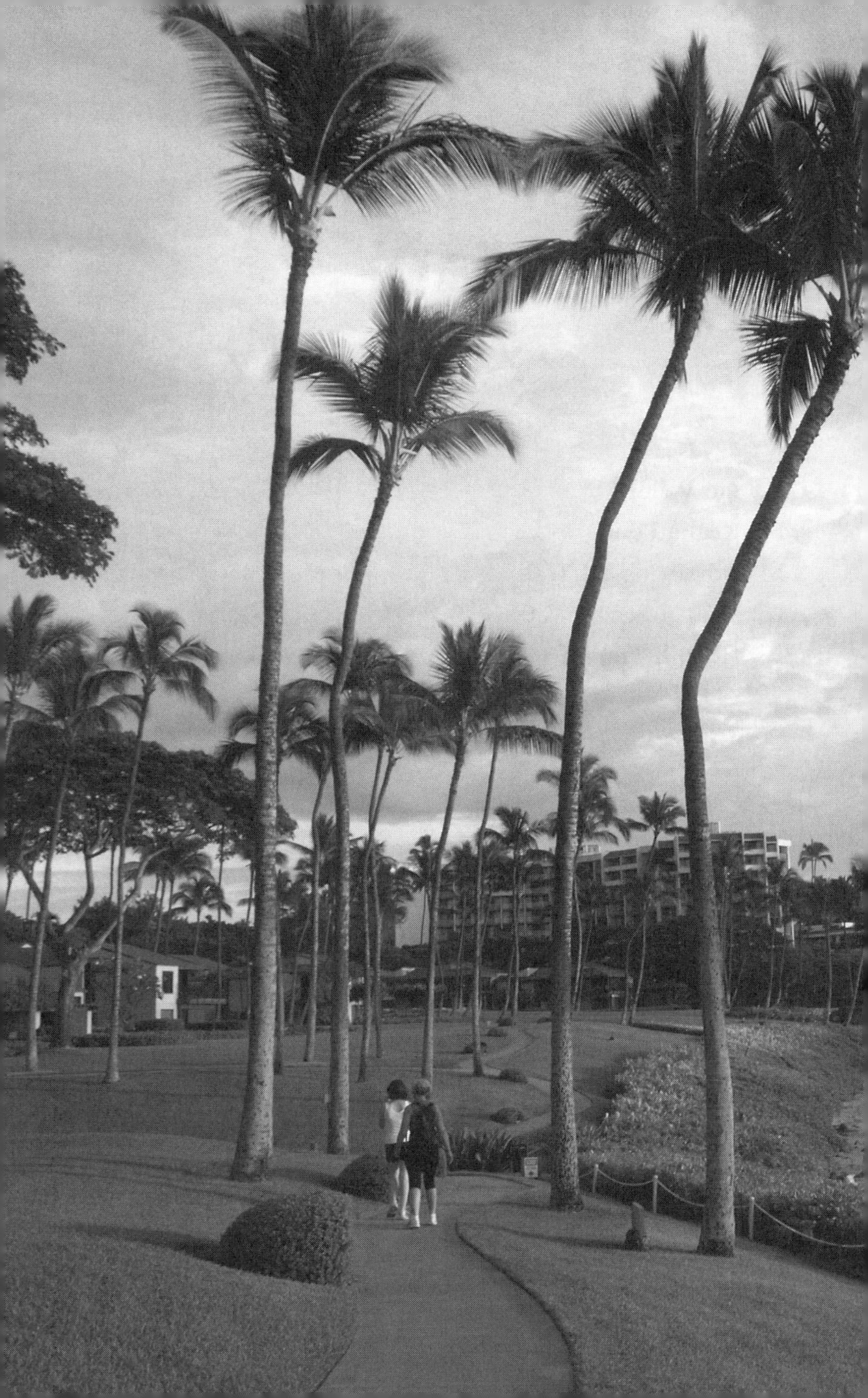

Central & South Maui

A narrow isthmus of land squeezed between the eroded West Maui Mountains and skyscraping Haleakala volcano, **Central Maui** is the island's business and administrative center. That might not sound too appealing for hiking, until you learn that Central Maui harbors one of the island's most famous viewpoints, of the Iao Needle, a rock spire forested in shaggy vegetation near the banks of a rushing stream. Down in Central Maui's more prosaic flatlands, hikers can see some of the last remaining coastal wetlands in all of Hawaii. Enthusiastic birders especially won't want to miss Kealia Pond National Wildlife Refuge facing Maalaea Bay, where sailboats and windsurfers scenically skim the waves.

In **South Maui**, the cookie-cutter "condovilles" of Kihei and Wailea's upscale beach resorts dominate the scene. Beside its rampant tourist development, South Maui has surprisingly fine beaches for swimming, snorkeling, surfing, kayaking, and all kinds of other water sports. Gentle recreational trails along the shoreline of Kihei and Wailea are perfect for both sunrise and sunset strolls. Although artificial buildings and traffic crowd the horizon, you can still soak up views of the Pacific Ocean and offshore islands. For more adventurous hikers, South Maui's La Pérouse Bay is the jumping-off point for a rugged trek along wild beaches and over rough *aa* lava flows to remote, windswept Kanaio Beach. Called the Hoapili Trail, this hike follows an ancient Hawaiian highway starting from inside Ahihi-Kinau Natural Area Reserve, where spinner dolphins rest in calm aquamarine bays and snorkelers can explore tide pools teeming with sea life.

Permits & Maps

No permits or fees are currently required to hike any of the trails described in this chapter. These dayhikes pass through lands managed by national, state, and county agencies, as well as private resort property. Overnight backpacking is prohibited, including along the Hoapili Trail; public campgrounds are not available anywhere in South Maui.

Overleaf and opposite: *Oceanside recreational paths are well-used in South Maui, especially by runners.*

To take the first four hikes described in this chapter, topographic maps aren't necessary. At Iao Valley State Monument and Kealia Pond National Wildlife Refuge, as well as at Kihei and Wailea, walking trails are clearly marked and basic trail maps are signposted along the way, including at trailheads. South Maui's remote Hoapili Trail is more challenging to find and to follow, although the written directions and basic trail map in this book should suffice. For a more detailed topographic map, the USGS 7.5-minute (1:24,000) *Makena* map shows the entire length of the Hoapili Trail.

See Appendix 3 (page 312) for more recommended topographical and driving maps, both digital and printed, to help you navigate around Maui.

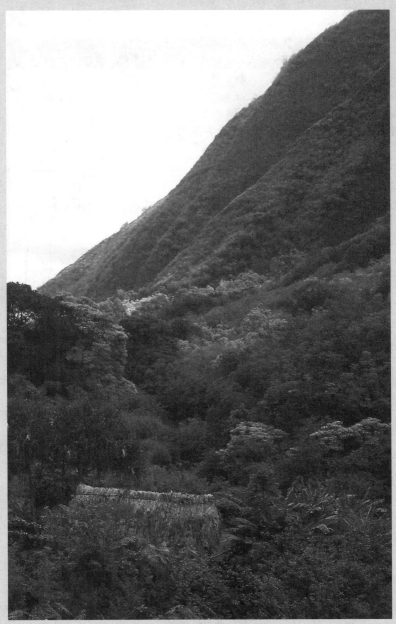

In Iao Valley, *short, family-friendly paths wind through tropical forest.*

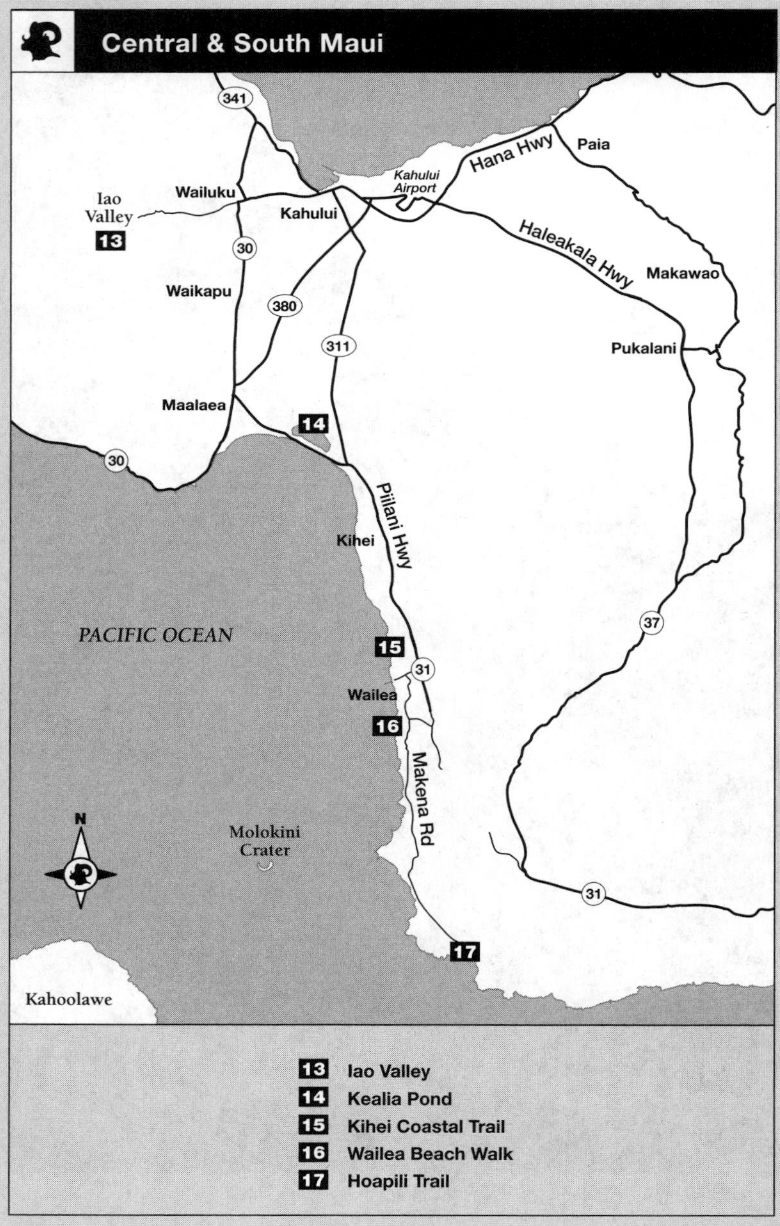
Central & South Maui
341
Hana Hwy
Paia
Kahului Airport
Iao Valley
13
Wailuku
Kahului
30
Haleakala Hwy
Makawao
Waikapu
380
311
Pukalani
Maalaea
14
30
Piilani Hwy
Kihei
37
PACIFIC OCEAN
15
31
Wailea
16
Makena Rd
N
Molokini Crater
31
17
Kahoolawe
13 Iao Valley
14 Kealia Pond
15 Kihei Coastal Trail
16 Wailea Beach Walk
17 Hoapili Trail

TRAIL FEATURES TABLE

Central & South Maui

TRAIL	Difficulty	Length	Type	USES & ACCESS	TERRAIN	FLORA & FAUNA	OTHER
13	1	0.6	Semiloop	Dayhiking, Child Friendly	Forest, Stream	Native Plants	Great Views, Swimming, Historic Interest
14	1	1.0	Out & Back	Dayhiking, Wheelchair Access, Child Friendly	Beach, Pond	Birds, Native Plants, Wildlife	Great Views
15	1	1.2	Out & Back	Dayhiking, Running, Child Friendly, Dogs Allowed	Beach	Birds, Native Plants, Tide Pools, Wildlife	Great Views, Swimming
16	1	3.0	Out & Back	Dayhiking, Running, Wheelchair Access, Child Friendly, Dogs Allowed	Beach	Birds, Native Plants, Tide Pools, Wildlife	Great Views, Swimming, Archaeological
17	3	4.0	Out & Back	Dayhiking	Beach, Lava Flow	Native Plants, Tide Pools, Wildlife	Great Views, Geologic Interest, Historic Interest, Archaeological, Secluded

USES & ACCESS
- Dayhiking
- Backpacking
- Running
- Biking
- Wheelchair Access
- Child Friendly
- Dogs Allowed
- Permit Required

TYPE
- Loop
- Out & Back
- Semiloop
- Point-to-Point

DIFFICULTY
- 1 2 3 4 5 +
less — more

TERRAIN
- Beach
- Forest
- Lava Flow
- Mountain
- Pond
- Summit
- Stream
- Waterfall

FLORA & FAUNA
- Birds
- Native Plants
- Tide Pools
- Wildlife

FEATURES
- Great Views
- Swimming
- Camping
- Geologic Interest
- Historic Interest
- Archaeological
- Secluded
- Shady
- Steep

Central & South Maui

TRAIL 13

Dayhike, Child Friendly
0.6 mile, Semiloop
Difficulty: **1** 2 3 4 5

Central Maui's most popular tourist stop, this state park offers exhilarating views of Iao Needle against a painterly backdrop of the West Maui Mountains, often veiled by rain clouds and mist. Stroll past native Hawaiian plants in the streamside botanical garden.

TRAIL 14

Dayhike,
Wheelchair Access,
Child Friendly
1.0 mile, Out & Back
Difficulty: **1** 2 3 4 5

A sunny coastal boardwalk leads you along one of Hawaii's only remaining natural wetlands along the shores of Maalaea Bay. It's a rare opportunity to spot endangered Hawaiian waterbirds, as well as migratory species from as far away as Alaska and Asia.

TRAIL 15

Dayhike, Run,
Child Friendly,
Dogs Allowed
1.2 miles, Out & Back
Difficulty: **1** 2 3 4 5

Come at dawn, around sunset, or on full-moon nights for a scenic walk beside Kihei's southern beaches, with their golden sands and gentle swimmable waves. This child-friendly oceanfront recreational trail also accommodates runners.

Wailea Beach Walk 137

A paved, wheelchair-accessible coastal path winds past Wailea's beach resorts, facing some of South Maui's best beaches. Come at sunset for sneak peeks at Hawaiian music and hula performances, or try your luck spotting whales offshore during winter.

TRAIL 16

Dayhike, Run,
Wheelchair Access,
Child Friendly,
Dogs Allowed
3.0 miles, Out & Back
Difficulty: **1** 2 3 4 5

Hoapili Trail 143

From La Pérouse Bay, where surf slaps the rocky shoreline, trek across jagged lava fields past archaeological sites to a secluded beach. Carry extra water and don't hike midday, when dehydration and heat exhaustion are serious risks. Hiking boots are helpful here.

TRAIL 17

Dayhike
4.0 miles, Out & Back
Difficulty: 1 2 **3** 4 5

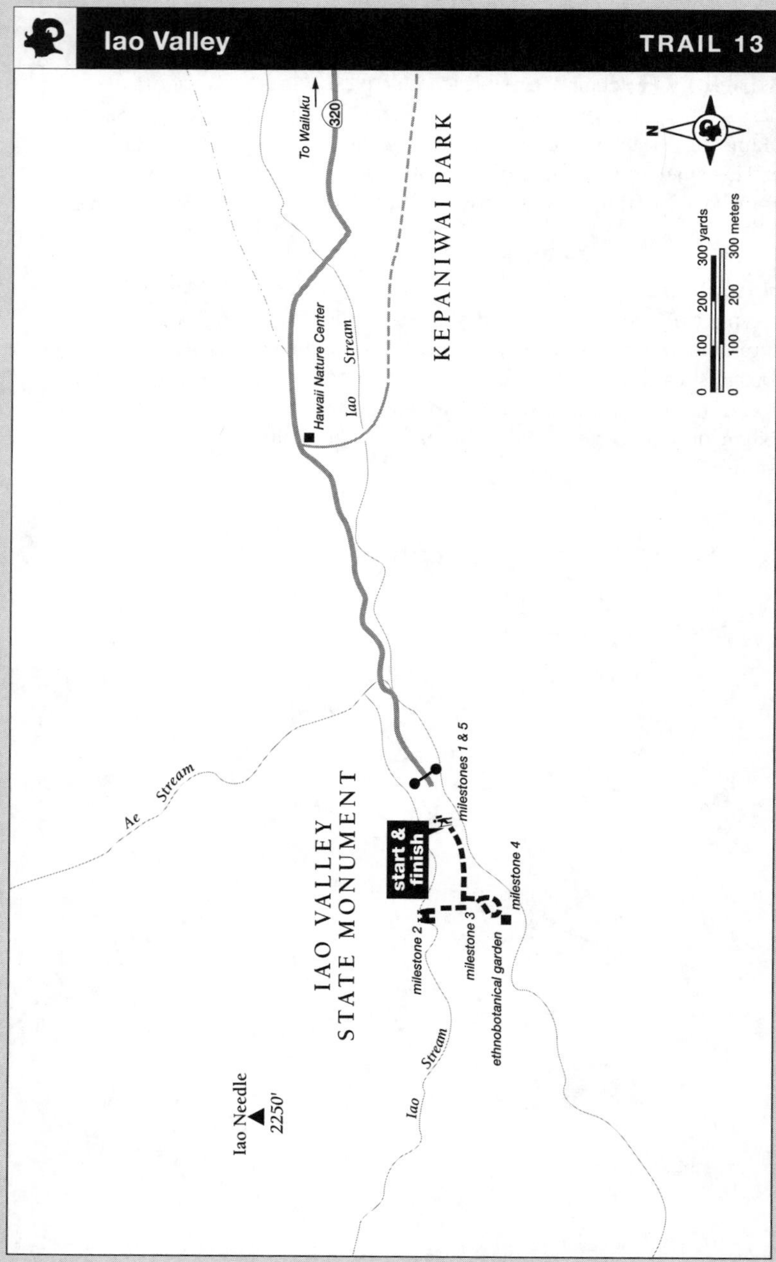
Iao Valley
TRAIL 13
To Wailuku
320
KEPANIWAI PARK
Hawaii Nature Center
Iao Stream
N
0 100 200 300 yards
0 100 200 300 meters
Ae Stream
IAO VALLEY STATE MONUMENT
start & finish
milestones 1 & 5
milestone 2
milestone 3
milestone 4
ethnobotanical garden
Iao Stream
Iao Needle
2250'

Iao Valley

Short and sweet, this paved walking path gets trampled by scores of tourists daily, but don't let the crowds deter you. Everyone wants to see the famous Iao Needle, jutting into the sky out of the verdant West Maui Mountains. Streamside swimming holes and an ethnobotanical plant garden await.

TRAIL USE
Dayhike, Child Friendly
LENGTH
0.6 mile, 15–30 mins.
VERTICAL FEET
±300′
DIFFICULTY
– **1** 2 3 4 5 +
TRAIL TYPE
Semiloop
SURFACE TYPE
Paved
START & END
N 20.88068°
W 156.54564°

FEATURES
Forest
Stream
Native Plants
Great Views
Swimming
Historic Interest

FACILITIES
Restrooms
Phone

Best Time

Iao Valley State Monument is open from 7 AM to 7 PM daily. Arrive early or late in the day to avoid the biggest crowds. Check the weather report before visiting here: Cloudy skies and drizzle frequently obscure the viewpoint. The valley is also subject to flash flooding whenever it rains, so use caution when hiking next to the stream or swimming.

Finding the Trail

From the intersection of Main and High streets in central Wailuku, drive 0.5 mile west on Main St. (Hwy. 32). At the fork in the road, veer right and follow Iao Valley Road for 2.2 miles over the bridge past Kepaniwai Park to Iao Valley State Monument. At press time, admission was free, although a vehicle entry fee of $5 had been proposed. Parking is available in a small, two-level paved lot. If that lot is full, backtrack east to find more parking at Kepaniwai Park, then walk 0.7 mile west along the road to the state monument entrance.

Trail Description

Note that although the park's trails are entirely paved, steep gradients and stairs make it inaccessible for wheelchairs.

On the west side of the parking lot's upper level is the **trailhead**, ▶1 next to the restrooms (no drinking water available). Almost immediately, you cross a footbridge over Iao Stream. Iao Needle is already visible uphill to your right. Follow the trail as it curves to the left, then stay to the right at each of the next trail junctions, which appear in quick succession. (You'll explore these alternate trails on your return trip to the trailhead.)

Great Views

Climb a short flight of steps that lead steeply up to the official **Iao Needle lookout**. ▶2 The small roofed, open-sided trail shelter comes in very handy during wet and windy conditions, a frequent state here in the rain shadow of the West Maui Mountains. According to Hawaiian legend, the iconic Iao Needle was once the suitor of Iao, the daughter of the demigod Maui, who turned his daughter's lover to stone. Today, this erosional feature thickly covered with native plants is one of the island's most-photographed spots. Rising 1200 feet above the valley floor, it's especially captivating when shrouded by mist and ringed by clouds, looking much like a classical Chinese or Japanese scroll painting.

Iao Stream also winds through nearby Kepaniwai Park, which has picnic tables and an interesting collection of buildings depicting Maui's multiethnic heritage, including Chinese, Japanese, Portuguese, and Native Hawaiian traditions.

When you've finished soaking up the dizzying views, head back down the steps from the lookout. At the first trail junction you meet, turn right and walk down a less steep flight of concrete steps. The trail meanders past fragrant guava trees whose ripe fruit falls on the paved path, approaching for a closer look at **Iao Stream**, ▶3 which carves this valley. Depending on the weather and the season, you may find the stream rushing along with incredible force or perhaps it will be no more than a trickle. Always exercise caution if you decide to take a dip in the water, as flash floods are a hazard and can occur

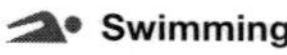

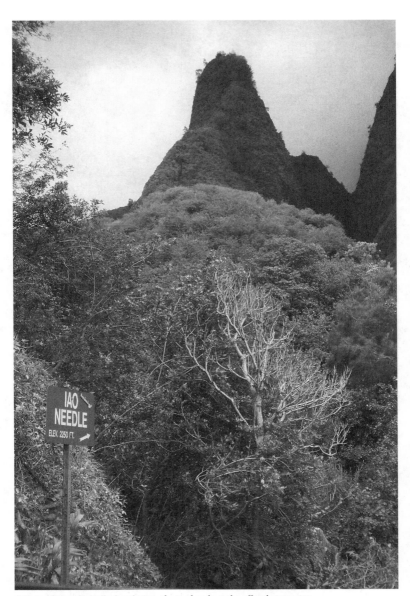

Although Iao Needle beckons, *the trail ends at the official viewpoint.*

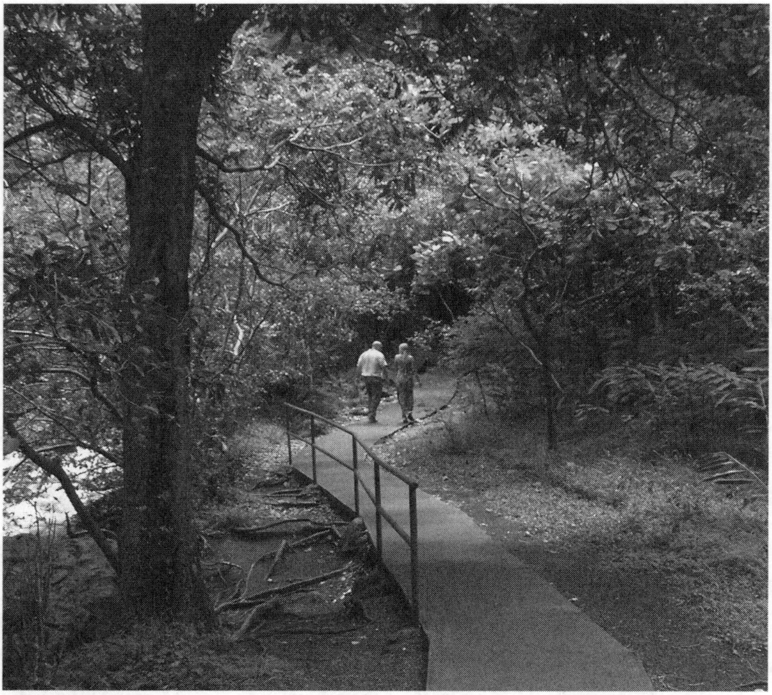

Side trails wind *beside Iao Stream, popular for its swimming holes.*

without warning. Diving is prohibited inside the state monument, especially from the bridge, because of the hidden danger of submerged rocks.

Very soon this streamside ramble ends as you ascend to meet the main trail on the far side of the bridge. The parking lot is a short walk ahead now. But after crossing the bridge, instead turn right and head downhill to the **ethnobotanical garden**. ▶4 This recently restored area offers visitors the chance to view stand-out examples of endemic Hawaiian flora, all clearly labeled and growing alongside a series of interconnected paved paths. Wander down by the stream, stopping to touch the green heart-shaped leaves of a taro plant or to rest on one of the

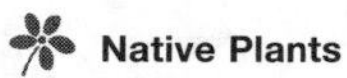
Native Plants

handy benches. When you're ready to leave, climb back uphill and turn right (away from the bridge) toward the parking lot, arriving back at the same **trailhead** ►5 you started from.

The Iao Valley's Hawaii Nature Center (808-244-6500, www.hawaiinaturecenter.org) offers kid-friendly ecology exhibits (open 10 AM to 4 PM daily) and leads guided rainforest walks (by reservation).

Notice

Iao Valley is where the forces of Kamehameha I triumphed over Maui's warriors in the 1790 Battle of Kepaniwai, which made way for the unification of the Hawaiian Islands. It is said that during this bloody battle, Iao Stream was choked by the bodies of fallen fighters (*kepaniwai* means "dammed waters" in Hawaiian). Today, Iao Valley is the focus of another fight, this time by environmentalists who want to restore the native watershed and stop Maui County from further draining the stream for the public water supply.

MILESTONES

►1	0.0	Start at trailhead near parking lot [N 20.88068°, W 156.54564°]
►2	0.2	Arrive at Iao Needle lookout [N 20.88048°, W 156.54677°]
►3	0.3	Descend along streamside loop
►4	0.5	Walk through ethnobotanical garden
►5	0.6	Arrive back at trailhead [N 20.88068°, W 156.54564°]

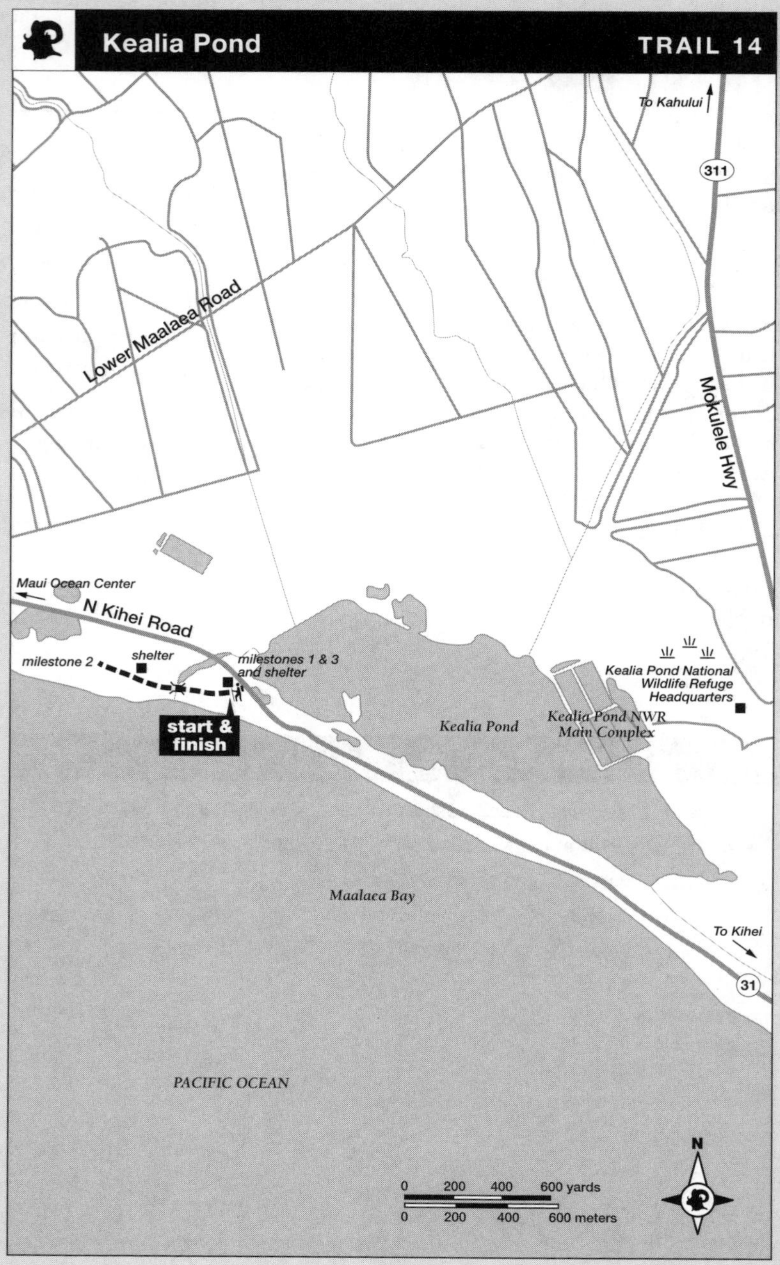
Kealia Pond
TRAIL 14
To Kahului
311
Lower Maalaea Road
Mokulele Hwy
Maui Ocean Center
N Kihei Road
milestone 2
shelter
milestones 1 & 3
and shelter
start &
finish
Kealia Pond National
Wildlife Refuge
Headquarters
Kealia Pond
Kealia Pond NWR
Main Complex
Maalaea Bay
To Kihei
31
PACIFIC OCEAN
N
0 200 400 600 yards
0 200 400 600 meters

Kealia Pond

The coastal boardwalk at this national wildlife refuge has made Central Maui's natural wetlands more accessible to the public. Although it's near busy highways, this wheelchair-accessible trail is still a pretty spot for bird-watching. Bring binoculars to spot endangered Hawaiian waterbirds and diverse migratory species.

TRAIL USE
Dayhike, Wheelchair Access, Child Friendly

LENGTH
1.0 mile, 30–45 mins.

VERTICAL FEET
Negligible

DIFFICULTY
– **1** 2 3 4 5 +

TRAIL TYPE
Out & Back

SURFACE TYPE
Boardwalk

START & END
N 20.79557°
W 156.48531°

FEATURES
Beach
Pond
Birds
Native Plants
Wildlife
Great Views

FACILITIES
None

Best Time

The parking lot gates for Kealia Pond National Wildlife Refuge's coastal boardwalk are open from 6 AM to 7 PM daily. Arrive early in the day to enjoy cooler temperatures and less windy conditions. The majority of migratory bird species land here sometime between late summer and early spring, roughly from August through April.

Finding the Trail

From Kihei, drive north on the Piilani Highway (Hwy. 31) or South Kihei Road, then continue driving northwest on North Kihei Road (Hwy. 310). The parking lot for the refuge's coastal boardwalk is on the *makai* (ocean) side of the road, 0.2 mile north of mile marker (MM) 2 on North Kihei Road.

Inconveniently, turning left off North Kihei Road directly into the parking lot is prohibited. Instead keep driving 1.8 miles northwest on North Kihei Road to the stoplight intersection with the Honoapiilani Highway (Hwy. 30). Turn right onto Highway 30, then make a U-turn at the next stoplight and backtrack south along the highway, turning left back onto North Kihei Road and driving 1.8 miles back southeast. Finally, turn right into the refuge's parking lot, which has 14 spaces. There is no admission fee.

As you leave the parking lot, only right turns are permitted, forcing you to drive southbound on North Kihei Road. If you're not going to Kihei, make a U-turn wherever possible along North Kihei Road, or else continue southeast to the junction with the Mokulele Highway (Hwy. 311), which connects north to Kahului Airport.

Trail Description

Although there is no staffed office at the coastal boardwalk, you can call Kealia Pond NWR headquarters at (808) 875-1582 or visit www.fws.gov for more information.

Kealia Pond National Wildlife Refuge (NWR) protects a unique treasure: It's one of the only natural wetlands left in the Hawaiian archipelago. Intermittent seasonal flooding occurs during winter (December to March), when migratory shorebirds and waterfowl are in residence here after flying in from far-flung places such as Canada, Alaska, and Siberia. When the refuge's water levels recede toward the end of summer (from August through October), it's easy to see how this place gets its name: roughly translated, *kealia* means "salt pan." Traditionally, ancient Hawaiians came here to harvest salt.

Don't forget to bring binoculars, drinking water, a hat, and plenty of sunscreen on this walk, which starts from the **trailhead** ►1 by the parking lot. At the trailhead, a roofed shelter gives helpful background on the refuge's ecology and wildlife. At any time of year, you can observe a variety of birds from the boardwalk, which leads northwest along the shoreline and over a small bridge.

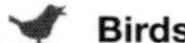 **Birds**

Keep a sharp eye out for the Hawaiian coot (alaekeokeo), Hawaiian stilt (aeo) and Hawaiian duck (koloa maoli); for a description of these rare endemic birds, see page 8. Cattle egrets, an introduced species of small white herons, aggressively

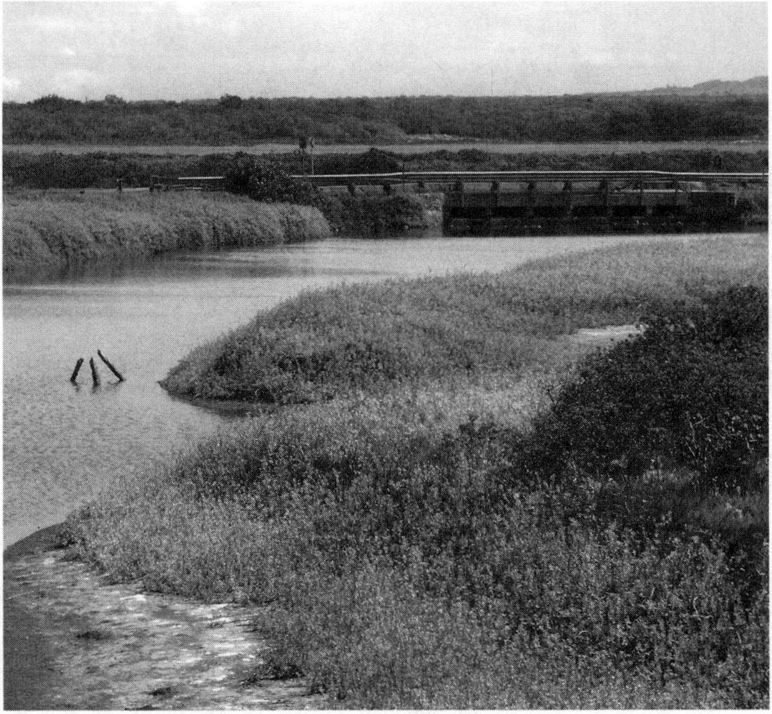

Maui's protected seasonal wetlands *are a haven for waterbirds.*

compete for food with native birds, sometimes eating their chicks, which also fall prey to mongooses and rats. Of all the migratory shorebirds and waterfowl that can be spotted here during winter, the most famous is the Pacific golden plover (kolea), which can fly nonstop for up to two days to reach the Hawaiian Islands.

As you amble along the boardwalk toward the limited shade of the second roofed trail shelter, don't forget to gaze *makai* (toward the ocean), not just *mauka* (inland) at the marshy wetlands. During summer (May to September), endangered Hawaiian hawksbill turtles sometimes nest on the sands here.

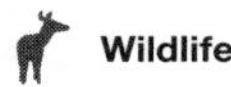

Wildlife

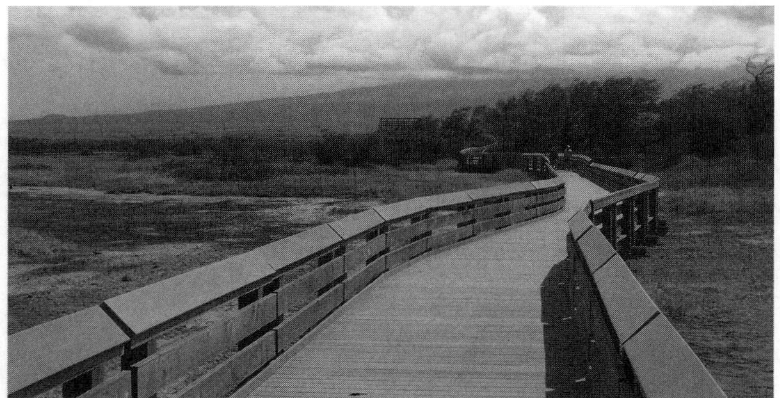

A coastal boardwalk *lets birders glimpse native and migratory species.*

Solitary by nature, these turtles prefer untrammeled beaches away from human habitation. Females sometimes dig nests in the thick vegetation that abounds along this beach. Much of the flora growing here is nonnative, although refuge managers are working hard to restore the natural ecosystem by pulling out mangrove and other invasive species.

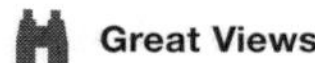

As you continue walking northwest along the exposed boardwalk, the West Maui Mountains rise ahead of you in the distance; notice the clean energy wind turbines atop the foothills. Soon you reach the shade of the trail shelter at the **end of the boardwalk**. ►2 Here you also get wide-open views of Maalaea Bay. In the afternoon, windsurfers, surfers, outrigger canoes, and sailboats all ply the waters

MILESTONES

►1	0.0	Start from trailhead next to parking lot [N 20.79557°, W 156.48531°]
►2	0.5	Reach the end of the boardwalk [N 20.79666°, W 156.49103°]
►3	1.0	Arrive back at trailhead and parking lot [N 20.79557°, W 156.48531°]

of the bay. Occasionally, North Pacific humpback whales can be spotted breaching and spouting offshore during winter. These migratory whales come to Hawaii to give birth, nurse their young, and mate, with their activity peaking between December and March.

When you're ready, turn around and retrace your steps along the boardwalk back to the **trailhead** ▶3 by the parking lot.

At Maalaea Harbor, Maui Ocean Center (808-270-7000, www.mauioceancenter.com) is a kid-friendly aquarium.

OPTIONS

Detour: Maui for the Birds

Enthusiastic birders will want to explore the dirt trails of **Kealia Pond NWR's main complex** (open 8 AM to 4 PM daily). The entrance is at mile marker (MM) 6 on the Mokulele Highway (Hwy. 311), 0.6 mile north of its intersection with the Piilani Highway (Hwy. 31). There is no entry fee, but hikers must self-register at the headquarters information office, located 0.5 mile along a dirt road from the highway entrance.

Near Kahului Airport, state-managed **Kanaha Pond Wildlife Sanctuary** is also worth a quick stop for birders. Park in the small roadside lot (open 6 AM to 6 PM daily), which has space for 12 cars. The lot is on the north side of the Haleakala Highway (Hwy. 37), just west of the intersection of Keolani Place and Dairy Road, north of the Hana Highway (Hwy. 36). Entry is free. From the parking lot, a short, wheelchair-accessible path leads out to a concrete blind. Avian species often spotted here include the Hawaiian coot, Hawaiian stilt, Hawaiian duck, and a variety of migratory shorebirds.

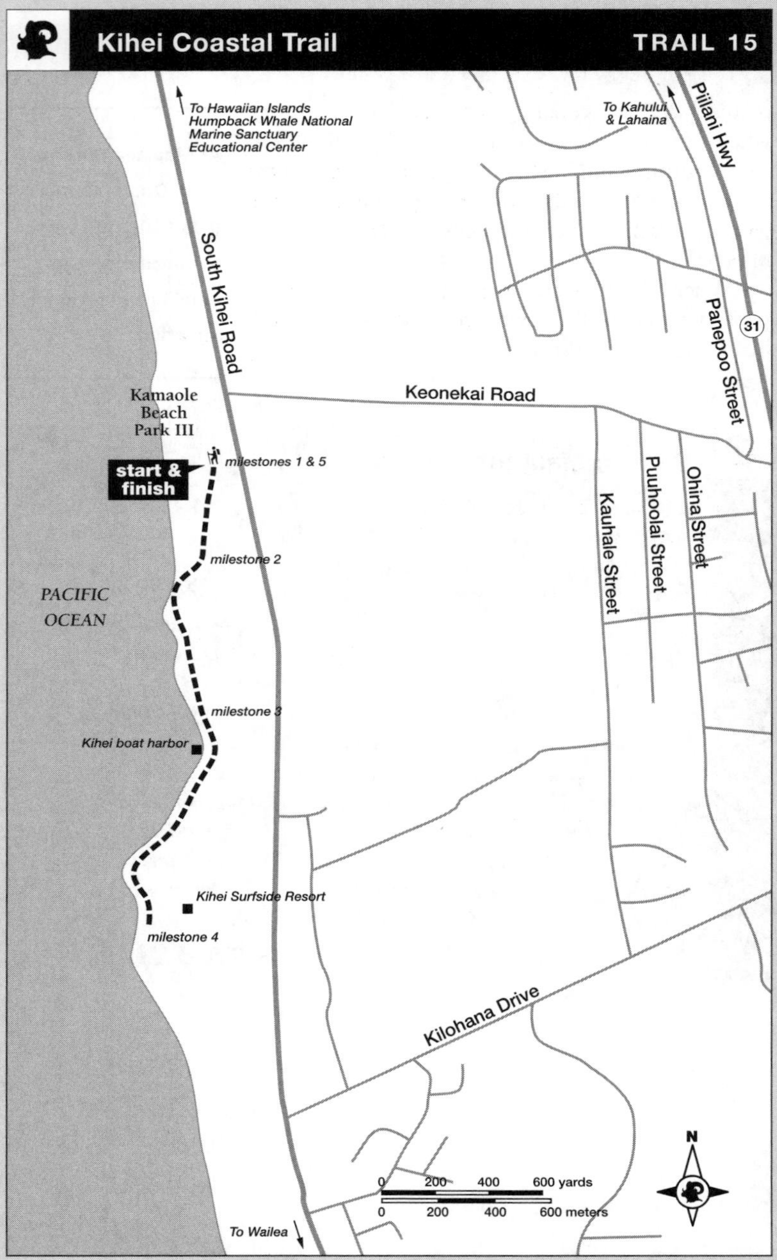

Kihei Coastal Trail
TRAIL 15
To Hawaiian Islands Humpback Whale National Marine Sanctuary Educational Center
To Kahului & Lahaina
Piilani Hwy
South Kihei Road
Panepoo Street
31
Keonekai Road
Kamaole Beach Park III
start & finish
milestones 1 & 5
Kauhale Street
Puuhoolai Street
Ohina Street
milestone 2
PACIFIC OCEAN
milestone 3
Kihei boat harbor
Kihei Surfside Resort
milestone 4
Kilohana Drive
N
0 200 400 600 yards
0 200 400 600 meters
To Wailea

Kihei Coastal Trail

Along South Maui's most developed coastal stretch—which puts it within easy reach of where many visitors stay—this Pacific path traces Kihei's southern golden-sand beaches. Panoramas of volcanic islands and sightings of migratory humpback whales will compete for your attention during a sunset beach stroll or early morning run.

TRAIL USE
Dayhike, Run, Child Friendly, Dogs Allowed
LENGTH
1.2 miles, 30–45 mins.
VERTICAL FEET
±50′
DIFFICULTY
– **1** 2 3 4 5 +
TRAIL TYPE
Out & Back
SURFACE TYPE
Dirt, Grass, Sand
START & END
N 20.71229°
W 156.44531°

FEATURES
Beach
Birds
Native Plants
Tide Pools
Wildlife
Great Views
Swimming

FACILITIES
Restrooms
Picnic Tables
Phone
Water

Best Time

This trail is walkable year-round. The Kamaole III Beach parking lot is officially open from 7 AM to 7 PM daily. Pedestrian access is 24 hours, although being on the beach after dark is not necessarily safe because of crime. The best times of day for hiking or running this trail are in the early morning or late afternoon, when temperatures are cooler.

Finding the Trail

County-run Kamaole Beach Park III (808-879-4364, 2800 South Kihei Road) is located at the southern edge of Kihei. The parking lot is on the *makai* (ocean) side of the town's main drag, Kihei Road, just south of the Keonekai Road intersection. Parking is free. Coming from Wailea, follow Wailea Alanui Road north to the four-way stop-sign intersection with Okolani Dr. Turn left and drive 0.4 mile, then turn right onto South Kihei Road and continue north for about a mile. The Kamaole III Beach parking lot will be on your left. From all other points on Maui, take the Piilani Highway (Hwy. 31) south to Keonekai Road, turn right and drive 0.6

mile *makai,* then turn left onto South Kihei Road and look for the parking lot almost immediately on your right.

Trail Description

Next to the county beach park's **parking lot,** ►1 you'll find restrooms, outdoor showers and drinking fountains. Tree-shaded picnic tables are scattered across the grass, while a lifeguard lookout tower stands at the edge of the beach, which is popular with local families for swimming. To find the official trailhead, either walk south along the beach or veer southwest across a grassy lawn area. Either way, you soon intersect with the signposted **northern end of the coastal trail.** ►2 In the mornings, snorkeling is also possible here at the southern end of Kamaole III Beach.

Swimming

Walking south on the official trail, the terrain is mostly sandy, but sometimes grassy or overlaid with gravel. The borders of the path are carefully defined by white coral rocks (which incidentally makes it easier to follow in the moonlight). From April 1 through December 1, wedge-tailed shearwaters (uau kani) lay their eggs in burrows hidden in the coastal dunes here. These birds are easily recognized by their dark-brown heads and backs with white plumage underneath. Their webbed feet are well adapted for swimming, but their legs are not strong enough to support them on land, so they crawl in the sand. Although once abundant in the main Hawaiian Islands, wedge-tailed shearwaters had almost disappeared from Maui until efforts were made to restore native vegetation here and control predators. Although locals often walk their leashed dogs here, it's better to leave your four-legged friend at home during the birds' nesting season to aid the recovery of this endangered native species.

At the Hawaiian Islands Humpback Whale National Marine Sanctuary Educational Center (808-879-2818, 726 South Kihei Road), check out the kid-friendly ocean exhibits (open 10 AM to 3 PM Monday to Friday), whale-spotting scopes and an ancient Hawaiian fishpond. Admission is free.

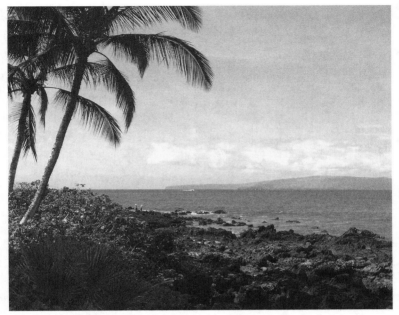

Hikers take in views of Kahoolawe, *an island rich in Native Hawaiian heritage sites.*

Continuing south, walk across the paved **Kihei boat ramp parking lot ▶3** approximately at the trail's halfway point. South of the boat ramp, the trail passes a bench and interpretive signs about protecting coral reefs and the restoration of Kahoolawe, that long, flat offshore island visible on the horizon. Kahoolawe was the place where ancient Hawaiian outrigger canoes began their long journeys to Tahiti, far away in the South Pacific. Over 500 Native Hawaiian archaeological sites have been found on that island, including many ceremonial and religious places. Kahoolawe is now uninhabited after being used as a bombing target by the U.S. military from World War II until 1990. Decades of Native Hawaiian political protests ended after the island was returned to the state of Hawaii in 1994.

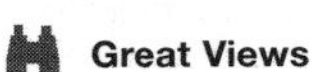
Great Views

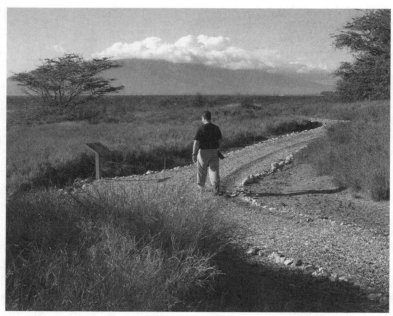

Interpretive signs *explain natural and cultural history along this scenic oceanfront path.*

Volunteers now work to restore native vegetation and repair the island's important cultural sites.

Panoramas of volcanic islands and sightings of migratory humpback whales will compete for your attention.

As you keep walking south along the coastal trail, look for another interpretive sign talking about the ancient Polynesian method of navigation, called wayfaring, which used only the sun, stars, and wind and wave patterns to cross the ocean. All too soon the trail nears the Kihei Surfside Resort condo complex. Skirt along the *makai* (seaward) side of the resort's manicured lawns, where reclining beach chairs are set up for guests. A paved parking lot is the abrupt, anticlimactic **southern end of the coastal trail**. ►4

Turn around and retrace your steps back to the Kamaole III Beach **parking lot**. ►5

MILESTONES

►1	0.0	Start from Kamaole III Beach parking lot [N 20.71229°, W 156.44531°]
►2	0.1	Pick up northern end of trail [N 20.71103°, W 156.44608°]
►3	0.3	Cross Kihei boat ramp parking lot [N 20.70848°, W 156.44594°]
►4	0.6	Reach southern end of trail [N 20.70507°, W 156.44701°]
►5	1.2	Arrive back at Kamaole III Beach parking lot [N 20.71229°, W 156.44531°]

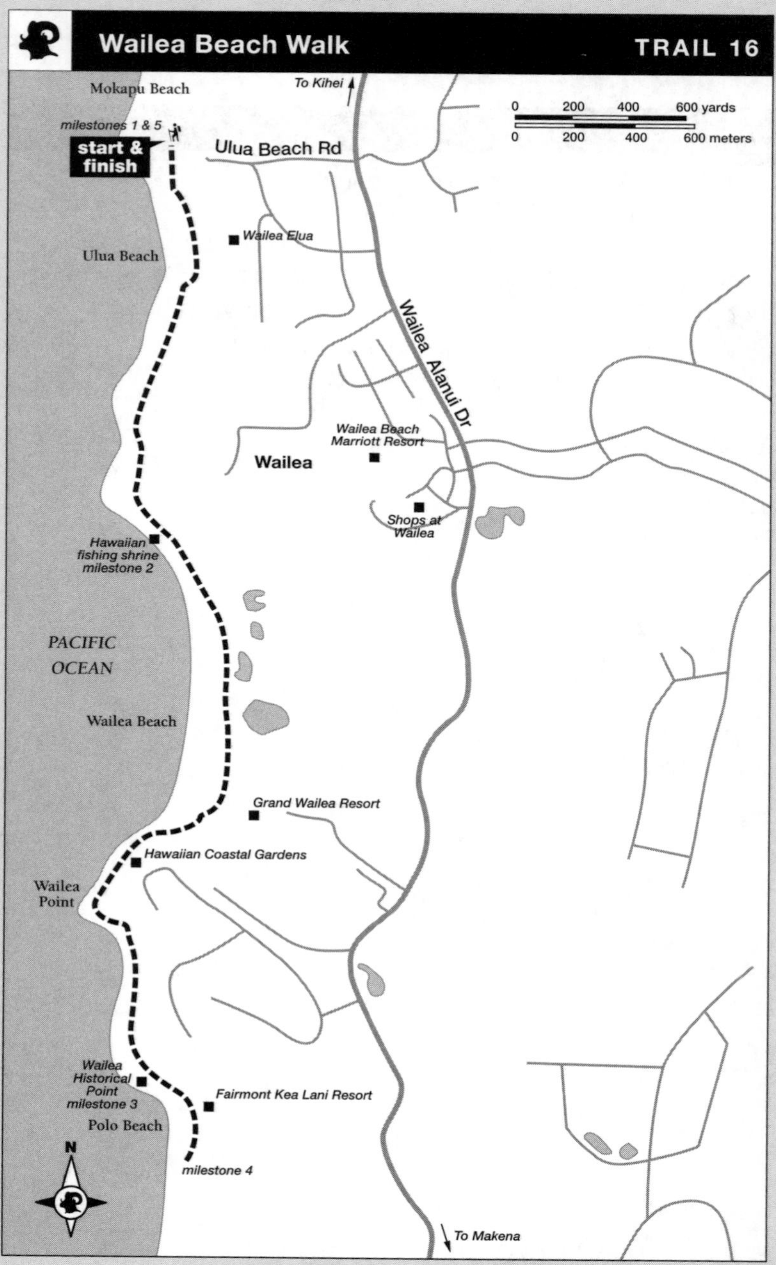

Wailea Beach Walk
TRAIL 16
Mokapu Beach
To Kihei
0 200 400 600 yards
0 200 400 600 meters
milestones 1 & 5
start & finish
Ulua Beach Rd
Wailea Elua
Ulua Beach
Wailea Alanui Dr
Wailea Beach Marriott Resort
Wailea
Shops at Wailea
Hawaiian fishing shrine milestone 2
PACIFIC OCEAN
Wailea Beach
Grand Wailea Resort
Hawaiian Coastal Gardens
Wailea Point
Wailea Historical Point milestone 3
Fairmont Kea Lani Resort
Polo Beach
N
milestone 4
To Makena

Wailea Beach Walk

Another mesmerizing sunset stroll, this trail winds past Wailea's condos and high-rise resort hotels, but still manages to preserve a natural sense of place. On this wheelchair-accessible paved path, you pass native plant gardens, Hawaiian archaeological sites, and places to spot migratory North Pacific humpback whales offshore during winter.

TRAIL USE
Dayhike, Run, Wheelchair Access, Child Friendly, Dogs Allowed

LENGTH
3.0 miles, 1–1½ hours

VERTICAL FEET
±150′

DIFFICULTY
– **1** 2 3 4 5 +

TRAIL TYPE
Out & Back

SURFACE TYPE
Paved

START & END
N 20.69163°
W 156.44292°

FEATURES
Beach
Birds
Native Plants
Tide Pools
Wildlife
Great Views
Swimming
Archaeological

FACILITIES
Restrooms
Water

Best Time

This trail is walkable year-round. The parking lot for Ulua and Mokapu beaches is officially open from 7 AM to 7 PM daily. Pedestrian access is 24 hours, although walking along the beach after dark is not always safe because of crime. The best time of day for walking or running is right before sunset, when temperatures are cooler and live Hawaiian music and hula dance performances are beginning at oceanfront resorts that line this path.

Finding the Trail

From Kihei, drive all the way south on South Kihei Road past Kilohana Dr., then veer left onto Okolani Dr. for 0.4 mile, following the signs toward Wailea. At the four-way stop-sign intersection, turn right onto Wailea Alanui Road and drive south for 0.4 mile. Look carefully for a small sign pointing to Ulua and Mokapu beaches on your right (if you reach the Wailea Beach Marriott Resort, you've gone too far). Turn right onto Ulua Beach Road, opposite Hale Alii Place. Drive 0.1 mile farther downhill to the public parking lot (free). If you're coming from anywhere farther south in Wailea or in Makena, drive north on Wailea Alanui Road past both the Shops at Wailea mall and the Wailea Beach Marriott Resort, looking for the Ulua Beach Road turnoff on your left.

Trail Description

Swimming

Ulua Beach is popular for swimming and snorkeling, especially in the morning before the winds pick up. An outcropping of lava rock separates it from twin Mokapu Beach, just north. At the lower end of the public parking lot for both beaches, you'll find restrooms, outdoor showers, and drinking fountains. To find the **trailhead**, ►1 look south of the restrooms for a paved path.

Wildlife

Walking southbound, the multiuse recreational trail hugs the coast, skirting the grassy oceanfront lawns of Wailea Elua Village condominium complex. After 0.3 mile, you pass an interpretive sign about North Pacific humpback whales. These whales migrate from Alaska to Hawaii's warmer coastal waters to mate and give birth during winter, usually between December and March. If you didn't bring binoculars, you can deposit 50 cents (quarters only) into the spotting scopes here.

Archaeological

Most of Wailea's beachfront resorts offer water-sports equipment rental for snorkeling, kayaking, surfing, and windsurfing, plus outrigger canoe tours.

The coastal trail winds south for another 0.2 mile to a small **Hawaiian fishing shrine**. ►2 Often draped with fresh flower leis, this phallic stone was placed here in ancient times to honor the god Kuula, worshipped by fisherfolk seeking an abundant catch. Today this site is still considered a *wahi pana*, or sacred place. Interestingly, the name *Wailea* can be loosely translated as "the waters of Lea," the Hawaiian goddess of canoe making.

The recreation trail next curves south onto the grounds of the Grand Wailea Resort. Around sunset, you might catch Hawaiian musicians and hula dancers performing here on an outdoor stage. Along this stretch of the main Wailea Beach, green sea turtles

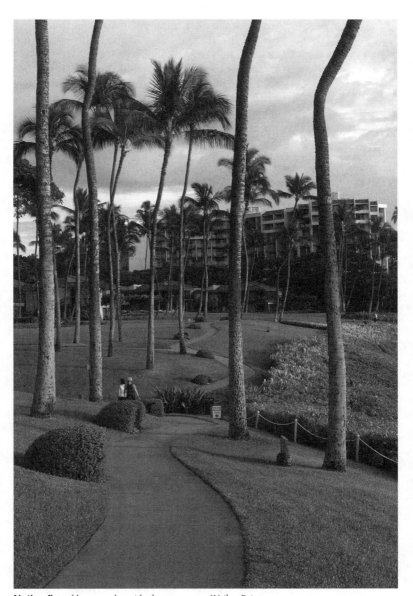

Native flora *blossoms alongside the ocean near Wailea Point.*

Wildlife

(honu) sometimes come ashore at night to rest and nest. Signs along the trail at the south end of the beach kindly ask visitors to SHOW TURTLES ALOHA by always keeping a respectful distance from these wild animals and not doing anything to disrupt their natural activities.

Native Plants

After passing through the resort's south gate, the recreational trail winds through the Hawaiian Coastal Gardens. This rocky coastal stretch around Wailea Point, now about a mile from this hike's starting point, has been thoughtfully replanted with dozens of native species, all helpfully identified on illustrated signboards alongside the trail. Look for a yellow-blossoming hibiscus called mao, as well as beach naupaka, which has white flowers that look as if they've been torn in half.

Archaeological

Before reaching the Fairmont Kea Lani Resort grounds, the trail circumambulates **Wailea Historical Point**. ►3 Here stand the stone foundations of ancient Hawaiian houses, called hale, that are thought to have been inhabited starting in the 1300s BC. Today this point is also one of South Maui's most popular sunset-watching spots. The trail winds just 0.2 mile farther through the grounds of the Fairmont Kea Lani Resort fronting idyllic Polo Beach. Around sunset, you might catch Hawaiian

Great Views

Swimming

MILESTONES

►1	0.0	Trail starts near Ulua Beach parking lot [N 20.69163°, W 156.44292°]
►2	0.5	Pass a small Hawaiian fishing shrine [N 20.68551°, W 156.44389°]
►3	1.3	Arrive at Wailea Historical Point [N 20.67714°, W 156.44397°]
►4	1.5	Turn around at the Fairmont Kea Lani Resort [N 20.67573°, W 156.44345°]
►5	3.0	Return to Ulua Beach parking lot [N 20.69163°, W 156.44292°]

music and hula dancers performing near the beach in the resort's pan-Polynesian luau.

The coastal trail ends at the **south side of the Fairmont Kea Lani Resort grounds**, ►4 about 1.5 miles from where you started. Here on the south side of Polo Beach, the rocky outcropping is a favorite place for families to go tide pooling. When you're ready, turn around and retrace your steps back to the **trailhead** ►5 at Ulua Beach. During the northbound trip, the views of the West Maui coast are postcard-perfect, with palm trees waving beside the coastal path.

It's free to walk inside the Grand Wailea Resort and peruse its multimillion-dollar art collection, including works by contemporary island artists.

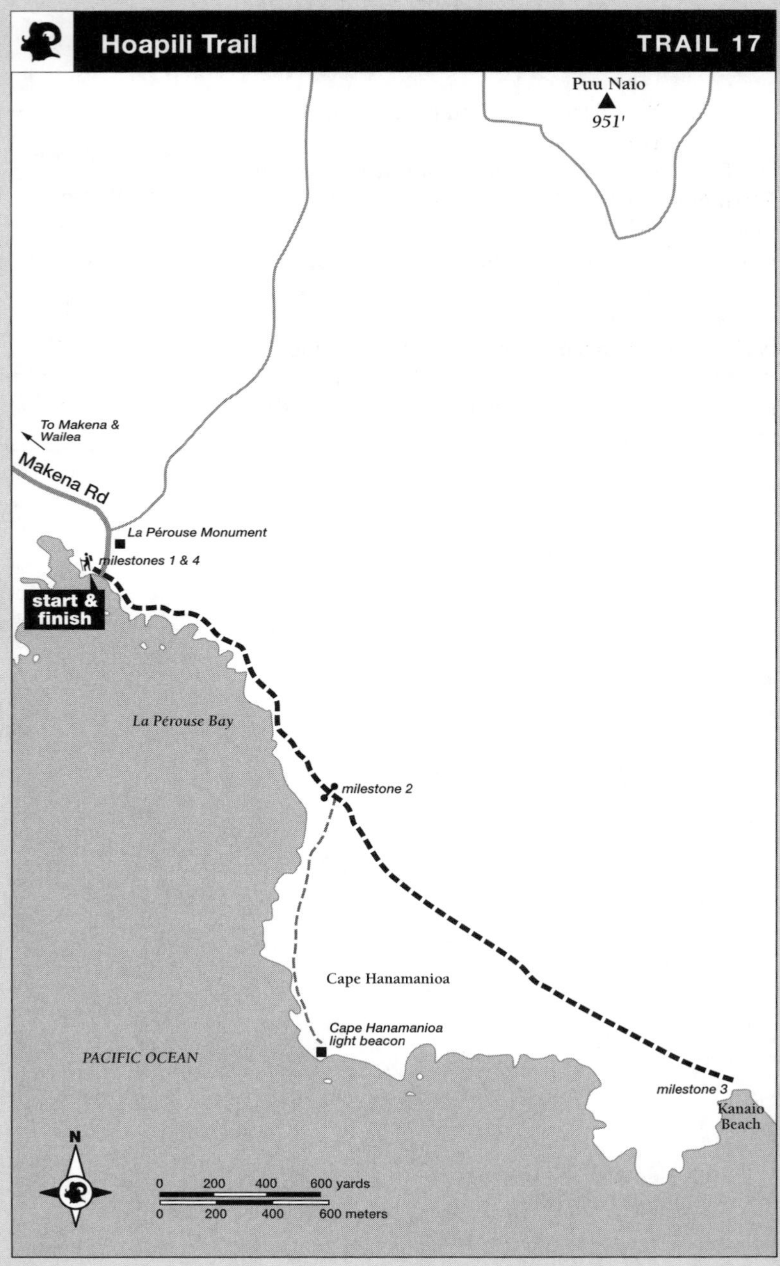
Hoapili Trail
TRAIL 17
Puu Naio
951'
To Makena & Wailea
Makena Rd
La Pérouse Monument
milestones 1 & 4
start & finish
La Pérouse Bay
milestone 2
Cape Hanamanioa
Cape Hanamanioa light beacon
PACIFIC OCEAN
milestone 3
Kanaio Beach
N
0 200 400 600 yards
0 200 400 600 meters

Hoapili Trail

Looking for a challenge? South Maui's toughest shoreline hike follows an ancient Hawaiian footpath over rocky lava flows through a nature preserve, bordered by tide pools and archaeological sites, to find hidden Kanaio Beach. Dramatic views of Haleakala volcano compete with panoramas of nearby islands and wildly tossing surf.

TRAIL USE
Dayhike
LENGTH
4.0 miles, 2–2½ hours
VERTICAL FEET
±250′
DIFFICULTY
– 1 2 **3** 4 5 +
TRAIL TYPE
Out & Back
SURFACE TYPE
Dirt, Lava, Sand
START & END
N 20.59950°
W 156.42000°

FEATURES
Beach
Lava Flows
Native Plants
Tide Pools
Wildlife
Great Views
Secluded
Geologic Interest
Historic Interest
Archaeological

FACILITIES
Restrooms

Best Time

This trail is best during the cooler winter months. Try to start hiking soon after sunrise. Avoid strenuous exertion midday. Dehydration, heat exhaustion, and heatstroke are all serious risks. Carry plenty of water and wear sunscreen, a hat, and sun-protective clothing—being reflected off dark-colored lava intensifies the sun's UV radiation. If you're hiking solo on this remote, little-traveled trail, know that emergency services are far away.

Finding the Trail

From Kihei, drive south on South Kihei Road or the Piilani Highway (Hwy. 31), then follow the signs toward Wailea. In Wailea, continue south on Wailea Alanui Dr., which becomes Makena Road. Approximately 2.2 miles south of the entrance to Makena Beach & Golf Resort, you'll notice signs for Ahihi-Kinau Natural Area Reserve (free entry). Drive 1.9 miles farther along the narrow, mostly paved road through the nature reserve. Rolling hills means limited sight distance for drivers, so watch out for oncoming traffic and cyclists. Beyond Makena

Stables, turn right at the La Pérouse monument (a pyramid-shaped rock tower with a metal interpretive plaque) and drive *makai* (seaward) along a short, potholed dirt road that's usually passable by 2WD vehicles. Leave your car in the unpaved parking area next to the ocean.

Trail Description

North of La Pérouse Bay, Oneloa Beach ("Big Beach") is among Maui's longest stretches of sand. It's popular with sunbathers and swimmers, despite its dangerous shorebreak.

Start hiking southbound from the end-of-the-road **parking lot** ▶1 at La Pérouse Bay, named for the French explorer who became the first Westerner to step ashore on Maui here in 1786. Known for its perilously high surf, this rocky coast is one of the most ruggedly natural spots on the island, with jet-black lava, frothy white-capped waves and aquamarine coves and pools combining for a striking seascape. Although the area's too dangerous for swimming, while standing on the shore you might see pods of spinner dolphins coming into the bay to rest.

Heading south along the shoreline, several use trails confusingly crisscross as they wind over and around piles of jagged, black *aa* lava. As long as you keep heading generally along the ocean's edge and not inland, you'll be fine. After 0.3 mile, you skirt east around a small cove. Another 0.2 mile brings you to a bigger pocket beach with a backdrop of kiawe trees; snorkelers often come here to explore tide pools.

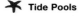

Walk south across this pocket beach and pick up the trail again, which traverses chunky brown *aa* lava. Look *mauka* (inland) for a clearly signposted pedestrian pass-through made of metal wire, about 0.7 mile from where you started. Turn left away from the ocean and **pass through the fence**. ▶2 Walk briefly *mauka* (inland), turning right to join the main Hoapili Trail, a broad, rolling highway of lava rock stretching southward. Ahead an official

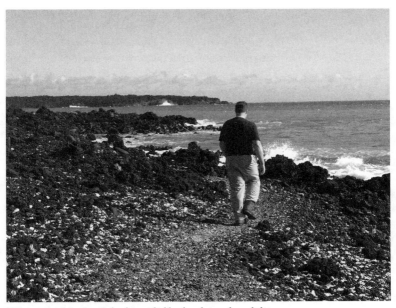

This ancient footpath *leads past hidden beaches and snorkeling coves.*

trail sign states that it's 2 more miles to Kanaio Beach, but don't worry, it's actually only about 1.3 miles farther.

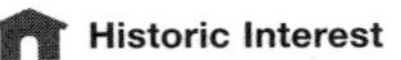

The Hoapili Trail that you're now laboring up and down on is part of an ancient lava road that once circled the entire island. This particular section of the trail was rebuilt by Maui's Governor Ulumaheihei Hoapili in the early 19th century, after a lava flow from the Haleakala volcano likely covered the original trail and the traditional Hawaiian village found here, whose residents had met La Pérouse just a few years prior. Today remnants of that village, for example, *hale* (Hawaiian house) foundations, can still be seen alongside the trail. Be careful not to climb on or disturb any of these ruins or rock piles, as they are protected archaeological and Hawaiian cultural sites.

Archaeological

As you hike along this roller coaster of a trail, expect loose lava rocks to keep rolling beneath your feet. It can be slow going along potentially ankle-twisting stretches, so take it easy and drink lots of water. A few wild axis deer skitter among the barren-looking lava fields. About 0.5 mile before Kanaio Beach, the rocky trail crests a small hill, where the Pacific Ocean spreads out before you. Looking left, you can see the colorful cinder cone Puu o Kanaloa (named after the Hawaiian god of the underworld) and the slopes scarred by Haleakala's most recent lava flow in 1790.

Great Views

Hungry? Roadside food trucks near Makena State Park sell fresh coconuts, fruit smoothies, and mixed-plate lunches to ravenous beachgoers and hikers, too.

The trail briefly dips into a gully with spiky hau trees, easily recognized by their huge prop-root systems. After climbing up out of the gully, the trail gradually descends to **Kanaio Beach**. ►3 You may see another official Hoapili Trail sign here that mistakenly gives the distance to Kanaio Beach as 2.0 miles. In fact, you're already here. Often lonely and deserted, the beach is too rough for swimming. Some kiawe trees provide welcome shade for a picnic lunch, as well as a wooden rope and bench swing. Since camping is not allowed, rest and relax, and then turn around and retrace your steps back to the **trailhead parking lot** ►4 at La Pérouse Bay.

MILESTONES

►1	0.0	Start from oceanside parking lot [N 20.59950°, W 156.42000°]
►2	0.7	Turn inland to pass-through [N 20.59158°, W 156.41193°]
►3	2.0	Arrive at Kanaio Beach [N 20.58229°, W 156.39815°]
►4	4.0	Return to oceanside parking lot [N 20.59950°, W 156.42000°]

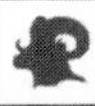

OPTIONS

Detour: Cape Hanamanioa

From the main Hoapili Trail, it's a 1.2-mile out-and-back detour to the modern light beacon at windy **Cape Hanamanioa** [N 20.58348°, W 156.41214°]. At the official Hoapili Trail sign southeast of the hikers' pass-through (Milestone 3 of the main hike), look for a rough 4WD road heading *makai* out to the point of land that's clearly visible jutting out into the ocean. Follow this rolling, rocky 4WD road out to the unsheltered tip of Cape Hanamanioa, where the sea views are stunningly unimpaired by tourist development. Watch for whales and dolphins offshore. When you're ready, retrace your steps to the main trail. Allow at least 30 minutes total for this out-and-back side trip.

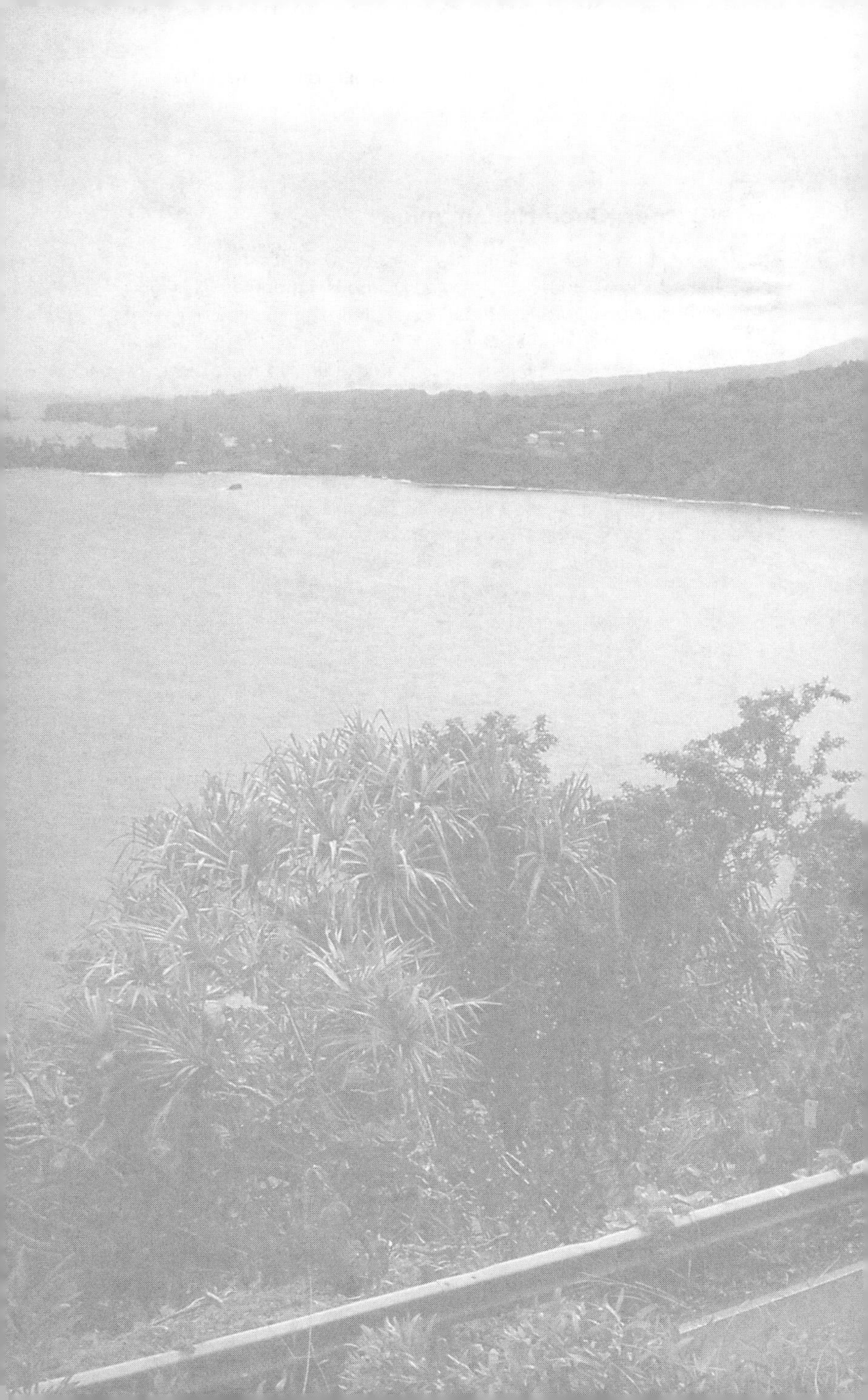

CHAPTER 3

East Maui & Upcountry

18. Waihou Spring
19. Twin Falls
20. Keanae Arboretum
21. Waianapanapa Coast & Caves
22. King's Highway North
23. King's Highway South

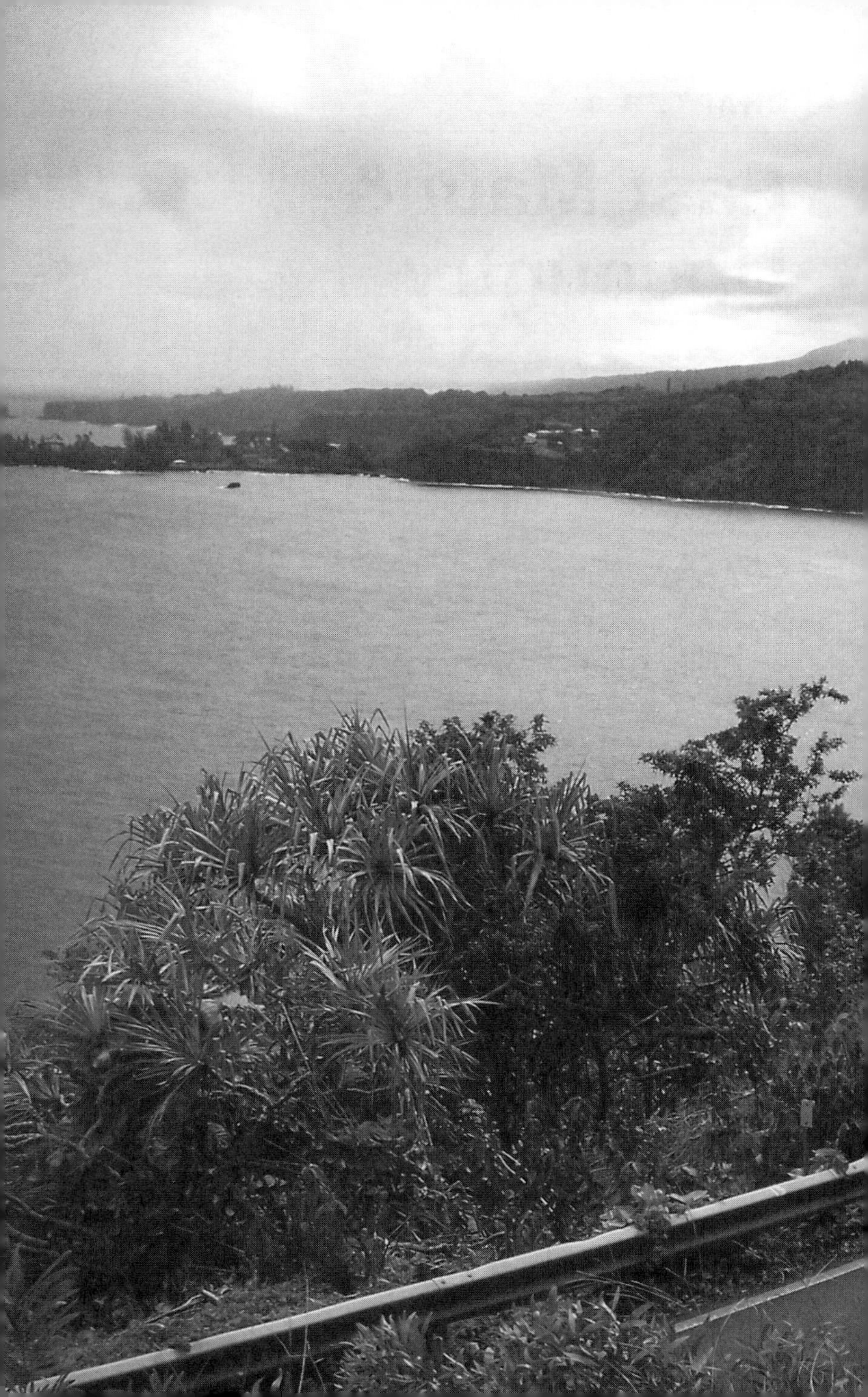

East Maui & Upcountry

Starting from the hang-loose surf town of Paia on the North Shore, **East Maui** hugs the island's windward coast. Frequent rain showers bring out tropical flowers along the famous Road to Hana, which traverses 54 one-lane bridges and winds around hairpin turns above towering sea cliffs. With the sleepy ranch town of Hana as your final destination, or even if you keep heading south to the tumbling waterfalls and bamboo forests of the Kipahulu coastal area of Haleakala National Park (see page 197), you can stretch your legs along the coastal trails described in this chapter. Roadside waterfalls tempt daytrippers to take cool dips, while lava flows and blowholes beckon to venturesome hikers eager to explore the rugged, mostly undeveloped coast. From Waianapanapa State Park's famous black-sand beach, you can walk on an ancient Hawaiian footpath bordered by glossy tropical foliage, giant-sized boulder beaches, lava-rock tide pools, and unusual sites from the island's history and legends.

Sprawling along the upper slopes of Haleakala volcano, Maui's **Upcountry** pierces the cloud-forest belt that hangs above the East Maui coast. Ranchers, farmers, gardeners, and *paniolo* (Hawaiian cowboys) make up the fabric of life in the island's Upcountry, a place many tourists don't go. Here, a pretty, peaceful forest walk to seasonal Waihou Spring makes a shady escape from sun-drenched trails down on the coast.

Permits & Maps

No permits are required for hiking any of the trails in this chapter, most of which cross state-owned lands. Only one trail—the hike to Twin Falls—passes over private property; heed any posted closure signs at that trailhead, as permission for hikers may be revoked at any time. All of the trips described in this chapter are dayhikes. Camping and rental housekeeping cabins are available near the trails inside Waianapanapa State Park (see page 16).

Overleaf and opposite: *The Road to Hana snakes along East Maui's lush windward coast.*

For the first four hikes described in this chapter, topographic maps are not necessary. At Waihou Spring and Waianapanapa State Park, trails are clearly signposted. The paved walk that winds through Keanae Arboretum is easy to find, as is the well-beaten path to Twin Falls. The King's Highway coastal trail, which runs north and south of Waianapanapa State Park, can be trickier to follow, although the written directions and basic trail maps in this book should suffice. Signs posted inside Waianapanapa State Park point out the starting sections of these trails. For a detailed topographic map, the USGS 7.5-minute (1:24,000) *Hana* map shows the entire King's Highway from Hana Bay north to Hana's commuter airport, passing through Waianapanapa State Park.

See Appendix 3 (page 312) for more recommended topographical and driving maps, both digital and printed, to help you navigate around Maui.

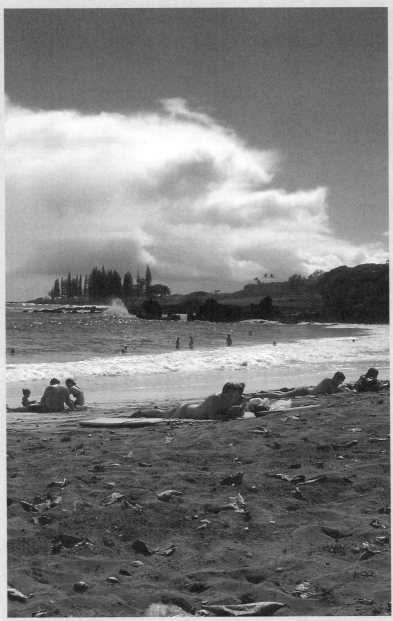

A luxurious strand of gray sands *awaits at Hamoa Beach outside Hana town.*

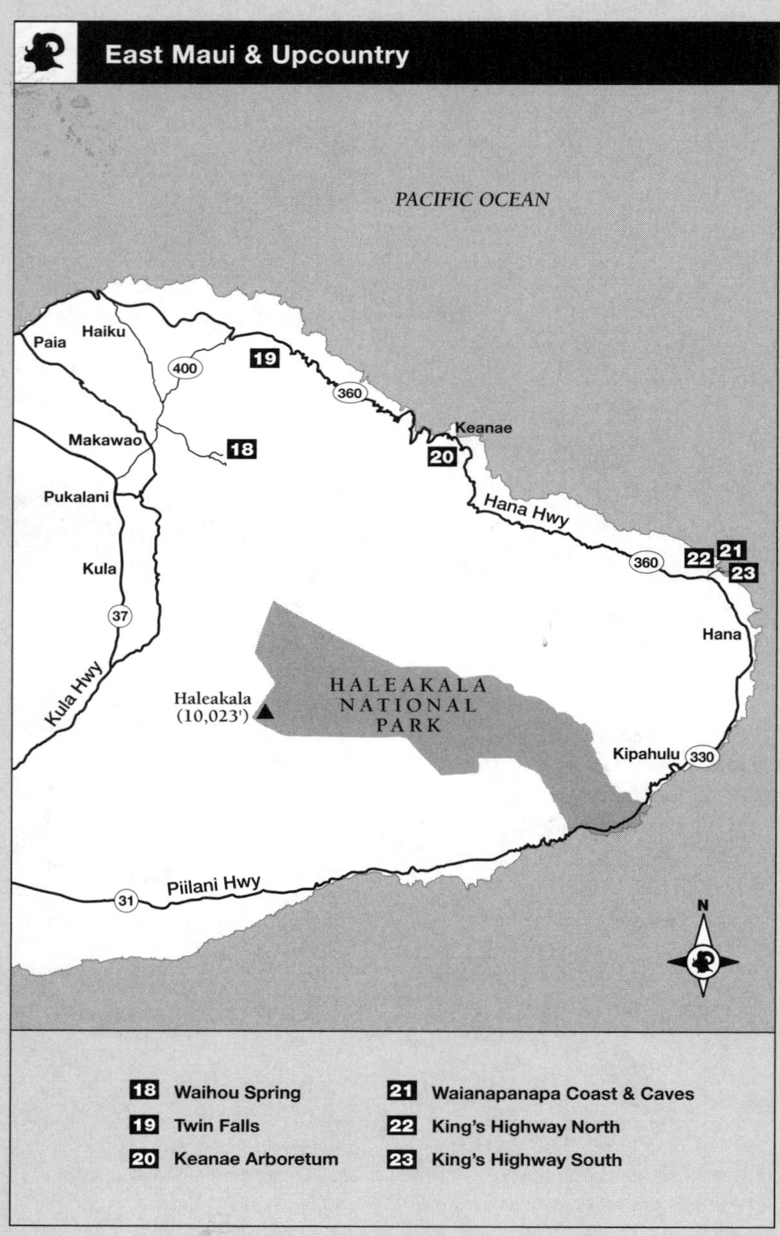
East Maui & Upcountry
PACIFIC OCEAN
Paia
Haiku
400
19
360
Keanae
Makawao
18
20
Pukalani
Hana Hwy
Kula
360
22
21
23
37
Hana
Kula Hwy
Haleakala
(10,023')
HALEAKALA
NATIONAL
PARK
Kipahulu
330
Piilani Hwy
31
N
18 Waihou Spring
19 Twin Falls
20 Keanae Arboretum
21 Waianapanapa Coast & Caves
22 King's Highway North
23 King's Highway South

East Maui & Upcountry

TRAIL	Difficulty	Length	Type	USES & ACCESS	TERRAIN	FLORA & FAUNA	OTHER
18	2	2.4	Semiloop	Dayhiking, Running, Child Friendly, Dogs Allowed	Forest, Stream	Birds, Wildlife	Great Views, Secluded, Shady, Steep
19	2	2.2	Out & Back	Dayhiking, Child Friendly, Dogs Allowed	Forest, Stream, Waterfall	Birds, Native Plants	Swimming, Shady
20	1	1.2	Out & Back	Dayhiking, Child Friendly, Dogs Allowed	Forest, Stream	Birds, Native Plants	Secluded, Shady
21	2	1.8	Semiloop	Dayhiking, Child Friendly	Beach, Lava Flow	Birds, Native Plants, Wildlife	Great Views, Swimming, Camping, Geologic Interest, Historic Interest, Archaeological
22	2	1.8	Out & Back	Dayhiking	Beach, Lava Flow	Birds, Native Plants, Tide Pools, Wildlife	Great Views, Historic Interest, Secluded
23	3	3.7	Point-to-Point	Dayhiking	Beach, Lava Flow	Birds, Native Plants, Tide Pools, Wildlife	Great Views, Historic Interest, Archaeological, Secluded

USES & ACCESS
- Dayhiking
- Backpacking
- Running
- Biking
- Wheelchair Access
- Child Friendly
- Dogs Allowed
- Permit Required

TYPE
- Loop
- Out & Back
- Semiloop
- Point-to-Point

DIFFICULTY
- 1 2 3 4 5 +
less more

TERRAIN
- Beach
- Forest
- Lava Flow
- Mountain
- Pond
- Summit
- Stream
- Waterfall

FLORA & FAUNA
- Birds
- Native Plants
- Tide Pools
- Wildlife

FEATURES
- Great Views
- Swimming
- Camping
- Geologic Interest
- Historic Interest
- Archaeological
- Secluded
- Shady
- Steep

East Maui & Upcountry

TRAIL 18

Dayhike, Run,
Child Friendly,
Dogs Allowed
2.4 miles, Semiloop
Difficulty: 1 **2** 3 4 5

Waihou Spring 159

Escape the heat in Maui's forested highlands, where this shady trail carpeted with pine needles winds around toward ocean views. A steep descent to a seasonal spring—and the hike back uphill from the streambed—will elevate your heart rate.

TRAIL 19

Dayhike, Child Friendly,
Dogs Allowed
2.2 miles, Out & Back
Difficulty: 1 **2** 3 4 5

Twin Falls 165

Not far from Paia, along the famous Road to Hana on Maui's windward coast, this popular detour visits two waterfalls, the latter most spectacular after rain. Expect to wade in the stream to reach the end of the trail.

TRAIL 20

Dayhike, Child Friendly,
Dogs Allowed
1.2 miles, Out & Back
Difficulty: **1** 2 3 4 5

Keanae Arboretum 171

A tame trail through a small, manicured garden lets you touch, sniff, and relax in the shade of dozens of native and nonnative flora species, from delicate ginger plants to sprawling palm trees. Often uncrowded, it's a hidden stop along East Maui's Hana Highway.

Waianapanapa Coast & Caves 177

East Maui's most popular state park is an inviting place to break your journey along the Road to Hana. Easy walking trails visit a black-sand beach, legendary caves, and a traditional Hawaiian *heiau* (temple). Watch out for the lava blowhole!

TRAIL 21

Dayhike, Child Friendly
1.8 miles, Semiloop
Difficulty: 1 **2** 3 4 5

King's Highway North 183

Starting at the state park's black-sand Pailoa Beach, explore the jagged lava flows along this historic Hawaiian footpath. Here the ocean bursts through lava-rock blowholes and the wind whips against outcroppings that make scenic perches for catching the sunrise.

TRAIL 22

Dayhike
1.8 miles, Out & Back
Difficulty: 1 **2** 3 4 5

King's Highway South 187

Ready for an adventure? From Waianapanapa State Park, follow the ancient King's Highway south along the dramatically rocky coast, passing archaeological sites and primitive beaches, all the way to crescent-shaped Hana Bay. This hike requires sturdy shoes.

TRAIL 23

Dayhike
3.7 miles, Point-to-Point
Difficulty: 1 2 **3** 4 5

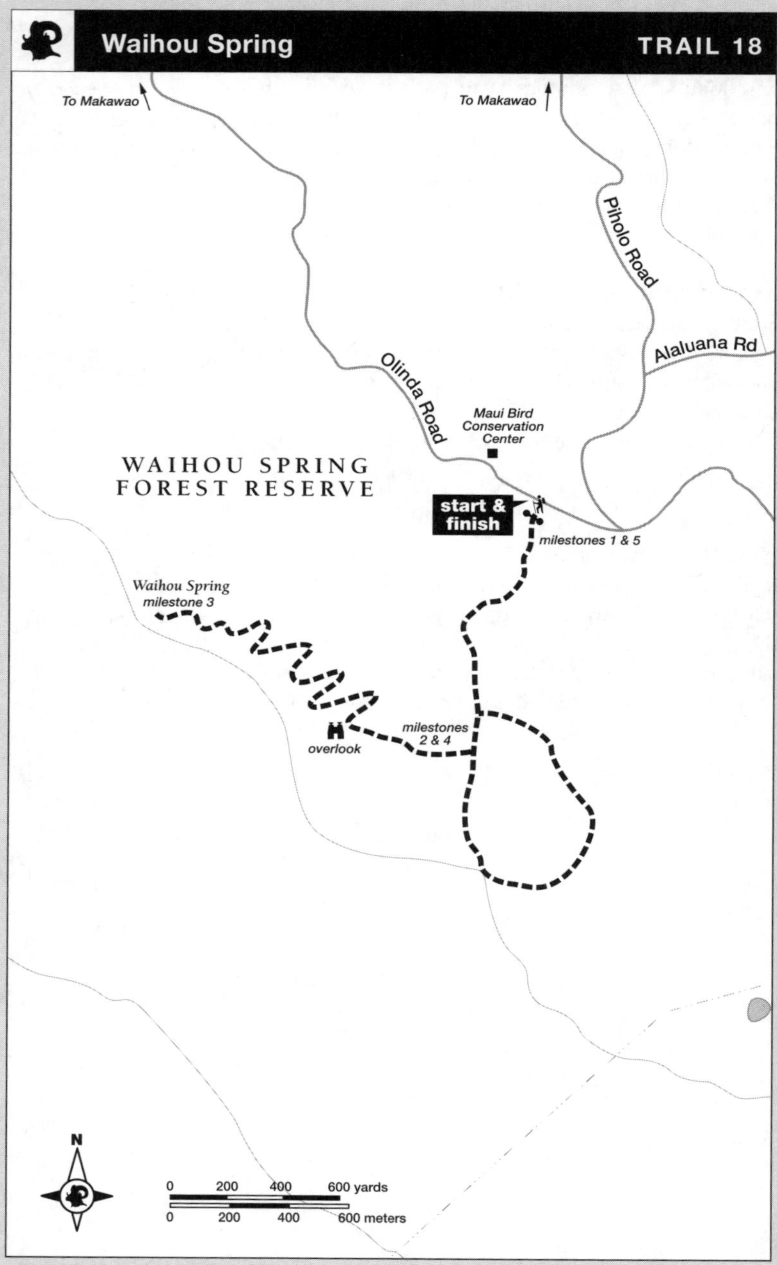
Waihou Spring
TRAIL 18
To Makawao
To Makawao
Piholo Road
Alaluana Rd
Olinda Road
Maui Bird Conservation Center
WAIHOU SPRING FOREST RESERVE
start & finish
milestones 1 & 5
Waihou Spring
milestone 3
milestones 2 & 4
overlook
N
0 200 400 600 yards
0 200 400 600 meters

Waihou Spring

Nestled among Upcountry ranch lands on the slopes of Haleakala volcano, this quiet path leads through an experimental forest filled with birdsong. Other rewards include peekaboo ocean views and a small streamside spring that flows during rainy months.

TRAIL USE
Dayhike, Run, Child Friendly, Dogs Allowed

LENGTH
2.4 miles, 1–1½ hours

VERTICAL FEET
±900′

DIFFICULTY
– 1 **2** 3 4 5 +

TRAIL TYPE
Semiloop

SURFACE TYPE
Dirt

START & END
N 20.80626°
W 156.27998°

FEATURES
Forest
Stream
Birds
Wildlife
Great Views
Secluded
Shady
Steep

FACILITIES
None

Best Time

This area of Waihou Spring Forest Reserve is open daily year-round from sunrise to sunset. Because the trail sits at a lower elevation than Maui's cloud-forest belt, both mornings and afternoons may offer clear ocean views, though later in the day tends to be mistier. During the driest months (e.g., May to October), the springs often do not flow, which makes this a better winter hike. Just watch out for steep, muddy trail sections.

Finding the Trail

From Paia, drive southeast on Baldwin Ave. for almost 6 miles to central Makawao. At the four-way stop-sign intersection with Makawao Ave., continue straight onto Olinda Road and wind another 4.7 miles uphill. Past the Maui Bird Conservation Center, look for the signposted trailhead gate on your right. Park at an angle to the forest reserve fence in the dirt pullout area next to the road, downhill from the gate.

From Kahului, take the Hana Highway (Hwy. 36) east to the Haleakala Highway (Hwy. 37), turn right and drive 7 miles uphill to Pukalani. Turn left onto Makawao Ave., then drive another 7 miles northwest to its intersection with Olinda Road. Turn right, and follow the directions above from central Makawao.

Trail Description

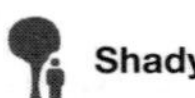

To find the **trailhead**, ►1 pass through the pedestrian gate off Olinda Road into Waihou Spring Forest Reserve, an experimental forest once deliberately planted with nonnative species. Today swamp mahogany *(Eucalyptus robusta)* trees flourish alongside Monterey cypress and stately pines that carpet an unusually broad walking trail with their soft needles.

On clear days, you'll enjoy views all the way down the slopes of Haleakala volcano to the ocean.

After ambling mostly downhill for less than 0.4 mile, you'll notice a 4WD road veers off to the left. Keep right to stay on the main loop trail. Soon you arrive at the first signposted trail junction, which correctly gives the distance to the overlook as 0.3 mile. Stay to the right here, too, and shortly you reach the **second marked trail junction**, ►2 about 0.5 mile from the trailhead. Follow the signposted arrows and veer right off the main loop trail to continue hiking toward the overlook and spring.

The trail continues rolling downhill, becoming more steep as it abruptly drops to the edge of a ridge. A little more than 0.7 mile from the trailhead and Olinda Road, you arrive at the official **overlook**.

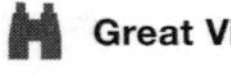

Here an ideally positioned bench gives winded hikers coming back up from the springs a quick respite. On clear days, you'll enjoy views all the way down the slopes of Haleakala volcano to the Pacific Ocean.

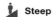

From the overlook, the trail switchbacks abruptly downhill, becoming narrow, rocky, and often muddy. After descending the steep cliffs, you arrive at **Waihou Spring** ►3, about a mile from the trailhead. The petite mossy cascade lies at the bottom of a boulder-strewn gulch. Whether or not

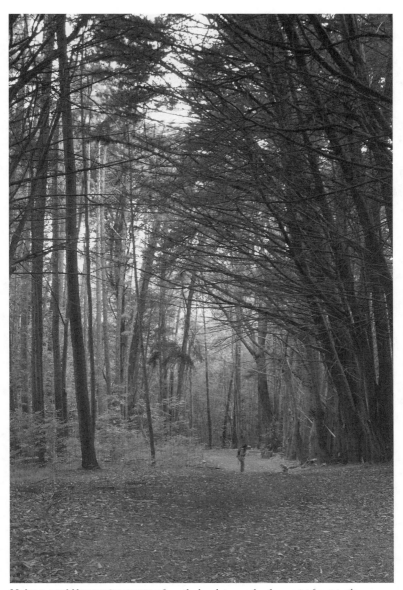

Make a cool Upcountry escape *from the beach to wander these quiet forest trails.*

Listen for the songs of the island's native forest birds, including bright-red honeycreepers endemic to Maui.

the spring is flowing partly depends on whether or not it has been raining recently. Looking up, you'll notice the other reason the spring is often dry: Several water diversion tunnels have been cut into the face of the rocks. Although the springs are not a dramatic sight, the coolness of the air is a sweet relief from Maui's hotter coastal climes.

Expect a short but pulse-pounding workout as you retrace your steps back uphill to the overlook. Continue backtracking to the last trail junction that you passed, the one with the sign marked OVERLOOK 0.25 MILES, SPRINGS 0.5 MILE. Turn right here to **rejoin the main loop trail**. ▶4 The trail once again becomes a broad path that rolls gently up and down through the forest. As you enjoy the peaceful walk, listen for the sounds of the island's native forest birds, such as the apapane and iiwi, both bright-red honeycreepers endemic to Hawaii (see page 6). You may also surprise a few axis deer along the trail.

Birds

Approximately 0.5 mile after rejoining the main trail, close the loop by arriving back at the first trailhead sign you passed, the one that says LOOP 0.6 MILE. Turn right here—otherwise , you'll end up walking the same loop twice—and start ascending underneath a verdant canopy of trees. After another 0.4 mile of walking uphill, you arrive back at the **gated trailhead** ▶5 by the dirt parking area alongside Olinda Road.

MILESTONES

►1	0.0	Start from trailhead gate off Olinda Road [N 20.80626°, W 156.27998°]
►2	0.5	Veer right off main loop trail toward overlook
►3	1.0	Finish descending switchbacks to reach spring [N 20.80460°, W 156.28669°]
►4	1.5	Turn right back onto main loop trail
►5	2.4	Return to trailhead gate off Olinda Road [N 20.80626°, W 156.27998°]

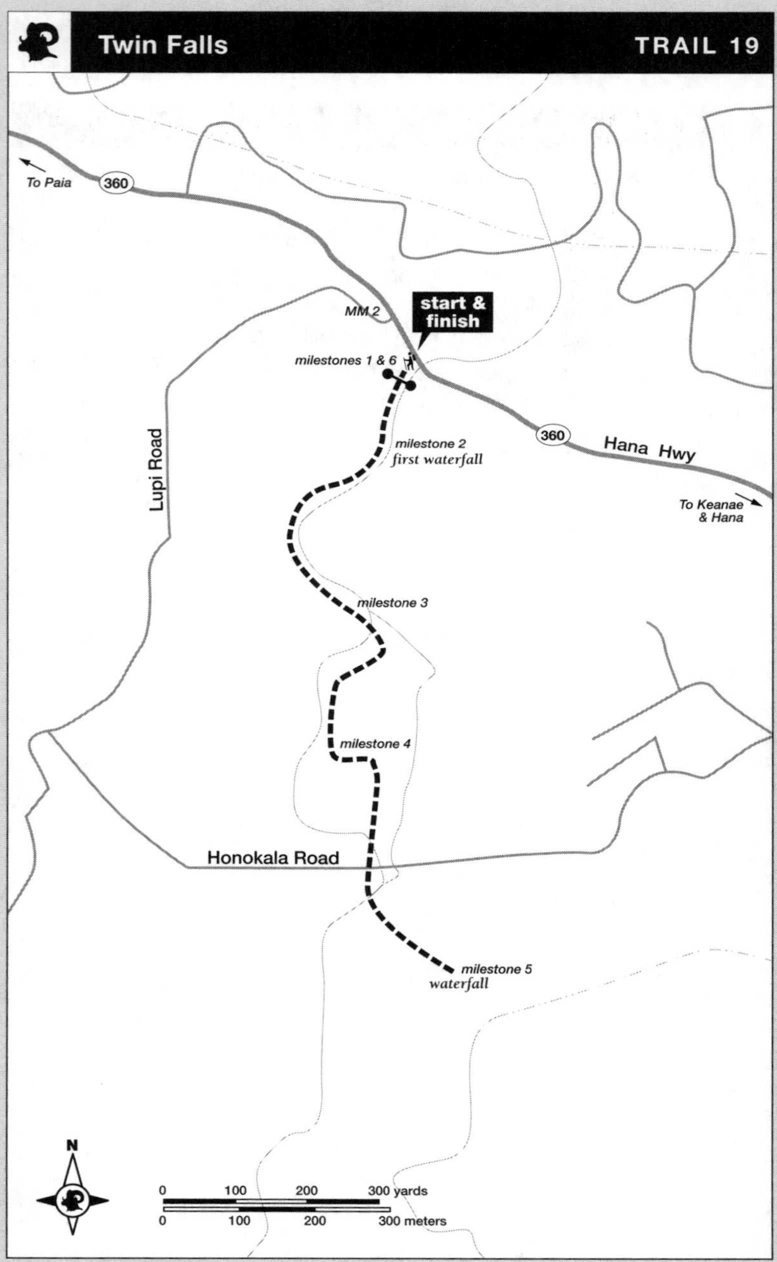
Twin Falls
TRAIL 19
To Paia
360
MM 2
start & finish
milestones 1 & 6
360
Hana Hwy
Lupi Road
milestone 2
first waterfall
To Keanae & Hana
milestone 3
milestone 4
Honokala Road
milestone 5
waterfall
N
0
100
200
300 yards
0
100
200
300 meters

Twin Falls

Along Maui's legendary Hana Highway, this mostly level streamside hike takes you to two waterfalls. The first is only a petite cascade, but the second can be breathtaking: Tucked inside a jungly forest, the misty waterfall drops over mossy rocks into a rippling pool, where you can swim.

TRAIL USE
Dayhike, Child Friendly, Dogs Allowed

LENGTH
2.2 miles, 1–1½ hours

VERTICAL FEET
±200′

DIFFICULTY
– 1 **2** 3 4 5 +

TRAIL TYPE
Out & Back

SURFACE TYPE
Dirt, Grass

START & END
N 20.91193°
W 156.24274°

FEATURES
Forest
Stream
Waterfall
Birds
Native Plants
Swimming
Shady

FACILITIES
Restrooms

Best Time

You can visit both falls year-round. The trail is least crowded in the early morning, before Hana-bound daytrippers arrive. Because the trail crosses private property, permission to hike may be revoked any time. Obey all posted signs at the trailhead gate. The valley is subject to flash floods, which can occur without warning. Check the weather forecast and do not start hiking if rain is predicted or dark clouds are visible.

Finding the Trail

From Paia, drive southeast on the Hana Highway (Hwy. 36) for about 19 miles. The roadside mile markers reset at zero where Highway 36 ends and Highway 360 (also called the Hana Highway) begins. Keep driving along Highway 360 for another 2 miles. Just past mile marker (MM) 2, look for a wide dirt parking area on your right. If it's full, do not park on the bridge just beyond it. Instead, drive across the bridge and park on the dirt highway shoulder farther uphill. Car break-ins and vandalism are common here—do not leave any valuables inside your vehicle. Some locals recommend leaving your car unlocked with windows rolled down, to deter thieves from damaging the vehicle simply to break in.

Trail Description

The Hana Highway abounds with roadside waterfalls, perfect for photos and sometimes swimming. Look for wherever cars are pulled off the highway, then follow the crowds.

From the dirt parking area next to the highway, head inland past the souvenir and snack stands. Start hiking from the **gated trailhead**. ►1 If the weather forecast predicts rain, or if it has been raining recently, this gate may be locked with signs posted that officially close the valley to hikers. Pay attention to these warnings, as the valley is prone to dangerous flash floods. On the far side of the gate, a few portable toilets are provided.

Twin Falls is one of the most popular dayhikes along the Hana Highway, so don't expect to have the trail to yourself. Since most daytrippers usually arrive after 10 AM, get here earlier than that if you want to have a shot at a private dip at the second waterfall. This streamside trail can also get very buggy, so bring some insect repellent. Sturdy shoes will help with stream crossings, although plenty of locals and tourists alike hike in rubbah slippah (flip-flops).

The trail starts out gently following a wide dirt road running between the stream to your left and fenced-off farm fields to your right. While some hikers choose a use trail through the farm fields, technically that's trespassing on private property. After about 0.4 mile of walking on the main dirt road, look off to your left for a short, often muddy path leading down to the stream's edge. Take it to find the **first waterfall**. ►2 A pretty small cascade, it's a family-friendly place to take a quick, cool dip. If the stream is flowing fast, it can be dangerous to enter the water—use your best judgment.

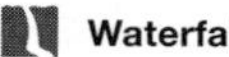

Clamber back up the side path leading to that first waterfall, then keep walking inland along the

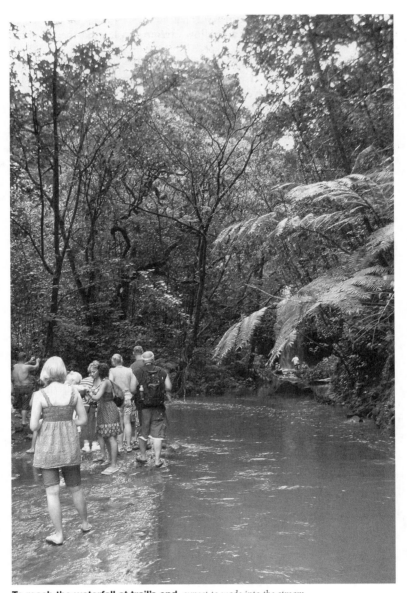

To reach the waterfall at trail's end, *expect to wade into the stream.*

Tucked inside a jungly forest, the misty waterfall drops over mossy rocks into a rippling pool, where you can swim.

same dirt road that you were hiking on previously. **Cross a shallow stream**. ►3 If it has been raining recently, expect to get at least your feet wet. About 0.8 mile from the trailhead, you reach a confusing intersection of dirt roads, some of which are private driveways. Make a 90-degree left turn at this **trail junction** ►4 onto a smaller path, which soon broadens again.

Pushing onward, you come to the remains of a concrete aqueduct. Climb the rungs up and over the obstacle, which sits atop the stream. Then take a deep breath before you start wading through the water to the base of the **second waterfall**, ►5 now clearly visible ahead and off to your right. Although it's only 100 yards or so, this final part of the hike might require extra time and some caution. Do not attempt to wade in the stream if it's flowing too fast or too high. Grabbing a downed tree branch to use as a makeshift hiking pole can improve your balance.

Swimming

When you reach the falls, a few dozen people may be swimming there already or swinging on the rope suspended from a tree at the pool's edge. Swimming underneath the falls is not recommended because of the ever-present danger of rockfall. Submerged rocks also make diving off the cliffs above foolhardy.

When you're ready, retrace your steps back to the major trail junction, making a 90-degree right turn back onto the dirt road that leads back to the **trailhead gate** ►6 by the highway.

MILESTONES

▶1	0.0	Start at trailhead gate [N 20.91193°, W 156.24274°]
▶2	0.4	Pass first waterfall
▶3	0.8	First stream crossing [N 20.90666°, W 156.24374°]
▶4	0.8	Turn left at trail junction [N 20.90498°, W 156.24332°]
▶5	1.1	Arrive at second waterfall
▶6	2.2	Return to trailhead gate [N 20.91193°, W 156.24274°]

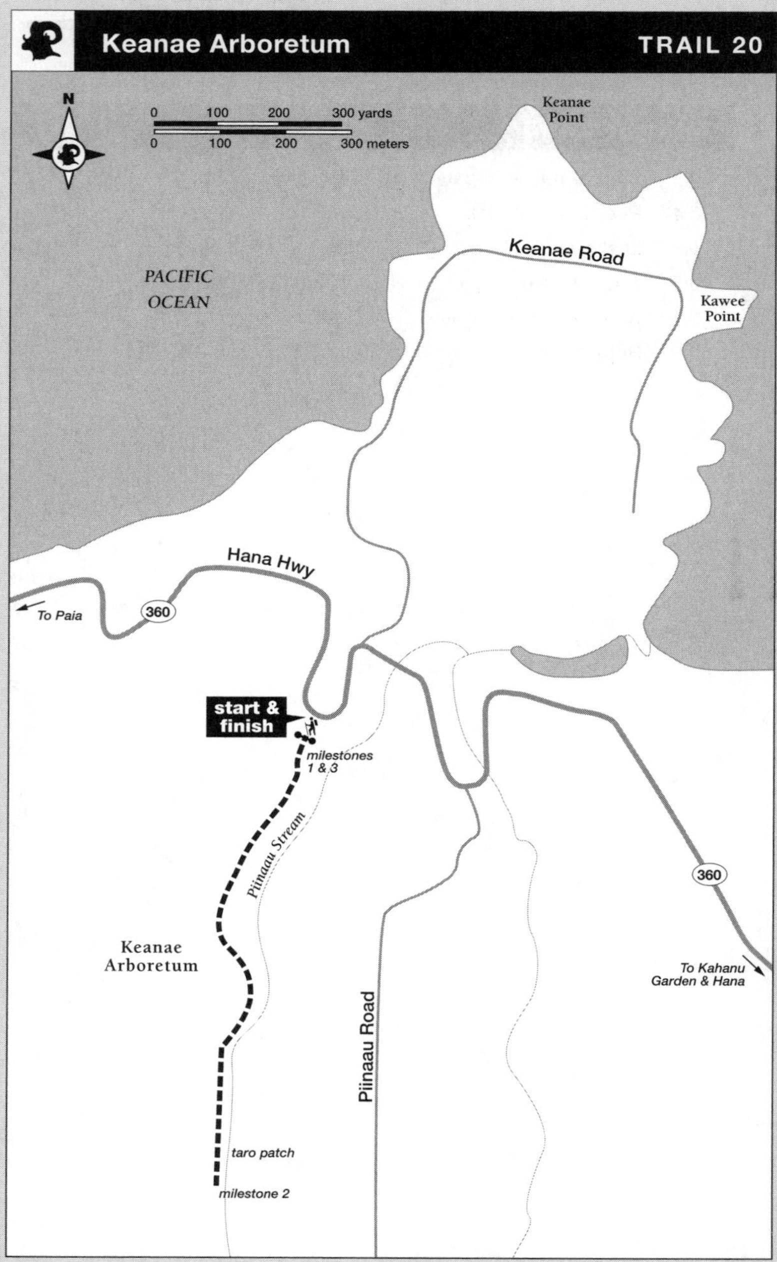
Keanae Arboretum
TRAIL 20
N
0 100 200 300 yards
0 100 200 300 meters
Keanae Point
PACIFIC OCEAN
Keanae Road
Kawee Point
Hana Hwy
To Paia
360
start & finish
milestones 1 & 3
Piinaau Stream
Keanae Arboretum
Piinaau Road
360
To Kahanu Garden & Hana
taro patch
milestone 2

Keanae Arboretum

The Road to Hana is more famous for its waterfalls, but this public arboretum is also worth a look along East Maui's rain-soaked coast. Wander along a gentle paved path among native and exotic plants, or bushwhack to a hidden streamside swimming hole.

TRAIL USE
Dayhike, Child Friendly, Dogs Allowed

LENGTH
1.2 miles, 30–45 mins.

VERTICAL FEET
±100′

DIFFICULTY
– **1** 2 3 4 5 +

TRAIL TYPE
Out & Back

SURFACE TYPE
Dirt, Paved

START & END
N 20.85734°
W 156.14926°

FEATURES
Forest
Stream
Birds
Native Plants
Secluded
Shady

FACILITIES
None

Best Time

You can visit the arboretum year-round. Most Hana-bound daytrippers arrive around lunchtime or in the early afternoon, when roadside parking pullouts may fill. Mornings are a better bet for solitude and clear skies, although walking in the mist can also be pretty. Do not start hiking when rain is forecast or if dark clouds are visible in the sky, because the stream is subject to dangerous flash flooding.

Finding the Trail

From Paia, drive southeast on the Hana Highway (Hwy. 36) for about 19 miles. The roadside mile markers reset at zero where Highway 36 ends and Highway 360 (also called the Hana Highway) begins. Keep driving along Highway 360 for another 16 miles. About 0.6 mile past mile marker (MM) 16, look for a dirt pullout parking area in front of a locked gate on the *mauka* (inland) side of Highway 360. You can also park on the dirt shoulder on the opposite *makai* (ocean) side of the highway. If you reach the signposted left turn for Keanae town, the Piinaau Road intersection, or MM 17, you've gone too far. Carefully make a U-turn near MM 17 and backtrack 0.4 mile to the arboretum entrance. Admission is free.

Trail Description

Pass through the roadside **entrance gate**, ▶1 which is marked by a white mailbox with a yellow label that reads KEANAE HUNTER CHECK STATION. Although there is no official sign for the Keanae Arboretum here, brown DLNR signs advise visitors that flash floods are possible in this area and that diving and jumping into the stream are prohibited. Walk uphill for a short distance along a dirt 4WD service road, which quickly turns to pavement as it passes the arboretum's official entrance sign.

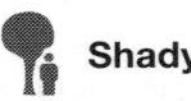

Shady

Maintained by the state, Keanae Arboretum runs alongside Piinaau Stream. In ancient times, Native Hawaiians cultivated taro plants here. Today, the arboretum harbors an incredible variety of both native and nonnative plant species, from tiny ornamental ginger plants to elegant tall palm trees that spread welcome shade. Timber and tropical fruit trees, including papaya, passion fruit, and guava, also thrive. Most of the plants are clearly labeled, and it's easy to spend a half hour or more here getting acquainted with myriad species you'll encounter on other hiking trails around the island. Keanae Arboretum is especially well regarded for its collection of Hawaiian medicinal and food plants, including examples of those brought over by the first Polynesian settlers.

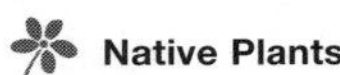

Native Plants

The aboretum's collection of Hawaiian medicinal and food plants includes species brought over by the first Polynesian settlers.

The arboretum's gently sloping, paved nature trail winds its way inland. After reaching a small grassy clearing, the trail turns to gravel and dirt mixed with grassy patches. Leaving the shady tall trees behind, the next exposed section of trail can be quite hot and sunny, depending on the weather. You can hear Piinaau Stream downhill to your left now. Soon you arrive at a wire hikers' pass-through. A small shed roofed with corrugated iron stands just beyond the gate. Now you are entering a traditional Hawaiian-style loi kalo (taro patch), or irrigated wetland terrace. Here the trail becomes indistinct

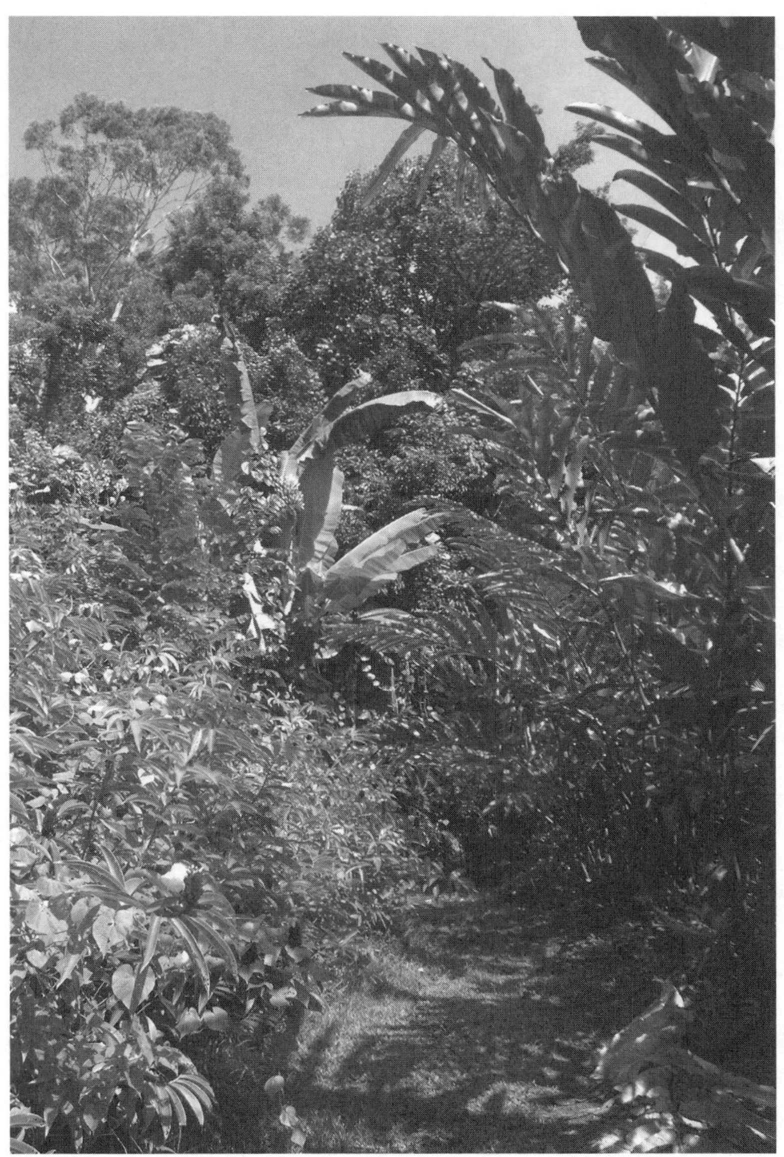

Get acquainted *with Hawaii's native and exotic flora at Keanae Arboretum.*

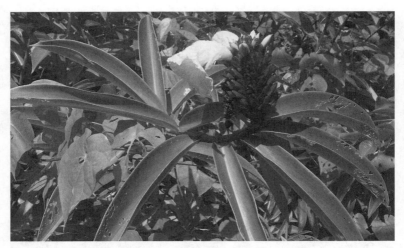

The exotic bromeliad family *is among the most diverse of Hawaii's introduced plants, blossoming in a rainbow of colors.*

and often thickly overgrown as it generally runs along the right side of the field.

On the far side of the taro patch, the **trail ends.** ▶2 If you venture beyond the white wire gate here, you can eventually access the stream. That's why you may notice other hikers carrying swimsuits and towels coming toward you. If you forge ahead, you're on your own, as reaching the stream usually requires some slippery bushwhacking through dense forest. It's worth it only if you're really gung-ho for a swim, or if none of the other waterfall pools along the Road to Hana have enticed you so far. Always exercise caution when getting in the water. If the stream is flowing too fast or high, skip it rather than get caught in a current that's too strong. Flash floods can occur without warning if it has been raining recently, either here or upstream.

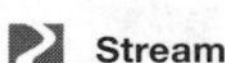 **Stream**

For heart-stopping views of the Keanae Peninsula, drive farther down the Hana Highway just past MM 17, where a roadside pullout on the *makai* (ocean) side of the highway offers postcard panoramas.

But your hike ends here. Retrace your steps through the taro patch and along the paved path through the arboretum to the **entrance gate** ▶3 next to the highway.

MILESTONES

- ▶1 0.0 Start at arboretum entrance gate [N 20.85734°, W 156.14926°]
- ▶2 0.6 Turn around on far side of taro patch
- ▶3 1.2 Return to arboretum entrance gate [N 20.85734°, W 156.14926°]

OPTIONS

Detour: Kahanu Garden & Piilanihale Temple

Plant lovers will want to make time for **Kahanu Garden** (open 10 AM to 2 PM daily, guided tour 10 AM Saturday). There you can walk among rare ethnobotanical Polynesian plants and the world's largest collection of breadfruit trees. Also on the property is Piilanihale, an ancient Hawaiian *heiau* (temple) built of lava rocks, now a national historic landmark. Admission to the garden costs $10 per adult, or $25 including a guided tour (reservations required); children under 13 are free. For more information, visit www.ntbg.org or call (808) 248-8912.

To find the garden, turn *makai* (toward the ocean) at the sign just past MM 31 on Highway 360, then drive 1.5 miles down the bumpy, partly paved Ulaino Road. A small stream crossing just before the garden entrance may make this road impassable to 2WD vehicles after heavy rains.

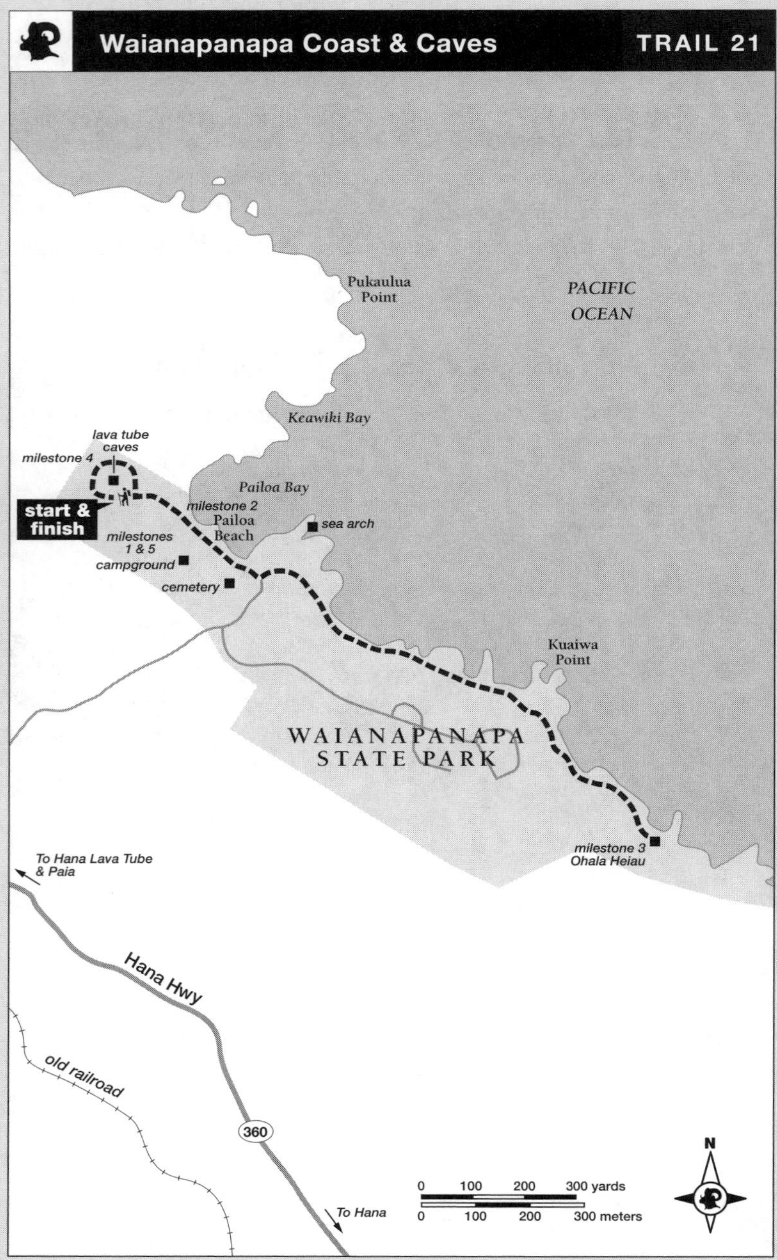
Waianapanapa Coast & Caves
TRAIL 21
Pukaulua
Point
PACIFIC
OCEAN
Keawiki Bay
lava tube
caves
milestone 4
Pailoa Bay
start &
finish
milestone 2
Pailoa
Beach
sea arch
milestones
1 & 5
campground
cemetery
Kuaiwa
Point
WAIANAPANAPA
STATE PARK
milestone 3
Ohala Heiau
To Hana Lava Tube
& Paia
Hana Hwy
old railroad
360
To Hana
0 100 200 300 yards
0 100 200 300 meters
N

Waianapanapa Coast & Caves

Soak up ocean vistas from black-sand Pailoa Beach, then pay your respects to an ancient Hawaiian *heiau* (temple) in Waianapanapa (roughly translated as "glistening waters") State Park. Detour to a natural lava-rock blowhole and caves made famous by island legends, too.

TRAIL USE
Dayhike, Child Friendly

LENGTH
1.8 miles, 45–60 mins.

VERTICAL FEET
±125′

DIFFICULTY
– 1 **2** 3 4 5 +

TRAIL TYPE
Semiloop

SURFACE TYPE
Dirt, Lava, Paved, Sand

START & END
N 20.78876°
W 156.00459°

FEATURES
Beach
Lava Flows
Birds
Native Plants
Wildlife
Great Views
Swimming
Camping
Geologic Interest
Historic Interest
Archaeological

FACILITIES
Restrooms
Picnic Tables
Phone
Water

Best Time

You can visit Waianapanapa State Park year-round. Most Hana-bound daytrippers arrive around lunchtime or in the early afternoon, when the parking lots often fill. Early morning is best for solitude. Late afternoon just before sunset can be another good time to hike here, unless East Maui's persistent rain clouds have already rolled in by then.

Finding the Trail

From Paia, drive southeast on the Hana Highway (Hwy. 36) for about 19 miles. The roadside mile markers reset at zero where Highway 36 ends and Highway 360 (also called the Hana Highway) begins. Keep driving along Highway 360 for another 32 miles. Just south of mile marker (MM) 32, turn left onto the signposted state park access road and drive 0.5 mile *makai* (toward the ocean), watching out for speed bumps and blind hills. Turn left at the T-intersection inside the park and continue driving 0.2 mile to the paved parking lot just north of the campground. Coming from the center of Hana town, drive north on Highway 360 for a little more than 2 miles, then turn right *(makai)* before MM 32.

Trail Description

Start on the east side of the state park's **north parking lot**. ▶1 The nearby camping area has restrooms and drinking water. Facing the ocean from the parking lot, walk along the paved trail leading to your right. Almost immediately, a trail junction appears, with a black-sand beach visible off to your left. The ocean views just from the railing here are stunning, especially at sunrise when the first rays of light break over the waves.

Great Views

Follow the signposted spur trail down to black-sand **Pailoa Beach**, ▶2 just 0.1 mile from your starting point. The beach itself is no bigger than a cove, but Pailoa Bay is a dramatic place, with crashing high surf and strong currents that swimmers should be wary of. Looking toward the south side of the bay, you spy a natural sea arch that experienced snorkelers can swim out to when the waters are calm. Most visitors enjoy lounging around on the soft, cindery black sands. (If you're curious what lies north of this pocket beach, take Trip 22, page 183, the next hike described in this chapter.)

Beach

Climb back up from the black-sand beach and rejoin the main trail by walking south above the park's shoreline. You'll pass a grassy camping area (see page 16) with picnic pavilions and a small Hawaiian cemetery on your right, as the trail alternates between paved sections and gravel. Keep near the coast so you don't miss the natural lava-rock blowhole—you'll know you've found it when you see the official signs warning you not to get too close. That's because the blowhole is very unpredictable—it might be blasting high into the air when you visit, or it might not be doing much of anything at all.

Camping

Hiking along the coast here can be buggy, especially around the lava tube caves and pools. Pack insect repellent.

Walk inland for a short distance to find a wide, grassy path beside hala (screwpine, or pandanus) trees, with their distinctive prop roots and long, green leaves traditionally used by Hawaiians for

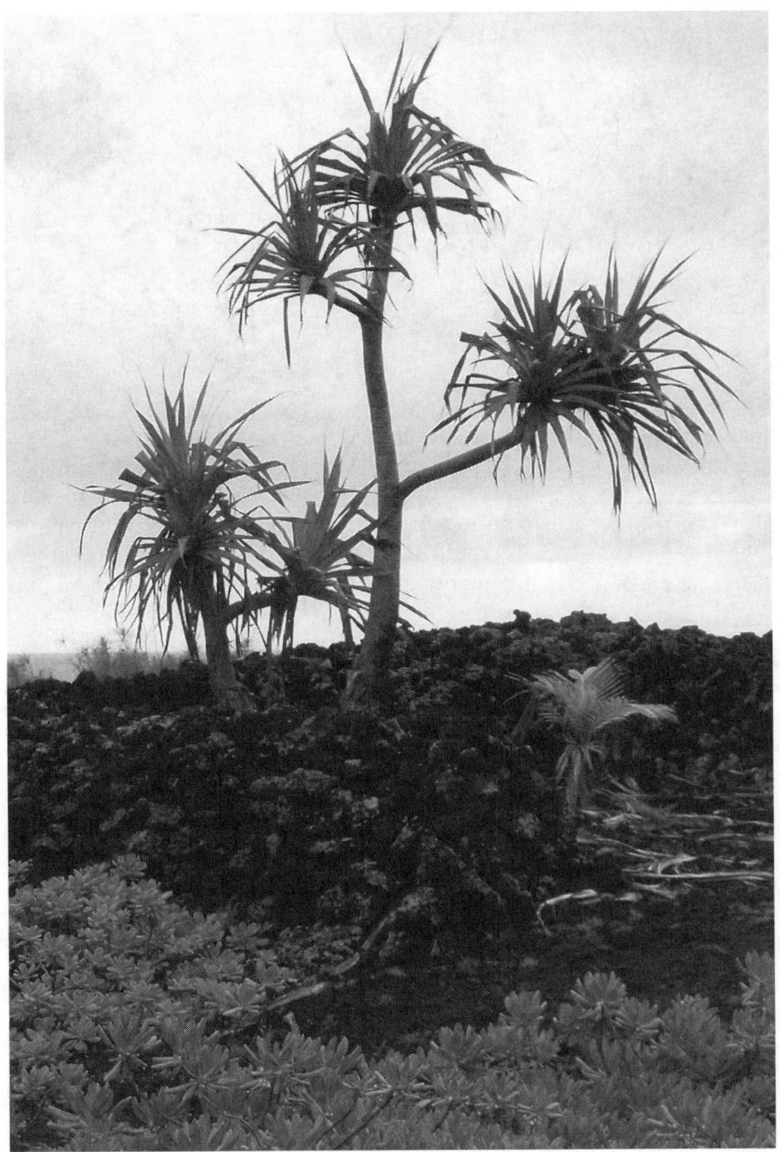

Native Hawaiian archaeological sites *are protected by Waianapanapa State Park.*

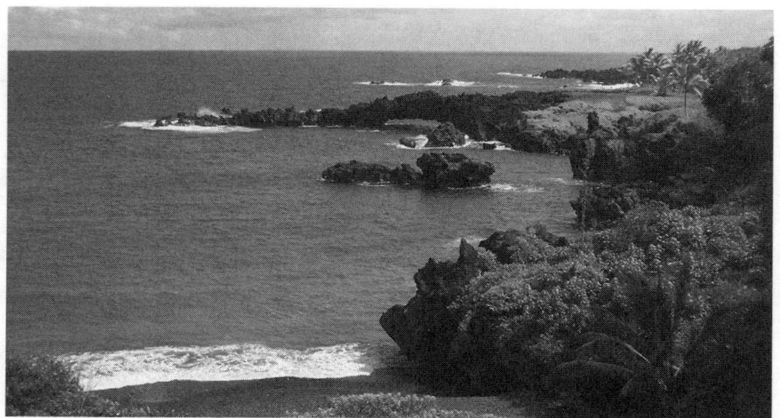

Hana daytrippers *detour for Pailoa Bay's dramatic black-sand beach.*

You'll spy a natural sea arch that experienced snorkelers can swim out to when ocean waters are calm.

lauhala weaving. A hiking pole or bamboo stick comes in handy here for knocking away any spiderwebs, especially if you're the first hiker here early in the morning. As the trail heads seaward to hug the coast again, look out at the ocean to spot another natural lava-rock arch. Uphill and off to your right, hidden by junglelike foliage, are the state park's rental housekeeping cabins (see page 16).

After about 0.6 mile, the trail crosses a footbridge, then turns to cinder as it heads out across dark-colored lava flows. Carefully follow the trail southbound across *aa* (rough, jagged) lava. You'll

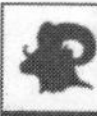

OPTIONS

Detour: Hana Lava Tube

If you're a caving fanatic, you'll want to explore one of Maui's largest known lava tube systems, about a mile north of Waianapanapa State Park. A self-guided tour of the privately owned **Hana Lava Tube** (open 10:30 AM to 4:30 PM daily) costs $12 per adult (children under 6 are free). For more information, visit www.mauicave.com or call (808) 248-7308. The entrance is on Ulaino Road, off Highway 360 just south of mile marker (MM) 31.

want to be wearing sturdy shoes with good traction and ankle support—flip-flops aren't useful here. About 0.9 mile from your starting point, the trail passes **Ohala Heiau**. ▶3 The remains of this small Hawaiian temple constructed of lava rocks are marked with a small interpretive plaque. Be careful not to disturb this sacred site or climb on it. From the temple, it's possible to continue hiking south all the way to Hana Bay (see Trip 23, page 187). This hike turns around at the temple, however. Retrace your steps for approximately 0.7 mile to the north parking lot.

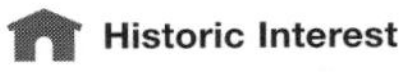

From the parking lot, it's a few minutes' walk north along a signposted paved path that descends to some **lava tube caves**. ▶4 The caves are draped with overhanging ferns and filled with cold, brackish water that nevertheless attract stout-hearted swimmers. On certain nights, usually during spring, the waters appear to flow red. Island legend attributes this to the spilled blood of a Hawaiian chieftess who was killed by her jealous husband. Scientists explain the phenomenon by a massing of tiny red-colored shrimp, called opae ula.

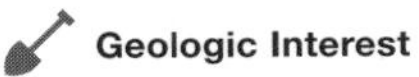

Continue walking counterclockwise around this short loop past the caves, climbing back up to the **north parking lot** ▶5 to finish this hike.

MILESTONES

▶1	0.0	Start from north parking lot [N 20.78876°, W 156.00459°]
▶2	0.1	Detour down to Pailoa Beach
▶3	0.9	Turn around at Ohala Heiau [N 20.78262°, W 155.99530°]
▶4	1.7	Arrive at lava tube caves
▶5	1.8	Return to north parking lot [N 20.78876°, W 156.00459°]

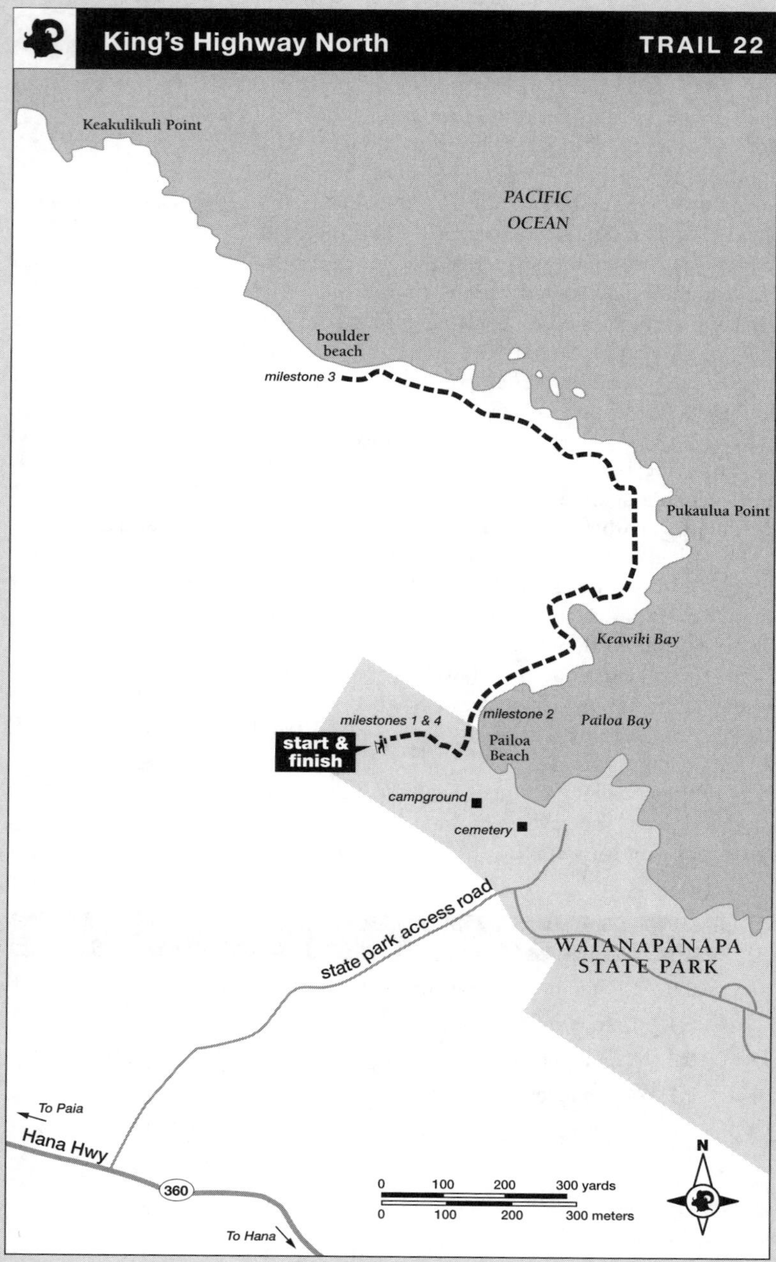
King's Highway North
TRAIL 22
Keakulikuli Point
PACIFIC OCEAN
boulder beach
milestone 3
Pukaulua Point
Keawiki Bay
milestones 1 & 4
milestone 2
Pailoa Bay
start & finish
Pailoa Beach
campground
cemetery
state park access road
WAIANAPANAPA STATE PARK
To Paia
Hana Hwy
360
To Hana
0 100 200 300 yards
0 100 200 300 meters
N

King's Highway North

Many visitors to Waianapanapa State Park walk only as far as the scenic black-sand beach. This hike tackles a section of the ancient King's Highway heading farther north along a wild, dramatic coastline flush with primal scenery. Wear shoes with good traction for walking over craggy lava flows.

TRAIL USE
Dayhike

LENGTH
1.8 miles, 1–1½ hours

VERTICAL FEET
±350′

DIFFICULTY
– 1 **2** 3 4 5 +

TRAIL TYPE
Out & Back

SURFACE TYPE
Dirt, Lava, Paved, Sand

START & END
N 20.78876°
W 156.00459°

FEATURES
Beach
Lava Flows
Birds
Native Plants
Tide Pools
Wildlife
Great Views
Historic Interest
Secluded

FACILITIES
Restrooms
Picnic Tables
Phone
Water

Best Time

You can visit Waianapanapa State Park year-round. Most Hana-bound daytrippers arrive around lunchtime or in the early afternoon, when the parking lots often fill. Early morning is best for solitude. Late afternoon just before sunset can be another good time to hike here, unless East Maui's persistent rain clouds have already rolled in by then.

Finding the Trail

From Paia, drive southeast on the Hana Highway (Hwy. 36) for about 19 miles. The roadside mile markers reset at zero where Highway 36 ends and Highway 360 (also called the Hana Highway) begins. Keep driving along Highway 360 for another 32 miles. Just south of mile marker (MM) 32, turn left onto the signposted state park access road and drive 0.5 mile *makai* (toward the ocean), watching out for speed bumps and blind hills. Turn left at the T-intersection inside the park and continue driving 0.2 mile to the paved parking lot north of the campground. Coming from the center of Hana town, drive north on Highway 360 for a little more than 2 miles, then turn right *(makai)* before MM 32.

Trail Description

Start hiking from the *makai* (ocean) side of the state park's **north parking lot** ►1. Walk toward the shoreline, veering right along a paved trail. Almost immediately the trail affords panoramic views of the coast, including a tantalizing black-sand beach downhill off to your left. The clifftop railing here is itself a prime sunrise-watching spot, although not as spectacular as other perches farther north along the trail.

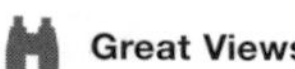

At the signposted trail junction, turn left and make your way down the spur trail to **Pailoa Beach**, ►2 about 0.1 mile from your starting point. This crescent-shaped beach may not be much bigger than a cove, but it's startlingly beautiful. Jet-black cinder sands reach out into azure waters capped by high frothy surf with a backdrop of jungly green foliage atop the lava flows surrounding the bay. Swimmers should be cautious of strong currents and only enter the water when conditions are reasonably calm.

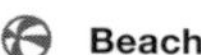

Jet-black cinder sands reach out into azure waters capped by high frothy surf with a backdrop of jungly green foliage.

Walk northeast across the sands to the far side of Pailoa Beach. Follow the faint trail that climbs up onto the lava-rock cliffs, pushing aside hala trees and twisted vines of beach naupaka, whose small white flowers look as if they've been torn in half. Atop the cliff, the trail winds over jagged *aa* lava and then quickly descends to the cove at Keawiki Bay, littered more with stones and lava rocks than soft, cindery sand.

Keep going across this small second cove and continue on the trail, which ascends onto rough, clinkered *aa* lava flows. From here, you trace a section of the King's Highway, a lava road built by ancient Hawaiians that once encircled Maui, allowing chiefs to travel around their domains. Today, only a few fragments of this historic island route can still be traveled by casual hikers (see also Trail 23, page 187).

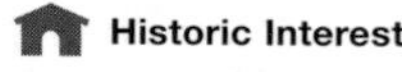

Watch your footing carefully as the trail twists through the lava, sometimes growing indistinct. Look for *ahu* (stone cairns) pointing out the true trail, which generally stays inland away from the coastal lava-rock blowholes and steep gullies. Ignore false spur trails leading *makai* (toward the ocean) and stay left at major trail junctions, heading generally northwest. After laboriously dipping into and out of a couple of gullies, you arrive at a **boulder beach**, ►3 made up of giant gray rocks polished by the tides. You're now almost 1 mile from the trailhead, although it might seem like you've hiked much farther because of the terrain's ruggedness.

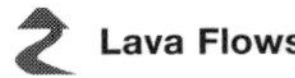

From here, the trail continues farther north along the coast, ending at the boundary fence of Hana's small commuter airport. But there is not much reward in hiking any farther up the coast, since the scenery is almost identical to what you've already seen and the trail becomes even harder to follow. Instead, turn around at the boulder beach. From there, retrace your steps back to Keawiki Bay and black-sand Pailoa Beach, ascending the trail on the latter's south side and turning right to return the **north parking lot**. ►4

To hike more of the historic King's Highway, South Maui's Hoapili Trail starts from La Pérouse Bay and traverses Haleakala's lava flows **(see page 143).**

MILESTONES

►1	0.0	Start from north parking lot [N 20.78876°, W 156.00459°]
►2	0.1	Head downhill to Pailoa Beach
►3	0.9	Turn around at boulder beach [N 20.79362°, W 156.00548°]
►4	1.8	Return to north parking lot [N 20.78876°, W 156.00459°]

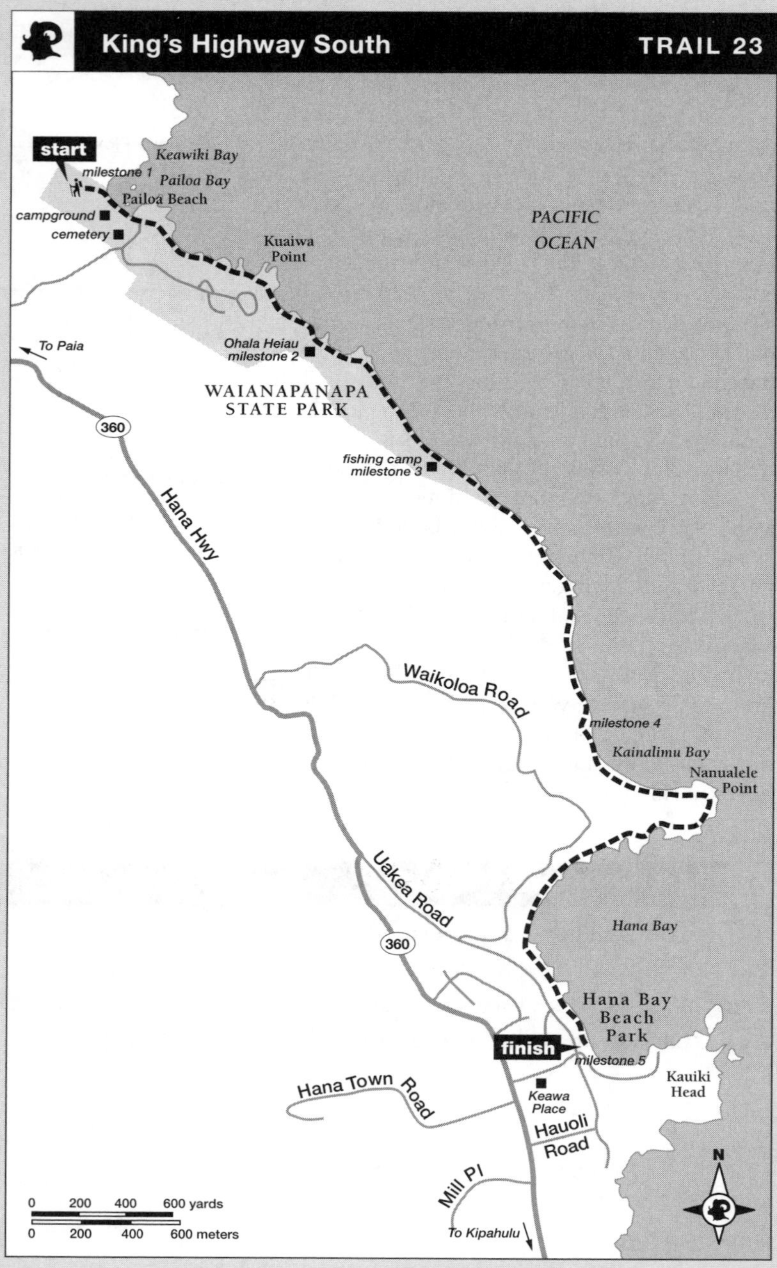
King's Highway South
TRAIL 23
start
Keawiki Bay
milestone 1
Pailoa Bay
Pailoa Beach
campground
cemetery
Kuaiwa Point
PACIFIC OCEAN
To Paia
Ohala Heiau milestone 2
WAIANAPANAPA STATE PARK
360
fishing camp milestone 3
Hana Hwy
Waikoloa Road
milestone 4
Kainalimu Bay
Nanualele Point
Uakea Road
Hana Bay
360
Hana Bay Beach Park
finish
milestone 5
Kauiki Head
Hana Town Road
Keawa Place
Hauoli Road
N
Mill Pl
0 200 400 600 yards
0 200 400 600 meters
To Kipahulu

King's Highway South

A whopper of a coastal walk, this challenging hike mostly follows a historic Hawaiian footpath along a rocky shoreline, peppered with lava flows and boulder beaches. To make it all the way from Waianapanapa State Park to picturesque Hana Bay, wear hiking boots with good traction and ankle support.

TRAIL USE
Dayhike

LENGTH
3.7 miles, 2–2½ hours

VERTICAL FEET
±250′

DIFFICULTY
– 1 2 **3** 4 5 +

TRAIL TYPE
Point-to-Point

SURFACE TYPE
Dirt, Lava, Paved, Sand

START
N 20.78876°
W 156.00459°

END
N 20.75602°
W 155.98466°

FEATURES
Beach
Lava Flows
Birds
Native Plants
Tide Pools
Wildlife
Great Views
Historic Interest
Archaeological
Secluded

FACILITIES
Restrooms
Picnic Tables
Phone
Water

Best Time

You can visit Waianapanapa State Park year-round. Most Hana-bound daytrippers arrive around lunchtime or in the early afternoon, when the parking lots often fill. Make sure you give yourself enough time to finish the entire hike, so that you arrive in Hana (or back at Waianapanapa State Park, if you're hiking round-trip) before sunset. Take a look at local tide charts—the southern section of this hike may be impassable at high tide.

Finding the Trail

From Paia, drive southeast on the Hana Highway (Hwy. 36) for about 19 miles. The roadside mile markers reset at zero where Highway 36 ends and Highway 360 (also called the Hana Highway) begins. Keep driving along Highway 360 for another 32 miles. Just south of mile marker (MM) 32, turn left onto the signposted state park access road and drive 0.5 mile *makai* (toward the ocean), watching out for speed bumps and blind hills. Turn left at the T-intersection inside the park and continue driving 0.2 mile to the paved parking lot just north of the campground. Coming from the center of Hana town, drive north on Highway 360 for a little more than 2 miles, then turn right *(makai)* before MM 32.

Because this is a point-to-point hike, you'll need to arrange a shuttle pick-up from the south end of the trail at Hana Bay. Alternatively, you can walk back to the state park's trailhead by retracing your steps all the way along the coastal trail or by cautiously walking on the shoulder of the paved highway north, either of which will double your total distance.

Trail Description

Start your hike on the *makai* (ocean) side of the state park's **north parking lot**. ►1 Facing the water, follow the paved path that veers off to your right. Almost immediately a signposted junction appears, where black-sand Pailoa Beach is visible downhill to your left. The views of Hana's wild, undeveloped coast don't get much better than at the railing right here, with green foliage creeping atop jet-black lava flows and deep aquamarine waters powdered by white-capped surf. To take the side trail down to Pailoa Beach and follow the King's Highway north along the coast of Waianapanapa State Park, see Trail 22, page 183.

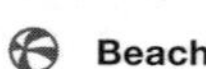

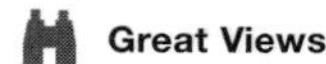

To follow the King's Highway south, this trip turns right at the junction. The trail, which alternates between paved and gravel sections, roughly parallels the shoreline. You pass a grassy camping and picnicking area on the right, as well as a small cemetery. To the left, look out for a natural lava-rock blowhole. As the warning signs advise, keep back a safe distance from the blowhole. Sometimes it's a dramatic sight as surf blasts dozens of feet into the air, while at other times, there's little or no action to be seen. After passing the blowhole, the trail ducks inland beside some hala (screwpine, or pandanus)

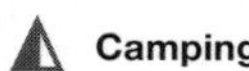

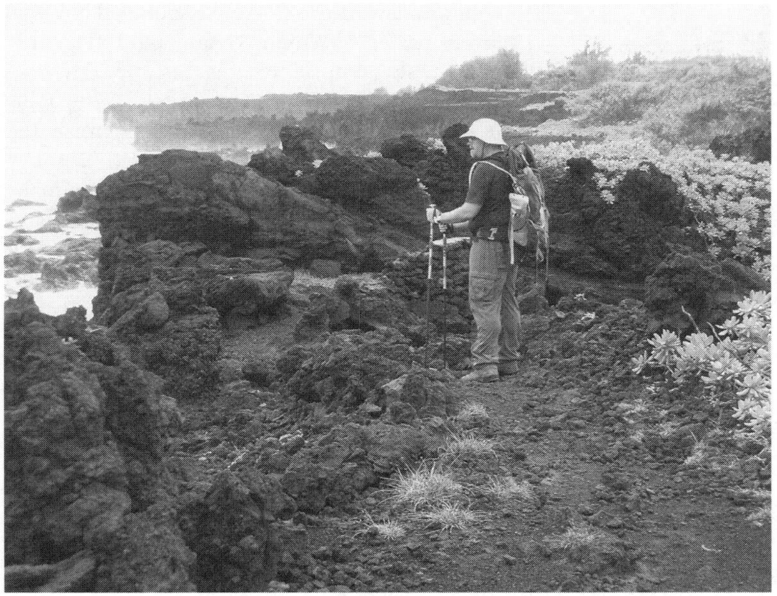

This rocky route *traces an ancient Hawaiian footpath beside dramatic surf.*

trees, then returns toward the coast. Uphill to your right, hidden by natural landscaping, are the state park's rental cabins (see page 16).

About 0.6 mile from your starting point, the trail passes over a footbridge, then becomes more cindery and strikes out across jagged *aa* lava flows. Shoes with good traction and thick soles are necessary here; flip-flops just won't cut it. The trail now follows the historic King's Highway, an ancient Hawaiian lava road that once stretched around Maui's entire 120-mile shoreline. The road allowed *alii* (royalty) to travel overland to visit their subjects, notably during the annual fall harvest festival, called the Makahiki, when taxes were collected from *makaaina* (commoners). Today, the King's Highway exists only in fragments, making this one of only a few opportunities to follow the historic route.

To explore more of the King's Highway, South Maui's Hoapili Trail traverses Haleakala's most recent lava flows (see page 143).

Great Views

Lava Flows

Native Plants

After a few minutes' walk south, the King's Highway passes by **Ohala Heiau**. ▶2 Today, only the lava-rock platform of this historic Hawaiian *heiau* (temple) remains. Be careful not to disturb this sacred site or climb upon it. Beyond the temple, the trail clambers up and down over rough, crunchy fields of *aa* lava, where rolling rocks underfoot make it necessary to plant your feet carefully. Beach naupaka vines, whose small white flowers that look as if they've been torn in half, are some of the lone plant colonists glimpsed on these lava flows.

A little more than 1 mile from your starting point, the trail passes along cliffs by a locals' **fishing camp**, ▶3 where a private shack is labeled FISHING HALE. A small wooden trail sign just beyond the camp incorrectly gives the distance to Hana as 2 miles; it's actually closer to 3 miles. Shaggy ironwood trees with their drooping needles overhang the lava flows as the trail laboriously continues picking its way up and down along the coast, always trending south. Ignore any confusing use trails or side roads leading inland. Helpful rock cairns and smooth stones set in the *aa* and *pahoehoe* (smooth) lava fields keep you on the right path.

About 2 miles from your starting point, the trail descends to **Kainalimu Bay**. ▶4 Here the wide crescent beach is made up almost entirely of large boulders, which take time to pick your way across. Because this beach runs adjacent to private property, watch out for unleashed guard dogs that may run out onto the beach, barking to announce your presence and looking fearsome. If you decide to turn around here, it's a gorgeous hike north along the coast back to Waianapanapa State Park.

Otherwise, scramble up onto the shoreline cliffs on the south side of Kainalimu Bay and keep following the King's Highway southbound. At the next cove south comes your first glimpse of Hana Bay, which will hopefully provide inspiration for all

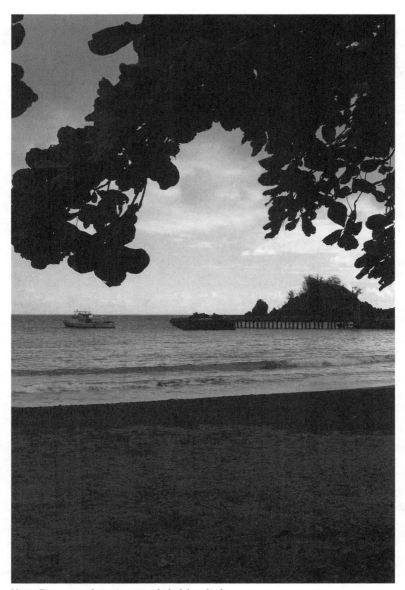

Hana Bay *is one of Maui's quietest little fishing harbors.*

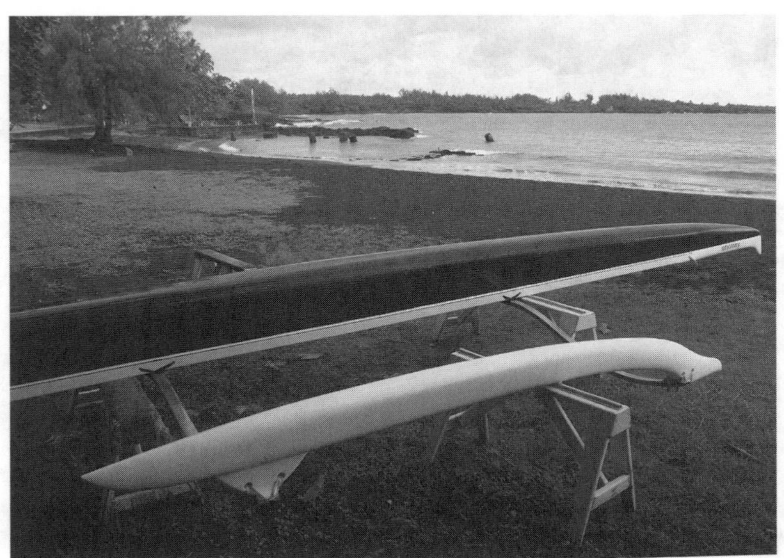

Many water sports, *including outrigger canoeing, are practiced at Hana Bay Beach Park.*

Caution

Beach

the lava-rock outcroppings and tide pools you soon have to hop across. There isn't much, if anything, left of the historic King's Highway by now—negotiate your own coastal path. At high tide, you may have to wade or swim short sections of the route. If you can, time your trip so that you traverse this last part of the hike at low tide.

Approximately 3.5 miles from your starting point, you reach the last lava-rock outcropping separating you from **Hana Bay Beach Park,** ►**5** just south. (If you'd rather not scale the outcropping, you can walk up the stairs and through the parking lot of the vacation-rental complex directly above you, then turn left onto paved Uakea Road and walk 0.3 mile downhill to reach Hana Bay.) The county beach park has picnic tables, barbecue grills, outdoor showers, restrooms, a pay phone, and a snack bar serving burgers, plate lunches, and shave ice.

Hana Bay is a popular spot for fishing, surfing, and outrigger canoeing, but swimmers should beware of strong currents.

If you haven't arranged for a shuttle ride to pick you up at Hana Bay, you have two choices, either of which will double your total hiking distance to almost 8 miles. Your first option is to retrace your steps along the coastal hiking trail all the way back to Waianapanapa State Park. Alternatively, walk uphill from Hana Bay Beach Park along Uakea Road for almost a mile to the Y-intersection with the Hana Highway (Hwy. 360), then turn right and walk another 2.5 miles north along the narrow shoulder of this treacherously winding highway. Pedestrian safety is a concern here, especially after dark. Still, it's a less exhausting return trip than doubling back on the coastal trail.

Kauiki Head overlooks Hana Bay. On the south side of this eroded cinder cone lies hidden red-sand Kaihalulu Beach.

MILESTONES

►1	0.0	Start from north parking lot [N 20.78876°, W 156.00459°]
►2	0.7	Arrive at Ohala Heiau [N 20.78262°, W 155.99530°]
►3	1.1	Pass by fishing camp [N 20.77840°, W 155.99089°]
►4	2.0	Reach Kainalimu Bay [N 20.76816°, W 155.98468°]
►5	3.7	Finish at Hana Bay Beach Park [N 20.75602°, W 155.98466°]

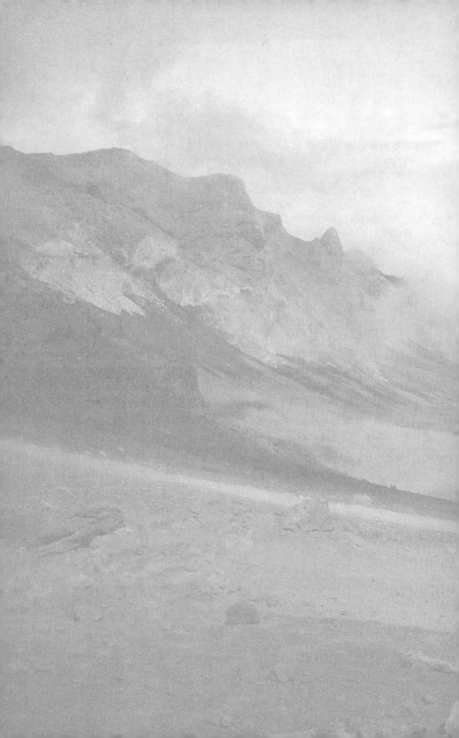

CHAPTER 4

Haleakala National Park

24. Hosmer Grove
25. Halemauu Trail to Holua
26. Halemauu Trail & Silversword Loop
27. Halemauu Trail to Paliku
28. Sliding Sands Trail to Ka Luu o ka Oo
29. Sliding Sands Trail to Kapalaoa
30. Sliding Sands Trail & Cinder Desert Loop
31. Sliding Sands Trail to Paliku
32. Sliding Sands & Halemauu Trails
33. Haleakala Grand Loop
34. Kaupo Gap
35. Skyline Trail
36. Kuloa Point Trail
37. Pipiwai Trail

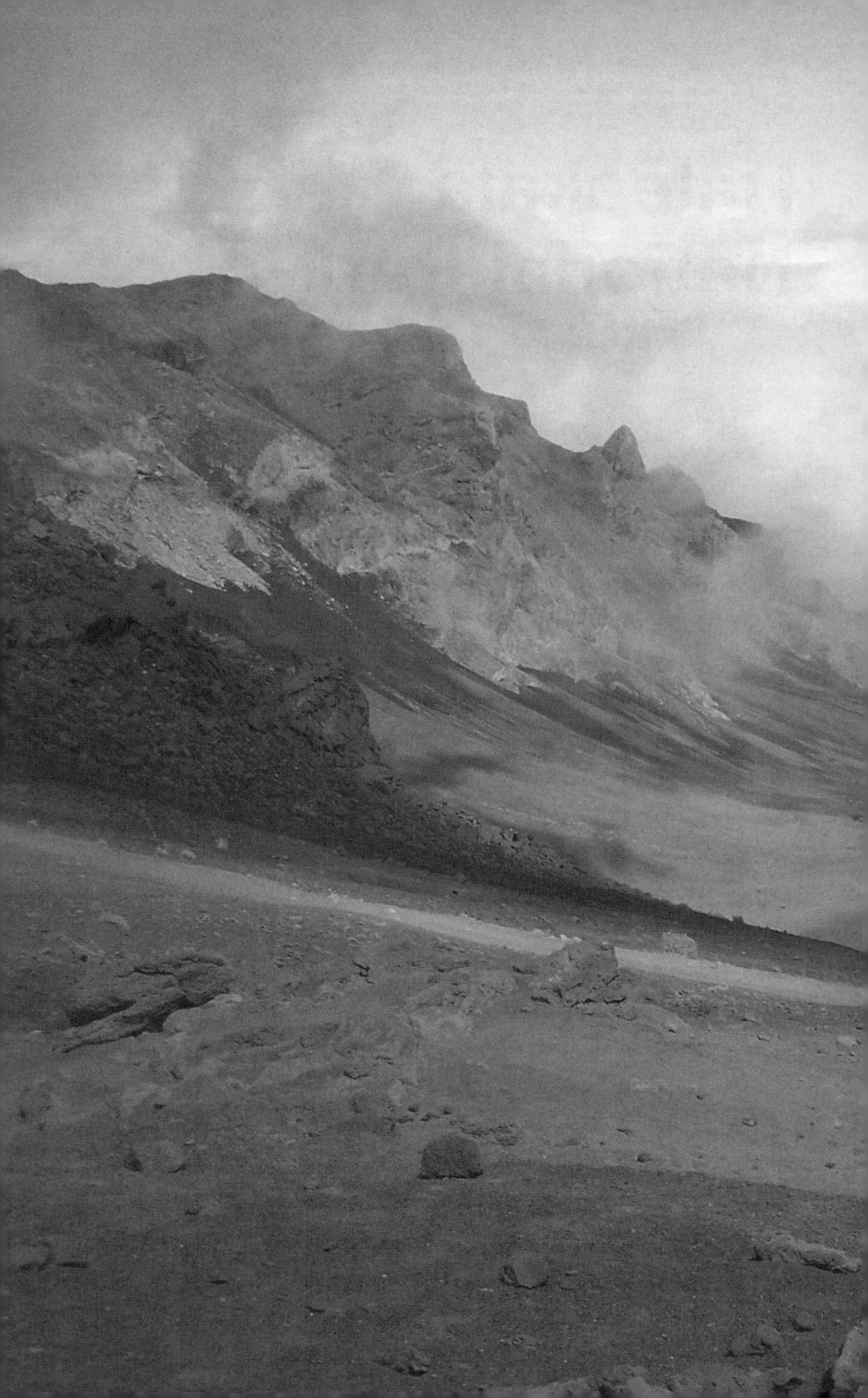

Haleakala National Park

Maui's premier hiking destination, **Haleakala National Park** dominates the landscape. The park's namesake volcano forms the eastern part of the island, sprawling from sea level to a summit elevation of 10,023 feet. The winding drive up from the coast to the summit is epic—in fact, it's the biggest elevation gain over the shortest distance of any road on earth. You'll see Ironman triathletes in training cycling uphill, as well as tourists cruising downhill on mountain bikes just after sunrise. The biggest crowds of park visitors gather at the volcano's summit just before dawn. Stepping onto almost any of the nearby hiking trails will engulf you in solitude and serenity. There are plenty of dayhikes around the summit region and down into the volcano itself. Come prepared for all kinds of weather and steep climbs at breathtakingly high altitudes. For backpackers, the park's historic wilderness cabins make overnight trip logistics easier.

In the park's **summit area**, the incredible volcanic landscape is composed of colorful cinder cones, dramatic volcanic vents and lava tubes, a cloud forest, and arid lava flows. What many people call Haleakala's "crater" is not actually a crater (those are only formed by volcanic explosions, scientifically speaking). What sits atop Haleakala is an erosional valley, cut slowly by ancient streams that once flowed from the summit to the sea through what is now the Koolau and Kaupo gaps. These two gaps are breaks in the volcano's walls that allow clouds to move through, creating changeable weather patterns, but also granting unmatched sunrise views. At first glance the volcano's summit area may look barren, but its unique ecosystem protects some of the most rare and endangered species in all of the Hawaiian Islands. Among the iconic flora and fauna found here are shiny-leafed silversword plants, which may live for up to a half century but only bloom once in a lifetime, and the endangered nene (Hawaiian goose). After almost going extinct, nene were reintroduced into the national park in 1962 when Boy Scouts carried geese that had been raised in captivity down into Haleakala volcano in their backpacks.

Overleaf and opposite: *Misty clouds overhang the lava rocks and cinder deserts of Haleakala's volcano summit.*

Full of geologic marvels and unique flora and fauna, the park's summit area tells only part of the story, however. Near the ocean at the bottom of the volcano's southern slopes lies the park's **Kipahulu area**. Famous for its waterfalls and the pools of Oheo Gulch, this coastal area of the park covers a remote section of Maui's south coastline. Note there is no road (or public access hiking trail) connecting the two areas of the park. To get to Kipahulu, first drive the scenic Road to Hana, a narrow, twisting piece of pavement that crosses 54 one-lane bridges as it winds slowly from the surf town of Paia down Maui's windward coast (see Chapter 3: East Maui & Upcountry, page 149). Beyond the rural town of Hana, it's another 10 miles of slow, winding highway driving passing more roadside waterfalls and blissful beaches, south to Kipahulu. Once you enter the national park's coastal area, you can follow a short nature loop leading to the idyllic waterfall pools of Oheo Gulch or climb uphill through a musical-sounding bamboo forest to view even more impressive falls.

Fees, Passes, Permits & Maps

At press time, entry to Haleakala National Park (808-572-4400, www.nps.gov/hale) cost $10 per vehicle ($5 for each motorcycle, cyclist, or pedestrian). This entrance pass is valid for three consecutive days in both the summit and coastal sections of the park, so hang on to your receipt. For multiple visits, a Hawaii Tri-Park Annual Pass costs $25 and allows free entry for 12 months from the date of purchase at Haleakala National Park, as well as Hawaii Volcanoes National Park and Puu Honua O Honaunau National Historical Park on the Big Island of Hawaii. If you're a frequent national parks visitor in Hawaii and on the U.S. mainland, an "America the Beautiful" annual pass costs $80 and allows unlimited access to all national parks and most federal recreational lands for one year; for U.S. citizens and permanent residents aged 62 or older, a lifetime Senior Pass costs $10, while a lifetime Access Pass for those with a permanent disability is free.

No permits are required for dayhiking in either the summit or coastal areas of the national park. Wilderness permits are required for all backpacking trips and any overnight stays at the wilderness cabins inside the volcano summit area. Overnight backpacking trips are prohibited in the coastal Kipahulu area of the park. Both the summit and coastal areas of the national park provide free dispersed drive-up camping areas. See page 15 for details about drive-up and backcountry camping and cabins in the park, including wilderness permits, fees, and reservations.

All but two of the trails described in this chapter are clearly outlined on the basic national park map brochure, freely available at national park entrance stations and visitor centers. For the Kaupo Trail or Skyline

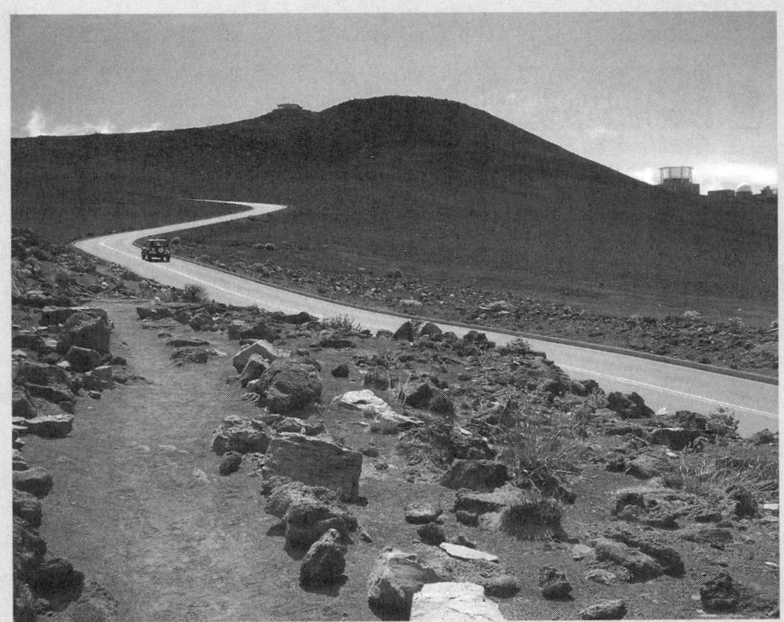

Winding Crater Road *leads up to the Haleakala's summit and Science City observatories.*

Trail, a topographic map will come in handy for determining distances and following the trails, which may be confusingly labeled and perhaps partly overgrown. National Geographic publishes *Haleakala National Park* ($11.95), a map scaled at 1:25,000 with a UTM grid for use with handheld GPS units. This waterproof, tear-resistant map (last updated in 2000) covers the entire national park from summit to sea. It may be sold at national park visitor centers, as well as at bigger bookstores elsewhere around the island (see page 312).

See Appendix 3 (page 312) for more recommended topographical and driving maps, both digital and printed, to help you navigate around Maui.

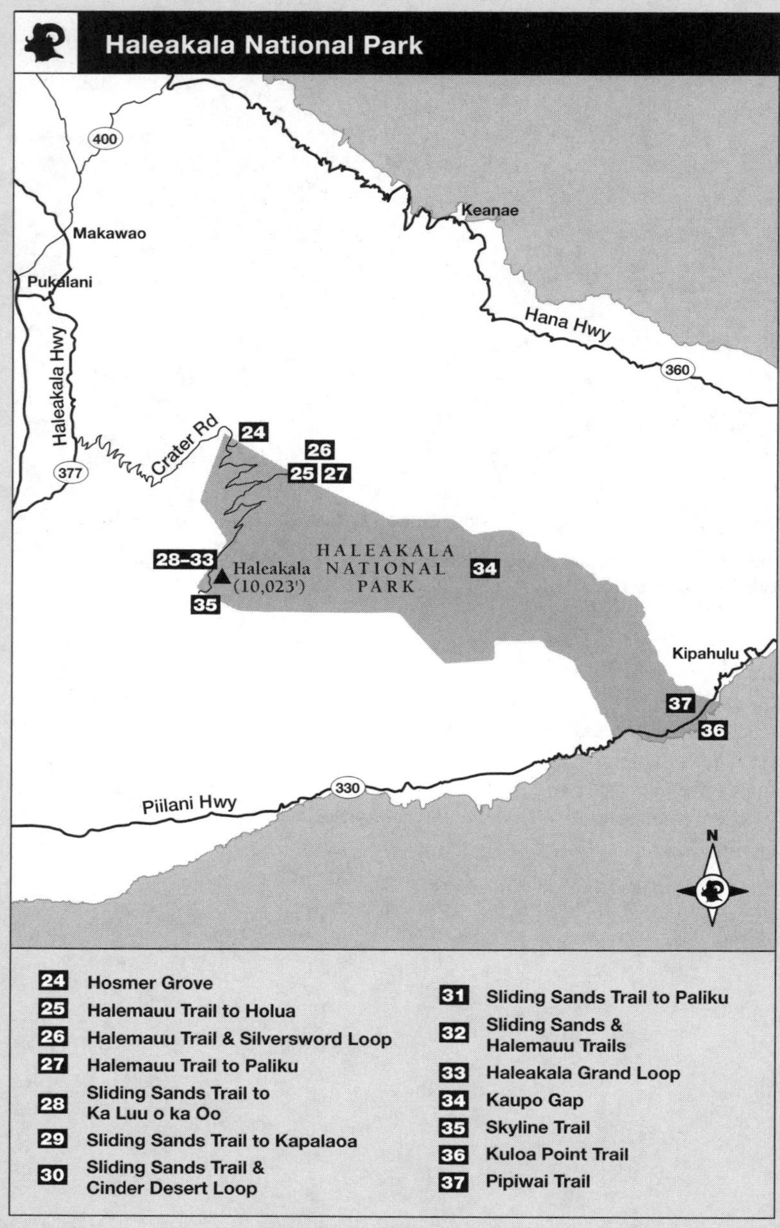
Haleakala National Park
400
Keanae
Makawao
Pukalani
Hana Hwy
360
Haleakala Hwy
Crater Rd
377
24
26
25
27
HALEAKALA
NATIONAL
PARK
28–33
Haleakala
(10,023')
34
35
Kipahulu
37
36
330
Piilani Hwy
N
24 Hosmer Grove
25 Halemauu Trail to Holua
26 Halemauu Trail & Silversword Loop
27 Halemauu Trail to Paliku
28 Sliding Sands Trail to Ka Luu o ka Oo
29 Sliding Sands Trail to Kapalaoa
30 Sliding Sands Trail & Cinder Desert Loop
31 Sliding Sands Trail to Paliku
32 Sliding Sands & Halemauu Trails
33 Haleakala Grand Loop
34 Kaupo Gap
35 Skyline Trail
36 Kuloa Point Trail
37 Pipiwai Trail

Haleakala National Park

TRAIL	Difficulty	Length	Type	USES & ACCESS	TERRAIN	FLORA & FAUNA	OTHER
24	1	0.5	Loop	Dayhiking, Child Friendly	Forest, Mountain, Stream	Birds, Native Plants, Wildlife	Camping, Shady
25	5	8.0	Out & Back	Dayhiking, Backpacking, Running	Forest, Lava Flow, Mountain	Birds, Native Plants, Wildlife	Great Views, Camping, Geologic Interest, Historic Interest, Steep
26	5	10.8	Semiloop	Dayhiking, Backpacking, Running	Forest, Lava Flow, Mountain	Birds, Native Plants, Wildlife	Great Views, Camping, Geologic Interest, Historic Interest, Steep
27	5	21.0	Out & Back	Backpacking, Permit Required	Forest, Lava Flow, Mountain	Birds, Native Plants, Wildlife	Great Views, Camping, Geologic Interest, Historic Interest, Archaeological, Secluded, Steep
28	3	5.0	Semiloop	Dayhiking	Lava Flow, Mountain	Birds, Native Plants, Wildlife	Great Views, Geologic Interest, Steep
29	5	11.8	Out & Back	Dayhiking, Backpacking	Lava Flow, Mountain	Birds, Native Plants, Wildlife	Great Views, Geologic Interest, Historic Interest, Steep
30	5	13.6	Semiloop	Dayhiking, Backpacking	Lava Flow, Mountain	Birds, Native Plants, Wildlife	Great Views, Geologic Interest, Historic Interest, Archaeological, Steep
31	5	18.4	Out & Back	Backpacking, Permit Required	Lava Flow, Mountain	Birds, Native Plants, Wildlife	Great Views, Geologic Interest, Historic Interest, Secluded, Steep
32	5	11.8	Point-to-Point	Dayhiking, Backpacking, Running	Forest, Lava Flow, Mountain	Birds, Native Plants, Wildlife	Great Views, Camping, Geologic Interest, Historic Interest, Steep
33	5	20.9	Point-to-Point	Backpacking, Permit Required	Forest, Lava Flow, Mountain	Birds, Native Plants, Wildlife	Great Views, Camping, Geologic Interest, Historic Interest, Archaeological, Secluded, Steep
34	5	7.2	Point-to-Point	Dayhiking, Backpacking	Forest, Lava Flow, Mountain	Birds, Native Plants, Wildlife	Great Views, Camping, Geologic Interest, Historic Interest, Archaeological, Secluded, Steep
35	5	10.5	Point-to-Point	Dayhiking, Backpacking, Biking	Forest, Lava Flow, Mountain, Summit	Birds, Native Plants, Wildlife	Great Views, Camping, Geologic Interest, Secluded, Shady, Steep
36	1	0.5	Loop	Dayhiking, Child Friendly	Stream, Waterfall	Birds, Native Plants, Wildlife	Great Views, Swimming, Archaeological
37	3	4.0	Out & Back	Dayhiking, Running, Child Friendly	Forest, Stream, Waterfall	Birds, Native Plants, Wildlife	Great Views, Shady

USES & ACCESS
- Dayhiking
- Backpacking
- Running
- Biking
- Wheelchair Access
- Child Friendly
- Dogs Allowed
- Permit Required

TYPE
- Loop
- Out & Back
- Semiloop
- Point-to-Point

DIFFICULTY
- 1 2 3 4 5 +
less more

TERRAIN
- Beach
- Forest
- Lava Flow
- Mountain
- Pond
- Summit
- Stream
- Waterfall

FLORA & FAUNA
- Birds
- Native Plants
- Tide Pools
- Wildlife

FEATURES
- Great Views
- Swimming
- Camping
- Geologic Interest
- Historic Interest
- Archaeological
- Secluded
- Shady
- Steep

Haleakala National Park

Halemauu Trail to Paliku 225

Trek from the volcano's rim down past Holua cabin and across a multicolored cinder desert to emerge in the misty rain shadow of the volcano's windward side. Linger overnight in Paliku's peaceful meadows, tucked underneath towering cliffs.

TRAIL 27

Backpack,
Permit Required
21.0 miles, Out & Back
Difficulty: 1 2 3 4 **5**

Sliding Sands Trail to Ka Luu o ka Oo 233

For a sampling of Haleakala's grandeur, follow the soft cinder switchbacks partway down from the summit toward the volcano floor, then detour around a magnificent cinder cone before huffing and puffing back up this steep—and aptly named—trail.

TRAIL 28

Dayhike
5.0 miles, Semiloop
Difficulty: 1 2 **3** 4 5

Sliding Sands Trail to Kapalaoa 239

Descend on switchbacks among the colorful giant cinder cones in Haleakala's literally breathtaking summit area. Then strike out across jet-black lava flows to Kapalaoa's historic wilderness cabin, where endangered nene (Hawaiian geese) often hang out.

TRAIL 29

Dayhike, Backpack
11.8 miles, Out & Back
Difficulty: 1 2 3 4 **5**

Sliding Sands Trail & Cinder Desert Loop 245

Follow the crowds down the popular Sliding Sands Trail, then detour onto untrammeled paths past cinder cones, volcanic vents, and an ancient Hawaiian archaeological site. This adventurous volcano summit dayhike doesn't require shuttling cars or hitchhiking.

TRAIL 30

Dayhike, Backpack
13.6 miles, Semiloop
Difficulty: 1 2 3 4 **5**

Skyline Trail 287

Trek from near the summit down the volcano's back side, starting in a wonderland of cinder cones, then dropping through Maui's misty cloud-forest belt. This challenging one-way hike finishes inside remote, little-visited Polipoli Spring State Recreation Area.

TRAIL 35

Dayhike, Backpack, Bike
10.5 miles, Point-to-Point
Difficulty: 1 2 3 4 **5**

Kuloa Point Trail 295

Beyond Maui's famous Road to Hana lies the coastal Kipahulu area of Haleakala National Park. Swimming is popular in the famous waterfall pools of Oheo Gulch, which tumble down a natural staircase of lava rocks to the sea. Beware of flash floods.

TRAIL 36

Dayhike, Child Friendly
0.5 mile, Loop
Difficulty: **1** 2 3 4 5

Pipiwai Trail 301

In Haleakala National Park's coastal Kipahulu area, this family-friendly jungle path climbs past waterfall lookouts through a bamboo forest where trees rustle musically in the wind. Swimming is not safe anywhere along this route—fatalities have occurred.

TRAIL 37

Dayhike, Run, Child Friendly
4.0 miles, Out & Back
Difficulty: 1 2 **3** 4 5

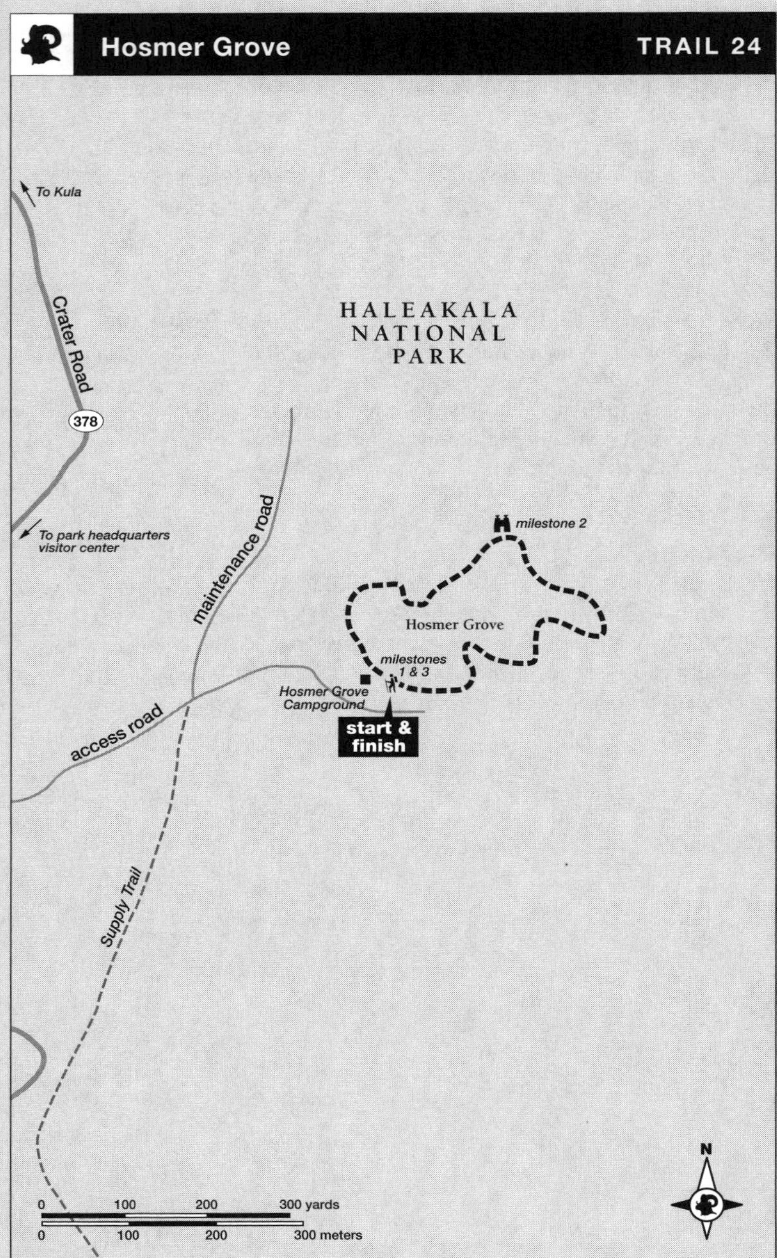
Hosmer Grove
TRAIL 24
To Kula
Crater Road
378
To park headquarters
visitor center
HALEAKALA
NATIONAL
PARK
maintenance road
milestone 2
Hosmer Grove
milestones
1 & 3
Hosmer Grove
Campground
start &
finish
access road
Supply Trail
0
100
200
300 yards
0
100
200
300 meters
N

Hosmer Grove

In the cloud forest below Haleakala volcano's summit, this child-friendly nature trail is practically an outdoor botanical classroom. Bring rain gear and binoculars for bird-watching. Also give yourself time to acclimate (e.g., start off walking slowly) if you've driven up the volcano directly from the coast.

TRAIL USE
Dayhike, Child Friendly

LENGTH
0.5 mile, 15–30 mins.

VERTICAL FEET
±200′

DIFFICULTY
– **1** 2 3 4 5 +

TRAIL TYPE
Loop

SURFACE TYPE
Dirt, Grass, Lava

START & END
N 20.76843°
W 156.23801°

FEATURES
Forest
Mountain
Stream
Birds
Native Plants
Wildlife
Camping
Shady

FACILITIES
Restrooms
Picnic Tables
Water

Best Time

You can hike this trail any time of year. Early morning is the best time for bird-watching. Daytime highs range from 50°F to 65°F year-round, but winter experiences more rainstorms and cooler temperatures. Bring a rainproof jacket and a warm hat, as this often muddy trail is thickly forested and the weather is notoriously changeable at this elevation.

Finding the Trail

From Kahului, follow the Hana Highway (Hwy. 36) southeast past the airport turnoff, then turn right onto the Haleakala Highway (Hwy. 37). Drive uphill for almost 8 miles, then turn left, continuing on the Haleakala Highway (Hwy. 377). Drive about 6 more miles uphill toward Kula, turning left on Hwy. 378, which becomes Crater Road. Continue for a little more than 10 winding, slow-moving miles uphill through open range for grazing livestock to the park's entrance station. Just 0.1 mile past the entrance, turn left onto the Hosmer Grove access road and drive 0.5 mile to the campground's paved parking lot.

Trail Description

Less than a mile uphill from the summit area entrance station, the park headquarters visitor center (open 6:30 AM to 4 PM daily) has educational nature displays.

At an elevation of almost 8000 feet above sea level, Hosmer Grove sits in Maui's cloud-forest belt, which encircles the upper slopes of Haleakala volcano like the rings of Saturn. The weather here is quite unpredictable, with rain showers always a possibility, especially later in the afternoon. High annual rainfall makes the forest cover thick, and both native and exotic botanical species thrive here. Shady Hosmer Grove comes alive with birdsong, especially just after sunrise. Colorful native honeycreepers and other birds can often be glimpsed right alongside this nature trail.

To find the trailhead, walk downhill from the parking lot shelter, which has informational signboards, toward **Hosmer Grove Campground**. ▶1 (For details about the park's free dispersed camping here, see page 15). There you'll also find picnic tables and potable water spigots. Look for the signposted trailhead off to your right, on the east side of the camping area. Start walking along the trail toward the forest. Almost immediately you cross a wooden bridge over a small stream, which may or may not be flowing, depending on recent rains.

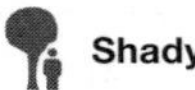

The trail quickly dives under the cover of an experimental forest, originally planted in the early 20th century by the Territory of Hawaii's first forester, Ralph Hosmer. Hosmer was curious about which exotic species could survive on Maui and eventually support a local timber industry. Most species he imported did not take root, but some thrived so well that today they are considered invasive (for example, rainbow-barked eucalyptus trees). Filling out the forest are a variety of cedar, spruce, and pine species, some of which are labeled along the trail. But it's not all exotic species along this gentle forest path. You also pass native Hawaiian foliage, such as shrubby ohia lehua, with its easily recognized red pom-pom blossoms; pukiawe, showing white

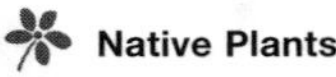

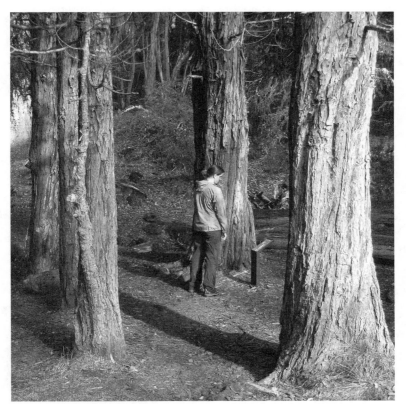

Experimental Hosmer Grove *grows thick with native and exotic arboreal species.*

five-pointed star-shaped flowers; akala (Hawaiian raspberry) plants; and mamane, an endemic hardwood tree with pale yellow flowers.

The grove's nature trail ambles gently up, down, and across a pine needle–carpeted forest floor before emerging back into the sunlight at a small clearing and **overlook**, ▶2 about 0.2 mile from the trailhead. Take a break by the railings here. With some patience (a pair of binoculars is also helpful), you are likely to spot quite a few species of native birds flitting among the trees down in the gully. Commonly

Birds

On select evenings between May and September, Hosmer Grove hosts guided stargazing and Hawaiian storytelling programs; call (808) 572-4400 for current schedules. Bring a flashlight, warm clothes, and a blanket.

seen species include crimson-colored apapane and also iiwi, another bright red-colored bird with a signature orange bill. Both birds are endemic species of Hawaiian honeycreeper, a diverse group that has evolved spectacularly in the islands through adaptive radiation.

The trail by now has mostly broken free of the forest cover as it presses past the overlook and onward through native shrubs and wet ferns. At the first minor trail junction you meet, stay to the left. Keep following the main trail as it briefly ascends a rocky section, then tumbles back downhill. Ignore any spur trails or confusing use trails along the way. Just before reentering the forest, turn right at a major trail junction, then veer left as the trail heads back through the trees to **Hosmer Grove Campground**. ▶3

MILESTONES

▶1	0.0	Start at Hosmer Grove Campground [N 20.76843°, W 156.23801°]
▶2	0.2	Arrive at overlook
▶3	0.5	Return to Hosmer Grove Campground [N 20.76843°, W 156.23801°]

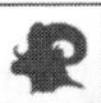

OPTIONS

Alternate Hikes on Haleakala for Birders

Many enthusiastic birders will want to head up the **Supply Trail**, which climbs steeply along the slopes of Haleakala volcano, starting off Hosmer Grove access road. Look for a small trailhead signpost on your right soon after turning off the main park highway. After climbing 2.3 miles with an elevation gain of more than 800 feet, the Supply Trail joins the Halemauu Trail (see Trail 25, page 213). Early morning is best for bird-watching and avoiding intense midday sun exposure on this trail.

Birders also won't want to miss the Nature Conservancy's **Waikamoi Preserve**, a protected area of cloud forest where native plants and birds thrive. Public access is only allowed via a three-hour, 3-mile guided hike starting at Hosmer Grove. Guided hikes usually depart at 9 AM on Monday and Thursday morning, weather permitting. An extended five-hour, 5-mile Walk on the Wet Side guided hike into the Waikamoi Preserve is usually offered one Sunday afternoon each month. For either of these guided hikes, show up at least 15 minutes early, dress in warm, waterproof layers, and wear sturdy hiking shoes or boots. For the required reservations, call (808) 572-4459 up to a week in advance.

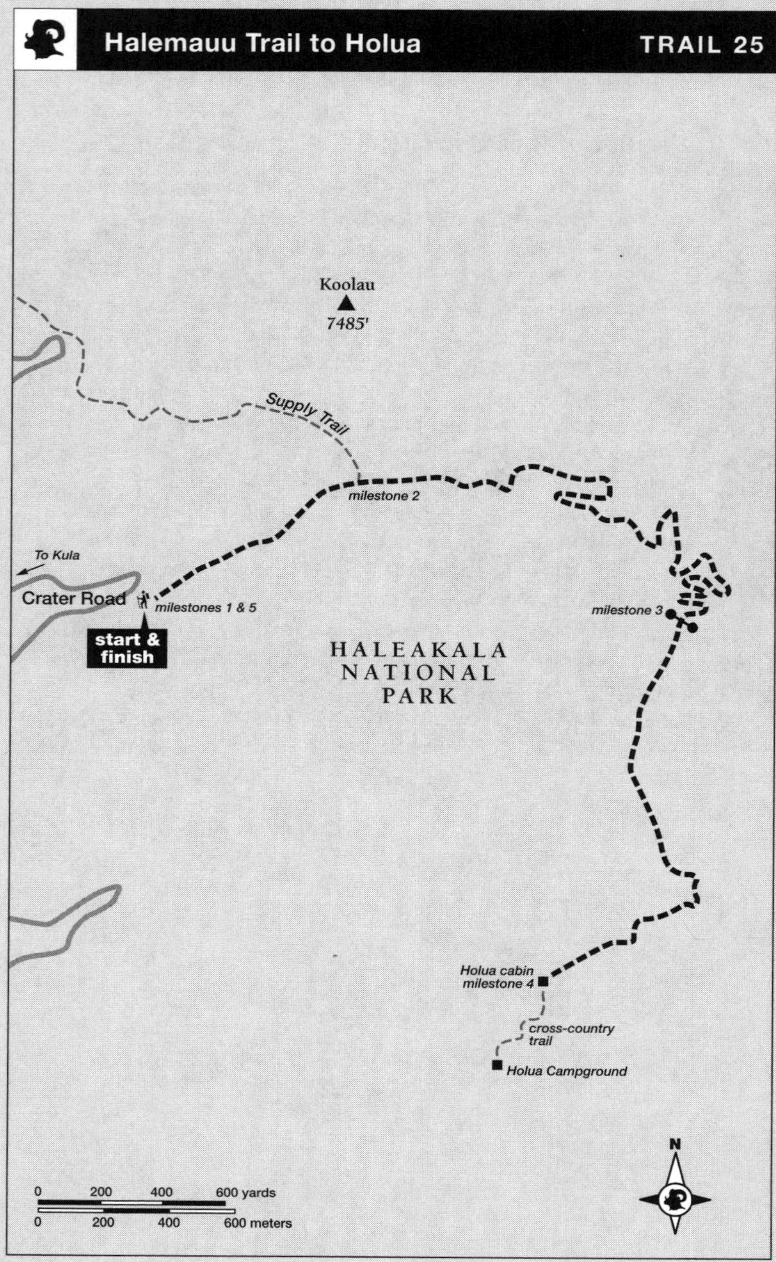
Halemauu Trail to Holua
TRAIL 25
Koolau
7485'
Supply Trail
milestone 2
To Kula
Crater Road
milestones 1 & 5
start & finish
milestone 3
HALEAKALA NATIONAL PARK
Holua cabin milestone 4
cross-country trail
Holua Campground
N
0 200 400 600 yards
0 200 400 600 meters

Halemauu Trail to Holua

Among the most popular dayhikes in Haleakala's summit area, the Halemauu Trail descends through cloud forest and switchbacks down fern-covered cliffs to the volcano floor. Enjoy panoramic ocean and mountain views at eye level with the clouds—and if you stay overnight at Holua, unforgettable sunrises over the Koolau Gap.

TRAIL USE
Dayhike, Backpack, Run

LENGTH
8.0 miles, 4–5 hours

VERTICAL FEET
±3600′

DIFFICULTY
– 1 2 3 4 **5** +

TRAIL TYPE
Out & Back

SURFACE TYPE
Dirt, Grass, Lava, Sand

START & END
N 20.75240°
W 156.22845°

FEATURES
Forest
Lava Flows
Mountain
Birds
Native Plants
Wildlife
Great Views
Camping
Geologic Interest
Historic Interest
Steep

FACILITIES
Restrooms
Picnic Tables
Water

Best Time

You can hike this trail year-round. Weather in the high-altitude summit region of Haleakala is unpredictable, however; the trail can be hot and sunny one minute, freezing cold and rainy the next. Starting early in the morning increases your chances of avoiding late afternoon clouds, rain, and mist that sometimes obscure the views.

Finding the Trail

From Kahului, follow the Hana Highway (Hwy. 36) southeast past the airport turnoff, then turn right onto the Haleakala Highway (Hwy. 37). Drive uphill for almost 8 miles, then turn left, continuing on the Haleakala Highway (Hwy. 377). Drive about 6 more miles uphill toward Kula, turning left on Hwy. 378, which becomes Crater Road. Continue for a little more than 10 winding, slow-moving miles uphill through open range for grazing livestock to the park's entrance station.

After paying the entry fee or showing your pass, continue driving uphill for 4.4 more miles, turning left into the signposted Halemauu Trailhead parking lot. If you need overnight camping or cabin permits (see page 15), stop off en route at the park headquarters visitor center, less than a mile uphill from the entrance along the main road. Permits are only available between 8 AM and 3 PM daily.

Trail Description

Hawaiian honeycreepers such as bright red apapane and iiwi and yellow-green amakihi flit about the blossoming flowers.

The Halemauu Trailhead parking lot has restrooms and informational signboards. If you need drinking water, however, fill up first at the park headquarters visitor center en route to the trailhead. Also ask the visitor center staff if nonpotable water is currently available at Holua cabin. If so, bring a way to purify it. If not, pack in all of the water you'll need for this dayhike or overnight trip.

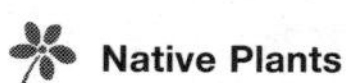

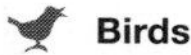

From the **trailhead parking lot**, ▶1 start walking down the clearly marked trail. On a rocky dirt surface, the trail slowly descends through native shrubland. Densely clustered endemic Hawaiian plants include lush green ferns, red-berried ohelo and pink-flowered pukiawe shrubs, and trees such as mamane, easily recognized by its yellow pea-blossom flowers. Early morning is a great time for bird-watching along this initial section of the trail. Hawaiian honeycreepers such as bright red apapane and iiwi and yellow-green amakihi flit about the blossoming flowers and the trees.

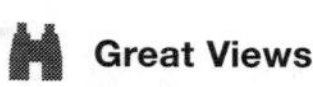

About 0.7 mile from the parking lot, the Halemauu Trail passes **the junction with the Supply Trail**, ▶2 which ruggedly descends to the Hosmer Grove access road (for details, see the "Options" box for Trail 24, page 211). At the junction, continue straight ahead on the Halemauu Trail (do not veer left onto the Supply Trail). Soon you are rewarded with your first views down the grassy slopes of Haleakala volcano all the way to the Pacific. About 0.3 mile past the Supply Trail junction, more views open up to your right, letting you

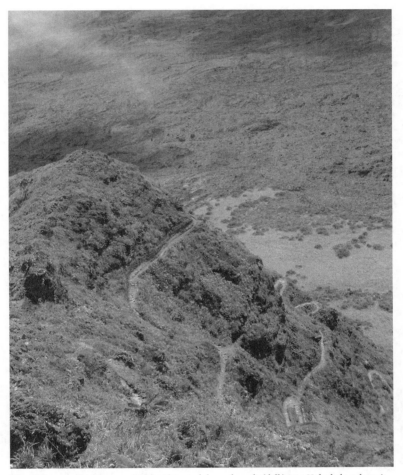

The Halemauu's steep switchbacks *wind down the pali (cliffs) into Haleakala volcano's cinder desert.*

peek into the volcano summit's vast erosional valley and its colorful cinder desert.

A little more than a mile from the parking lot, the Halemauu Trail begins to drop gently on long, lazy switchbacks that eventually become steeper and narrower. Contouring right around a ridge, Holua cabin comes into view at the bottom of the *pali* (cliffs). Take heart: By now you're more than halfway down the switchbacks, about 2 miles from the trailhead. Directly below, you can spy the trail ahead as it snakes its way down a shaggy green cliff with a triangular top. Keep descending on mostly exposed switchbacks, taking advantage of occasionally shady sections to rest. The lush ferns that grow on the cliffs all around include fringed amauu, which unusually change color from reddish pink to dark green as the plant ages.

Steep

On clear nights, the unobstructed views of the Milky Way from atop Haleakala are unmatched anywhere else on Maui.

Finally, the switchbacks tighten and steepen dramatically before you reach the **gate at the bottom of the cliffs**, ▸3 now approximately 2.7 miles from the trailhead parking lot. Shut the wooden gate securely behind you to keep out wild pigs and grazing livestock that would otherwise wreak havoc on the volcano's fragile ecosystem. From the bottom of the cliffs, it's around 1.3 miles farther to Holua cabin. The trail starts off grassy underfoot, but soon becomes a cindery path that rolls up and down through lava flows. This stretch of the hike can be quite exposed and hot on sunny days.

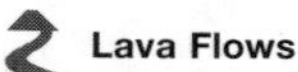
Lava Flows

Soon a rustic-looking wilderness cabin comes into view off to the west. Turn right off the main trail onto a short spurt trail that ends in front of **Holua**

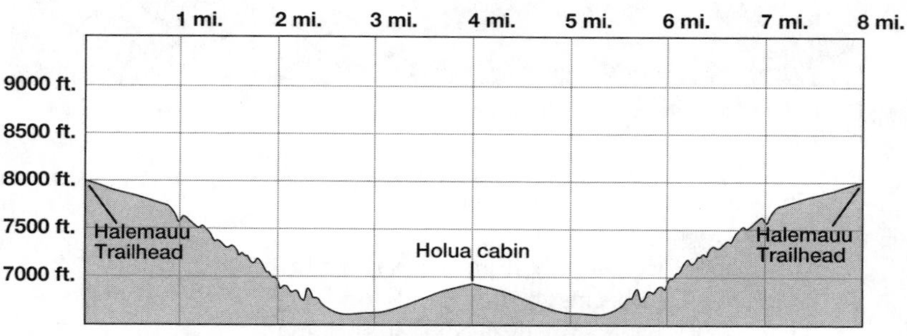

TRAIL 25 Halemauu Trail to Holua Elevation Profile

cabin, ▶4 built by the Civilian Conservation Corps in the 1930s. Barking nene (Hawaiian geese) often wander around outside, taking advantage of the shade provided by the cabin and its picnic table out front. Do not feed or give water to these endangered birds, to help them stay wild. When you're rested and ready, turn around and retrace your steps east of Holua cabin back to the main trail. Turn left and walk back toward the bottom of the cliffs, once again passing through the gate, then climbing nearly 1300 feet back up the switchbacks and along the snaking ridgeline to return to the **trailhead parking lot**. ▶5

If you're staying overnight at Holua, the dispersed camping area is directly south of the cabin. Follow a muddy use trail uphill, veering left around the (usually unstaffed) ranger cabin and a composting toilet to find a few already impacted campsites set on a small ledge overlooking the volcano floor. Whether you're pitching a tent or staying in the cabin, be sure to wake up before sunrise to catch the phenomenal play of light on the clouds rolling through the Koolau Gap, visible off to the east. On clear nights, the unobstructed views of the Milky Way from atop Haleakala are unmatched anywhere else on Maui, thanks in part to reduced light pollution at the summit.

Camping

MILESTONES

▶1	0.0	Start from trailhead parking lot [N 20.75240°, W 156.22845°]
▶2	0.7	Reach junction with Supply Trail [N 20.75611°, W 156.22070°]
▶3	2.7	Pass through gate at bottom of cliffs [N 20.75225°, W 156.21297°]
▶4	4.0	Arrive at Holua cabin [N 20.74163°, W 156.21796°]
▶5	8.0	Return to trailhead parking lot [N 20.75240°, W 156.22845°]

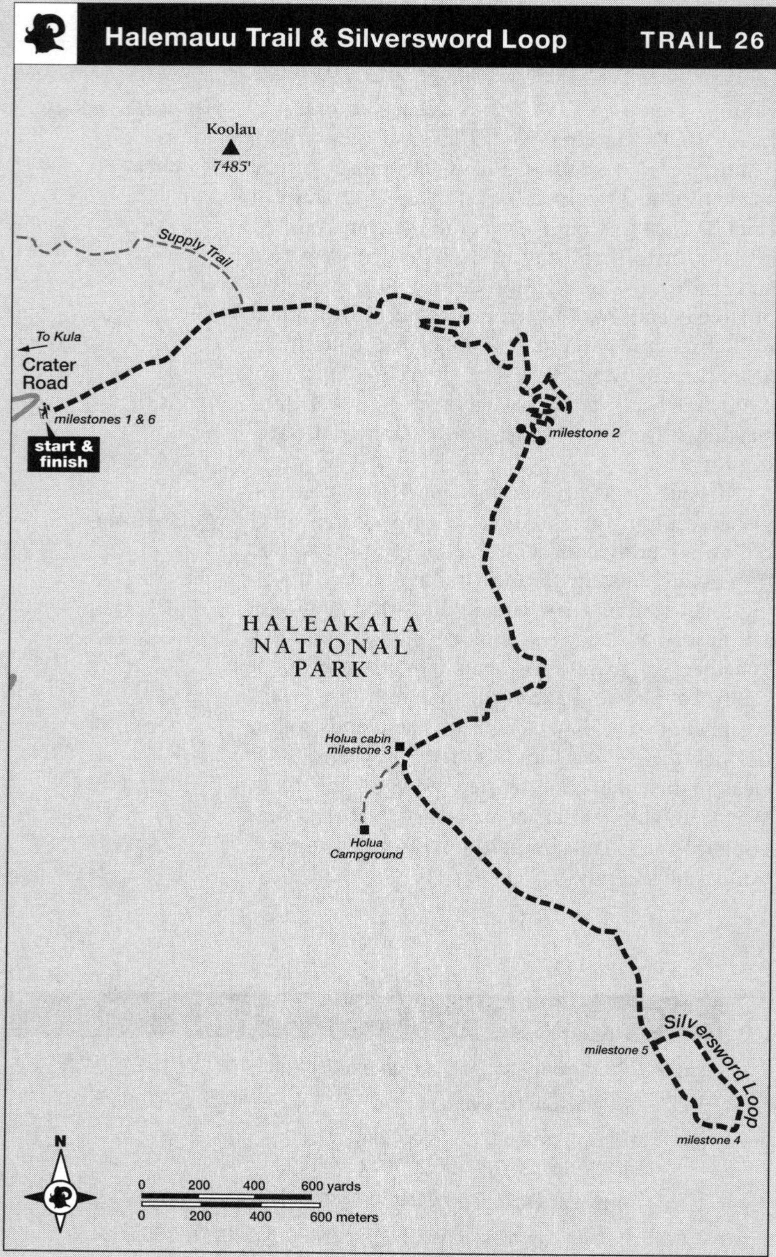

Halemauu Trail & Silversword Loop
TRAIL 26
Koolau
7485'
Supply Trail
To Kula
Crater Road
milestones 1 & 6
start & finish
milestone 2
HALEAKALA NATIONAL PARK
Holua cabin milestone 3
Holua Campground
Silversword Loop
milestone 5
milestone 4
N
0 200 400 600 yards
0 200 400 600 meters

Halemauu Trail & Silversword Loop

For hikers in good shape, this extended route follows more of the popular Halemauu Trail, which is the fastest way on foot into the erosional valley of Haleakala's summit area. Beyond Holua cabin, venture into the volcano's kaleidoscopic cinder desert to find rare, strangely beautiful silversword plants.

TRAIL USE
Dayhike, Backpack, Run

LENGTH
10.8 miles, 5–6½ hours

VERTICAL FEET
±4000′

DIFFICULTY
– 1 2 3 4 **5** +

TRAIL TYPE
Semiloop

SURFACE TYPE
Dirt, Grass, Lava, Sand

START & END
N 20.75240°
W 156.22845°

FEATURES
Forest
Lava Flows
Mountain
Birds
Native Plants
Wildlife
Great Views
Camping
Geologic Interest
Historic Interest
Steep

FACILITIES
Restrooms
Picnic Tables
Water

Best Time

You can hike this trail year-round. Weather in the high-altitude summit region of Haleakala is unpredictable, however; the trail can be hot and sunny one minute, freezing cold and rainy the next. Starting early in the morning increases your chances of avoiding late afternoon clouds, rain, and mist that sometimes obscure the views.

Finding the Trail

From Kahului, follow the Hana Highway (Hwy. 36) southeast past the airport turnoff, then turn right onto the Haleakala Highway (Hwy. 37). Drive uphill for almost 8 miles, then turn left, continuing on the Haleakala Highway (Hwy. 377). Drive about 6 more miles uphill toward Kula, turning left on Hwy. 378, which becomes Crater Road. Continue for a little more than 10 winding, slow-moving miles uphill through open range for grazing livestock to the park's entrance station.

After paying the entry fee or showing your pass, continue driving uphill for 4.4 more miles, turning left into the signposted Halemauu Trailhead parking lot. If you need overnight camping or cabin permits

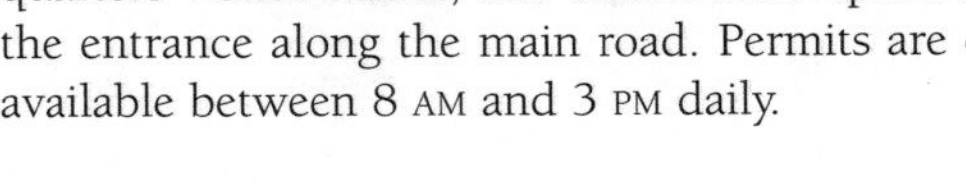
(see page 15), stop off en route at the park headquarters visitor center, less than a mile uphill from the entrance along the main road. Permits are only available between 8 AM and 3 PM daily.

A rocky trail leads across an otherworldly landscape of jagged lava, partially colonized by native Hawaiian plants.

Trail Description

The Halemauu Trailhead parking lot has restrooms and informational signboards. But if you need drinking water, fill up at the park's headquarters visitor center en route to the trailhead. Also ask the visitor center staff if nonpotable water is currently available at Holua cabin. If so, bring a way to purify it. If not, pack in all the water necessary for this strenuous hike or an overnight trip, plus some extra in case of emergencies.

Start at the **trailhead parking lot**. ►1 The well-marked Halemauu Trail begins by descending through a native Hawaiian shrubland ecosystem. Early morning hikers stand a good chance of spotting many colorful native forest birds along this route, including a rainbow variety of Hawaiian honeycreepers. About 0.7 mile from the trailhead, walk straight past the intersection with the Supply Trail, a spur that leads steeply downhill toward Hosmer Grove (for details, see the "Options" box for Trail 24, page 211). About 1 mile from the parking lot, jaw-dropping ocean and volcano panoramas open up on both sides of the trail.

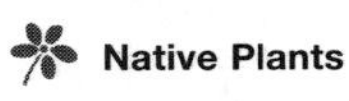

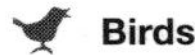

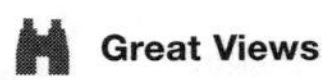

The trail curves right around a ridge and switchbacks steadily down the *pali* (cliffs). Around 2 miles from the trailhead, if it's a clear day, you can spy Holua cabin down on the volcano floor. As it winds ever more sharply down the steep, well-cut switchbacks, the Halemauu Trail moves in and out of shady spots, where native Hawaiian ferns sprout on the cliffsides thanks to water that seeps through the rocks. When the trail reaches the end of the switchbacks at the bottom of the cliffs, pass through

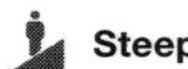

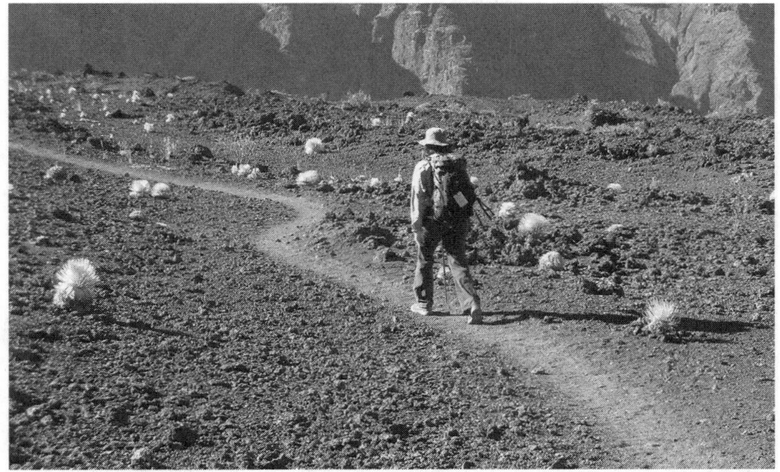

Hike past rare, shiny-leafed silversword plants *in Haleakala volcano's cinder desert.*

a wooden gate. ▶2 Close it securely behind you, to keep out wild pigs and grazing animals that could endanger the rare flora and fauna of the volcano's ecosystem.

On the other side of the gate, hike across grassy fields, which are quickly overtaken by lava flows as the path underfoot becomes cindery. It's an often sunny, even hot hike of about 1.3 miles to Holua cabin, which comes ever closer into view off to your right. At the spur trail T-junction, turn right and walk over to historic **Holua cabin**, ▶3 built by the Civilian Conservation Corps in the 1930s. There you can take a quick break and enjoy a little shade under the eaves of the cabin or at the picnic table out front. If you are staying in the cabin overnight, leave your pack inside. Campers can follow a short use trail directly south of the cabin, which climbs up a small ledge, veering left around the ranger cabin (usually unstaffed) and a composting toilet to reach a few already impacted campsites. Some sites are partly sheltered from the wind by low lava-rock walls.

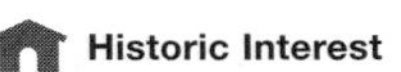

Historic Interest

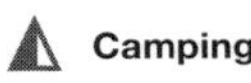

Camping

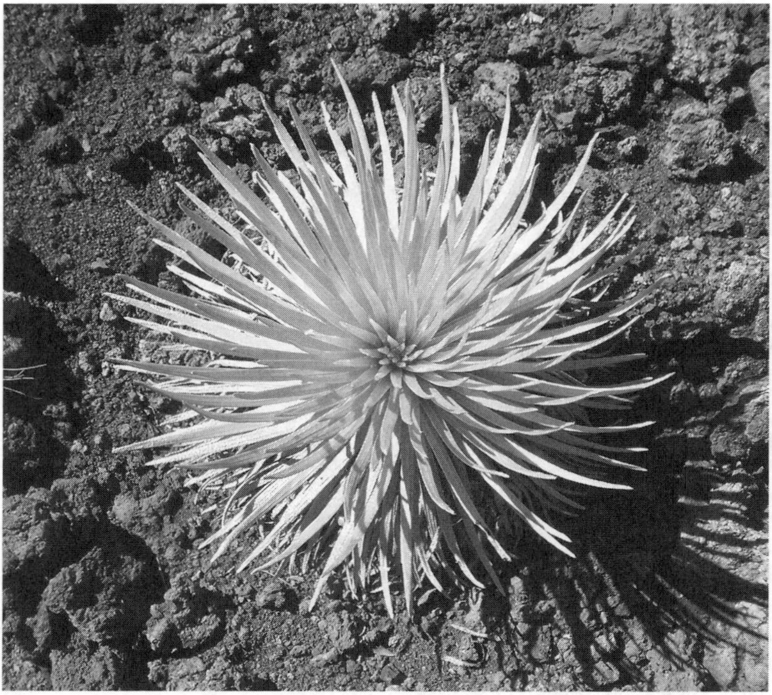

On Maui, the threatened native silversword *grows only in Haleakala's summit region.*

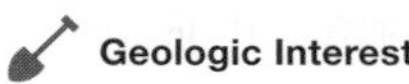

Geologic Interest

When you're rested and refreshed, retrace your steps from the cabin to the main Halemauu Trail, turning right at the T-junction to further explore the volcano's cinder desert. A rocky trail leads across an otherworldly landscape of jagged lava, partially colonized by native Hawaiian plants, including hardy ferns and shrubby *ohelo* plants, whose red berries are gobbled by nene (Hawaiian geese). You may have already encountered these endangered birds back at Holua cabin. Keep an eye out for these gentle, but wild creatures soaring on the winds across the volcano floor.

The trail's surface softens as you head deeper into the volcano's multicolored cinder desert. A little more than a mile from Holua cabin, you pass the northern terminus of the Silversword Loop. Ignore it and keep going another 0.3 mile along the Halemauu Trail, then turn left onto the **south end of the Silversword Loop**. ▶4 This gentle side trail rolls gently up and down through a naturally occurring "garden" of silversword plants. With their shiny silver leaves adapted to reflect the intense solar radiation near the volcano's summit, these threatened plants bloom only once in a lifetime. Don't stray off the trail here, as the plants' fragile root systems can be damaged severely by hikers who trample on the cryptobiotic soil crust, which supports life in this arid region.

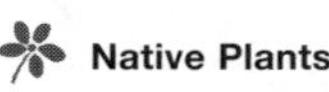

At the north end of the Silversword Loop, **turn right at the T-junction to rejoin the Halemauu Trail**. ▶5 It's a little more than a mile's hike back to the spur trail turnoff for Holua cabin and campground. If you're not staying overnight at Holua, instead keep following the main Halemauu Trail for 1.3 miles more to reach the bottom of the cliffs. Pass through the gate, then climb for 1.7 miles up the cliffs' steep switchbacks before striding the final mile uphill on a partly rocky path back to the **trailhead parking lot**. ▶6

With shiny silver leaves adapted to reflect intense solar radiation, the threatened silversword plants bloom only once in a lifetime.

MILESTONES

▶1	0.0	Start at trailhead parking lot [N 20.75240°, W 156.22845°]
▶2	2.7	Pass through gate at bottom of cliffs [N 20.75225°, W 156.21297°]
▶3	4.0	Arrive at Holua cabin [N 20.74163°, W 156.21796°]
▶4	5.4	Turn left onto Silversword Loop [N 20.73037°, W 156.20615°]
▶5	5.8	Turn right to rejoin Halemauu Trail [N 20.73298°, W 156.20892°]
▶6	10.8	Return to trailhead parking lot [N 20.75240°, W 156.22845°]

Halemauu Trail to Paliku

TRAIL 27

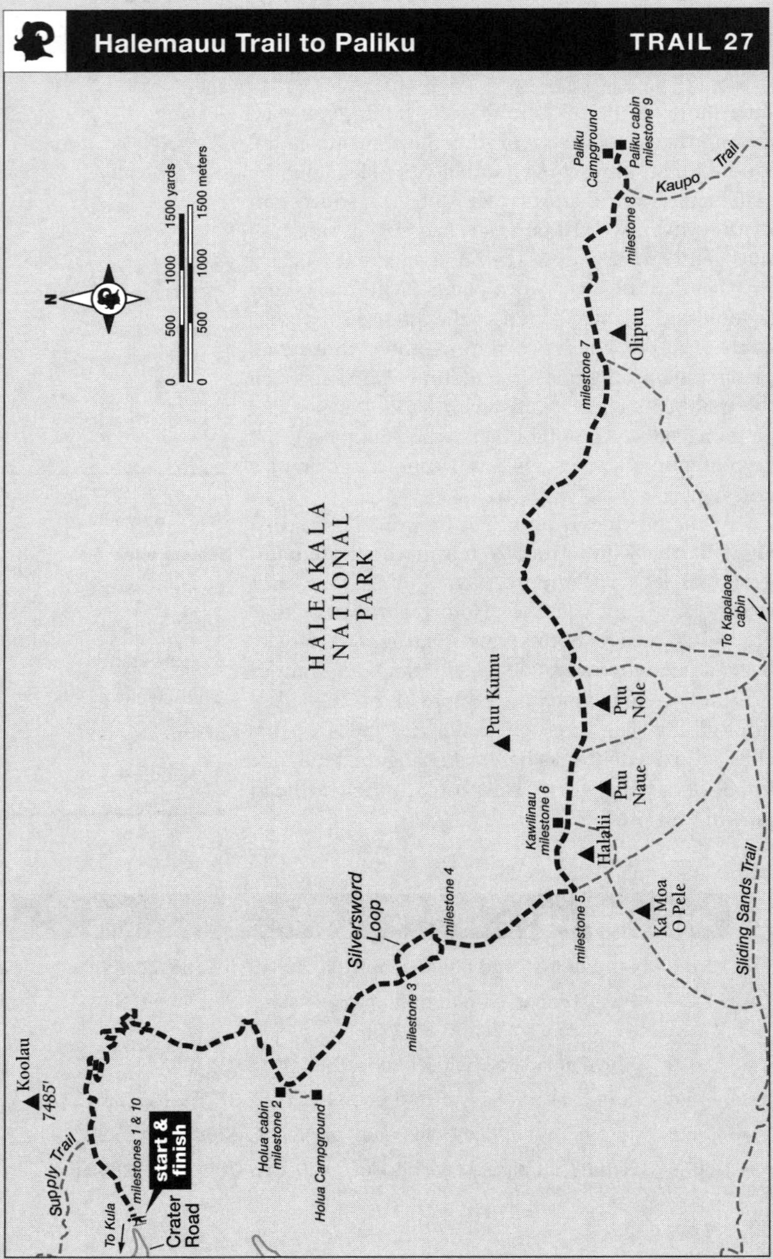

Halemauu Trail to Paliku

Mesmerized by the kaleidoscopic cinder desert of Haleakala's summit region, many hikers miss out on a side trip over to the volcano's more lush windward side. Above serene Paliku's grassy meadows and forested groves, mist-shrouded craggy cliffs draped with lacy waterfalls rise.

TRAIL USE
Backpack,
Permit Required

LENGTH
21.0 miles, 2 days

VERTICAL FEET
±7000′

DIFFICULTY
– 1 2 3 4 **5** +

TRAIL TYPE
Out & Back

SURFACE TYPE
Dirt, Grass, Lava, Sand

START & END
N 20.75240°
W 156.22845°

FEATURES
Forest
Lava Flows
Mountain
Birds
Native Plants
Wildlife
Great Views
Camping
Geologic Interest
Historic Interest
Archaeological
Secluded
Steep

FACILITIES
Restrooms
Picnic Tables
Water

Best Time

You can hike this trail year-round. Weather in the high-altitude summit region of Haleakala is unpredictable, however; the trail can be hot and sunny one minute, freezing cold and rainy the next. Starting early in the morning increases your chances of avoiding late afternoon clouds, rain, and mist that can obscure the views and make the final stretch of the trail to Paliku a mucky march.

Finding the Trail

From Kahului, follow the Hana Highway (Hwy. 36) southeast past the airport turnoff, then turn right onto the Haleakala Highway (Hwy. 37). Drive uphill for almost 8 miles, then turn left, continuing on the Haleakala Highway (Hwy. 377). Drive about 6 more miles uphill toward Kula, turning left on Hwy. 378, which becomes Crater Road. Continue for a little more than 10 winding, slow-moving miles uphill through open range for grazing livestock to the park's entrance station.

After paying the entrance fee or showing your pass, continue driving uphill for less than a mile along the main park road to the headquarters visitor center. Pick up wilderness permits for overnight trips inside (for details about camping and cabins, see page 15). Permits are only available between 8 AM and 3 PM daily. From the headquarters visitor center, drive 3.5 miles farther uphill on the main park road, turning left into the Halemauu Trailhead parking lot.

Trail Description

Blooming only once in a lifetime, the silversword's stalks of maroon blossoms are an arresting sight among the sere lava.

If you need drinking water, fill up en route to the trailhead outside the park headquarters visitor center. Also ask the visitor center staff if nonpotable water is available at Holua and Paliku. If so, bring a way to purify it. If not, you must pack in all of the water you'll need for your overnight trip, both for drinking and for cooking, plus some extra in case of emergencies.

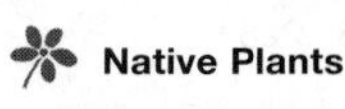

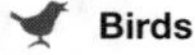

Start at the **Halemauu Trailhead ►1** at the east end of the parking lot. The trail starts gently enough, winding downhill through native shrubland where Hawaiian honeycreepers flit among the blossoming plants and trees, especially early in the morning. About 0.7 mile from the parking lot, walk straight past the intersection on your left with the Supply Trail, which heads ruggedly downhill to Hosmer Grove (see the "Options" box for Trail 24, page 211).

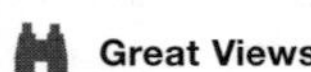

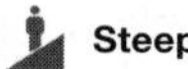

Sprawling views down the slopes of Haleakala volcano to the ocean and across the summit area's erosional valley start appearing about a mile from the trailhead. From this point, the trail contours right around a ridge and starts to drop in earnest on switchbacks down the *pali* (cliffs). A variety of native Hawaiian ferns grow on the cliffsides, fed by water seeps in the volcanic rock. About 2 miles from the trailhead, on clear days you can see Holua cabin down across the volcano floor.

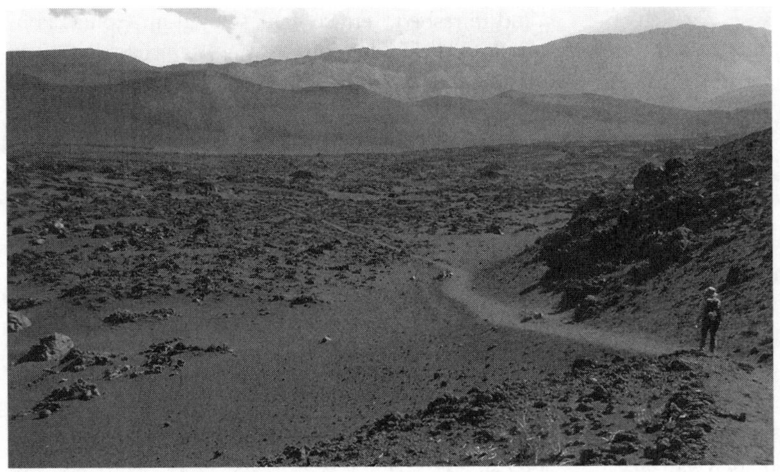

Striking out *across Haleakala's cinder desert between Holua and Paliku cabins*

Less than 3 miles from your starting point, the switchbacks narrow and steepen before abruptly stopping at the bottom of the *pali*. Walk through the wooden gate, closing it securely behind you to keep out wild pigs and grazing livestock that threaten the volcano's fragile ecosystem and its threatened native plants and animals. Keep following the Halemauu Trail across fields of grass that soon turn to lava flows with cinders crunching underfoot. It's a little more than a mile to the next T-junction, where you turn right onto a spur trail leading to **Holua cabin**, ▶2 nestled under cliffs in a grassy meadow.

Built by the Civilian Conservation Corps (CCC) in the 1930s, the cabin is the last shade you're likely to get for the next 5 miles, so take a break here and enjoy the company of the endangered nene (Hawaiian geese) that often rest under the picnic table out front. The camping area is reached via a short use trail that heads south and slightly uphill, then veers left around the (usually unstaffed) ranger cabin and a composting toilet. When you're rested

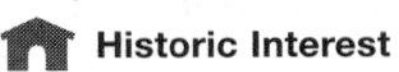

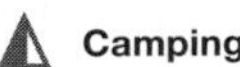

and refreshed, retrace your steps from Holua cabin back to the T-junction, turning right back onto the main Halemauu Trail.

It's a little more than a mile's walk through rolling lava fields to the northern terminus of the **Silversword Loop**, ►3 a 0.4-mile spur trail curving off to your left. It's worth taking, especially because it adds only negligible distance to your overall trip. Here the threatened silversword plant thrives in the arid volcanic environment, its shiny silver leaves reflecting the intense solar radiation. Blooming only once in a lifetime, the silversword's stalks of maroon blossoms are an arresting sight among the sere lava and cindery hills. Turn left at the loop's southern terminus to **rejoin the main Halemauu Trail**. ►4

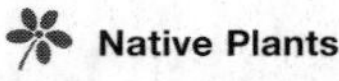

Above serene Paliku, mist-shrouded cliffs draped with lacy waterfalls rise.

You find yourself walking once more through barren-looking fields of jagged *aa* lava colored rust-brown and jet-black, with only a few ohelo shrubs and other native plants homesteading among the rocks and cinders. The Halemauu Trail makes a gradual descent of less than a mile to the next major junction, where you **veer left toward Paliku** ►5 instead of continuing straight ahead toward Kapalaoa cabin. Now you're finally walking in the heart of the volcano's cinder desert. The trail chugs uphill to a small saddle, then descends past a rainbow-colored volcanic vent. Off to your left, the triangular peak of Hanakauhi (elevation 8907 feet) pierces the sky.

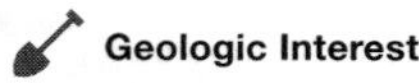

Archaeological

The trail descends on soft cinders, passing **Kawilinau** ►6 about 0.4 mile from the previous trail junction. Nicknamed the "Bottomless Pit," Kawilinau is actually 65 feet deep. In ancient times, some Hawaiians made pilgrimages here to drop the umbilical cords of newborn infants into the pit, believing it would make their children stronger. Past the pit, at each of the next four trail junctions, ignore any side trails leading south (off to your right) toward Kapalaoa cabin. Instead keep hiking

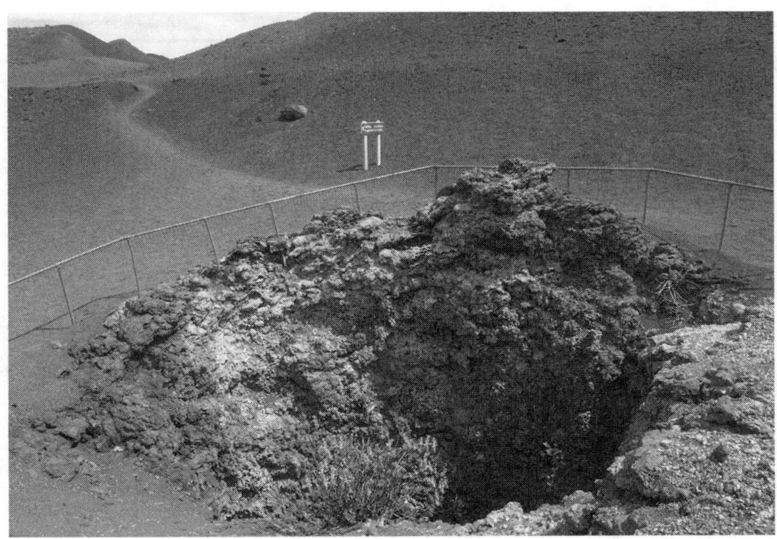

Nicknamed the "'Bottomless Pit," *Kawilinau is actually only 65 feet deep.*

straight ahead on the Halemauu Trail, following the signs pointing toward Paliku.

The trail steadily loses elevation as it changes from a cinder path into a rocky lava road. All around is a moonscape of cinder cones in a variety of shapes, sizes, and colors. Eventually you'll pass into a verdant landscape of grasslands and forest trees. About 2.6 miles from Kawilinau, you'll meet the last trail junction signposted for Kapalaoa at the base of **Olipuu cinder cone**, ►7 which has dominated the horizon for the last mile. From this junction, veer north (left) around the cinder cone.

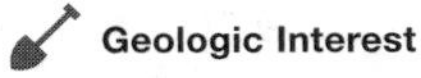

Geologic Interest

Beyond Olipuu, the trail continues dropping through native shrubland and over both rough *aa* and smooth *pahoehoe* lava. The atmosphere is often heavily laden with mist. Welcome to the rainy windward side of Haleakala's eroded summit region! It can be tricky to follow the trail in the fog, but official NPS signs and *ahu* (cairns) left by other hikers will

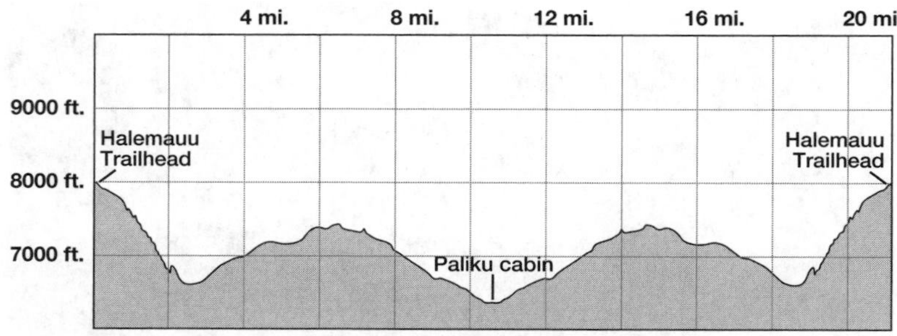

TRAIL 27 Halemauu Trail to Paliku Elevation Profile

help you with wayfinding. Be careful with your footing, as some dry washes and steep lava gullies right beside the trail are potentially ankle-wrenching.

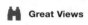

A little more than a mile from Olipuu, **veer left at the junction with the Kaupo Trail** ▶8 (see the "Options" box, opposite page). Continue 0.2 mile more through grassy meadows toward Paliku's overhanging cliffs, down the faces of which waterfalls often stream. A variety of native plants and trees flourish here, as do forest birds and curious nene who are likely waiting for your arrival at

MILESTONES

▶1	0.0	Start from Halemauu Trailhead [N 20.75240°, W 156.22845°]
▶2	4.0	Reach Holua cabin [N 20.74163°, W 156.21796°]
▶3	5.1	Detour onto Silversword Loop [N 20.73298°, W 156.20892°]
▶4	5.5	Rejoin main Halemauu Trail [N 20.73037°, W 156.20615°]
▶5	6.3	Veer left toward Paliku [N 20.72120°, W 156.20174°]
▶6	6.7	Pass Kawilinau
▶7	9.3	Reach Olipuu cinder cone [N 20.71809°, W 156.15982°]
▶8	10.4	Veer left at Kaupo Trail junction [N 20.71657°, W 156.14517°]
▶9	10.6	Arrive at Paliku cabin [N 20.71764°, W 156.14183°]
▶10	21.0	Return to Halemauu Trailhead [N 20.75240°, W 156.22845°]

Paliku cabin. ►9 Tucked nearly underneath the cliffs, this cabin, like Holua, was built by the CCC in the 1930s. A short spur trail before reaching the cabin leads off left to the designated camping area. A nonpotable water spigot and composting toilet are nearby.

 **Historic Interest**

Camping

Uphill farther east of the wilderness cabin, Paliku's ranger cabin is often unstaffed. If any emergencies arise, be prepared to hike all the way back out of the volcano. If you retrace your steps (but skip the Silversword Loop detour on the return trip), it's approximately a 10.5-mile trek back to the **Halemauu Trailhead.** ►10

Notice

Dress in warm, waterproof layers for this hike. You'll pass through different life zones and significantly change elevations, so be prepared for any kind of weather. In the same day, you might experience blistering high-altitude sunshine (wear sunscreen with a high SPF rating) and cold, wet, and windy conditions that can cause hypothermia. It's important to keep the interior of your backpack dry. That way, when you reach Paliku, your tent, sleeping bag, and change of clothes will be warm and dry.

If you're staying in the unheated wilderness cabins, do not rely on the pot-bellied woodstoves, your only external fuel source, to be in working order or to be stocked with enough fuel to make a fire.

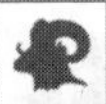

OPTIONS

Alternate Hikes to and from Paliku

You can extend this overnight hike into a three-day backpacking trip by spending the first night at Holua, either camping or staying in the cabin, before continuing to Paliku. If you have an extra day at Paliku, you could also hike partway down the Kaupo Gap for a strenuous, but beautiful side trip (see Trail 34, page 279).

Sliding Sands Trail to Ka Luu o ka Oo TRAIL 28

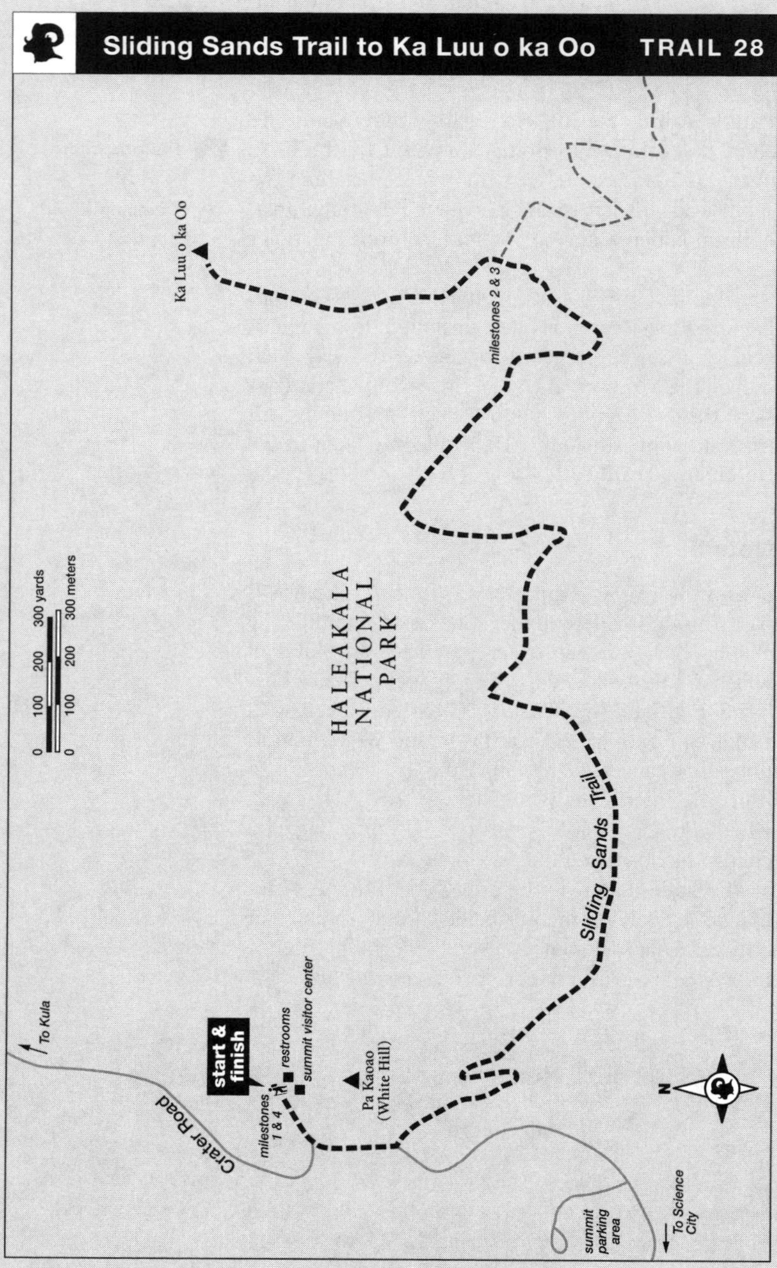

Sliding Sands Trail to Ka Luu o ka Oo

Starting above the lofty level of clouds near Haleakala's summit, this famous trail switchbacks on soft cinders down to the volcano floor. But you only need to follow it partway to be impressed by the panoramic views, especially on a spur trail around a colorful cinder cone.

TRAIL USE
Dayhike

LENGTH
5.0 miles, 2–3 hours

VERTICAL FEET
±3000′

DIFFICULTY
– 1 2 **3** 4 5 +

TRAIL TYPE
Semiloop

SURFACE TYPE
Dirt, Lava, Paved, Sand

START & END
N 20.71470°
W 156.25064°

FEATURES
Lava Flows
Mountain
Birds
Native Plants
Wildlife
Great Views
Geologic Interest
Steep

FACILITIES
Visitor Center
Restrooms
Phone
Water

Best Time

You can hike this trail year-round. Weather in the high-altitude summit region of Haleakala is unpredictable, however; the trail can be hot and sunny one minute, freezing cold and rainy the next. Starting soon after sunrise means that you'll stay ahead of the guided horseback tour groups on the way down. Avoid hiking midday, when the high-altitude sunshine is most intense.

Finding the Trail

From Kahului, follow the Hana Highway (Hwy. 36) southeast past the airport turnoff, then turn right onto the Haleakala Highway (Hwy. 37). Drive uphill for almost 8 miles, then turn left, continuing on the Haleakala Highway (Hwy. 377). Drive about 6 more miles uphill toward Kula, turning left on Hwy. 378, which becomes Crater Road. Continue for a little more than 10 winding, slow-moving miles uphill through open range for grazing livestock to the park's entrance station. After paying the entrance fee or showing your pass, keep driving uphill for a little more than 10 miles to a stop-sign intersection. Continue straight ahead into the paved parking lot for the summit visitor center (if you turn right, the main park road continues another 0.5 mile uphill to the volcano's actual summit).

Trail Description

> **At sunrise, you can escape some of the crowds by climbing Pa Kaoao (White Hill) or by hiking partway down the Sliding Sands Trail.**

The park's summit visitor center (open from 5:15 AM to 3 PM daily) sits at a exhilarating elevation of 9740 feet above sea level. Signs advise visitors to walk slowly and not overexert themselves until they become acclimated. Watch out for signs of altitude sickness (see page 14). If you show any symptoms that do not resolve, experts advise driving back down the mountain to lower elevations. Outside the visitor center are restrooms and drinking fountains. Note that water is not available anywhere along this hike.

Start from the west side of the **parking lot**, ▶1 farthest from the visitor center and closest to the main park road. Follow a paved sidewalk west toward the road, passing a metal hitching rail used by guided horseback tour groups. You'll feel the crunch of volcanic cinders underfoot as the trail winds south around the base of Pa Kaoao (White Hill). Pa Kaoao is a popular perch for sunrise watchers, who scramble up a short dirt trail from the parking lot to reach the top of the cinder cone.

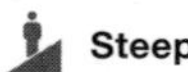
Steep

On the south side of Pa Kaoao, it quickly becomes obvious how the Sliding Sands Trail (called Keoneheehee in Hawaiian) got its name. Your feet will sink into the soft cinders along switchbacks that lead rather steeply downhill to the volcano floor. In many sections, however, the cinders are so compacted by hundreds of hikers' feet each day that there is little danger of literally sliding. The trail is broad enough that you're unlikely to find the drop-offs too dizzying either. As you drop easily and steadily on the trail's switchbacks, remember that the return trip may take you up to twice as long.

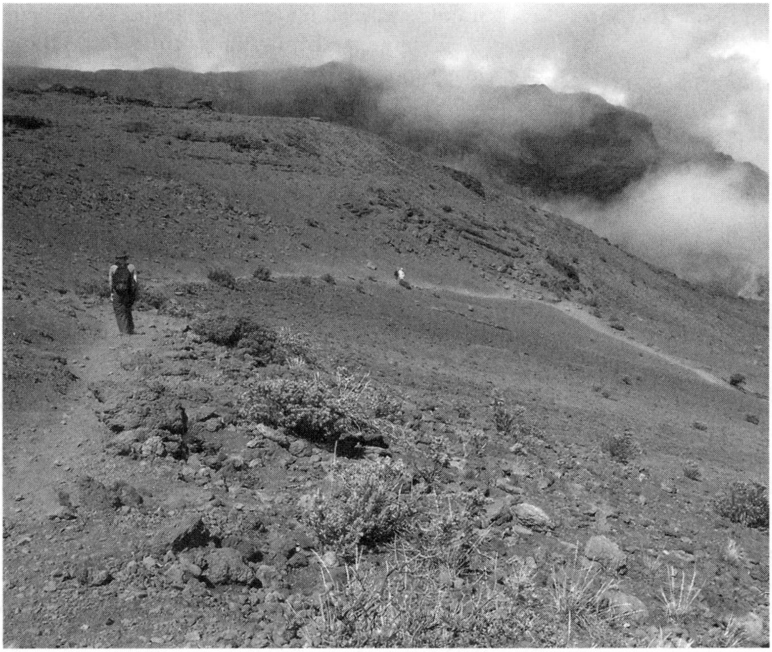

Hikers descend *from the volcano's summit area into a geologic wonderland.*

From the top of the switchbacks, the sweeping views of the volcano's playground of cinder cones are fantastic. It almost feels like walking on an alien planet at eye level with the clouds. Although there is not much vegetation in this stark lunar landscape, those shrubby green plants with yellow daisylike flowers growing alongside the trail are hardy kupaoa, members of the aster family. Lower down, the trail's switchbacks pass through rockier *aa* lava flows from centuries or even millennia ago. A few rare and threatened silversword plants, with their shiny silver leaves that reflect the solar radiation and tall stalks of maroon flowers, dot the sides of the trail.

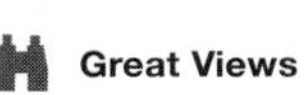

Great Views

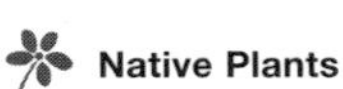

Native Plants

Almost 2 miles from your starting point, the trail reaches a **signposted junction with the Ka Luu o ka Oo spur trail**. ►2 Turn left onto this 1.2-mile semiloop side trip, which starts with a scramble down a short, but steep slope of crumbly lava. The narrow trail levels out and becomes more cindery as it heads north and slightly downhill toward Ka Luu o ka Oo. It climbs slightly as it approaches the cinder cone, which is splashed with a rainbow variety of colors, including rust red, emerald green, desert tan, chocolate brown, and jet black. As the trail circles clockwise around the knife edge of a volcanic vent, you are able to peer inside. This side trip ends a short distance beyond the dramatic vent at a sweeping viewpoint across the volcano's erosional valley.

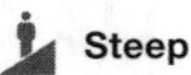

Geologic Interest

Although Haleakala last erupted in the 1790s, that's just a blink of an eye in geologic time—scientists classify it as an active volcano.

Steep

When you've taken plenty of photos, turn around and retrace your steps back to the **junction with the Sliding Sands Trail**. ►3 Turn right back onto the main Sliding Sands Trail and start hiking back up the switchbacks. If you're in good shape, it's only about an hour's hike uphill to the **summit visitor center parking lot**. ►4

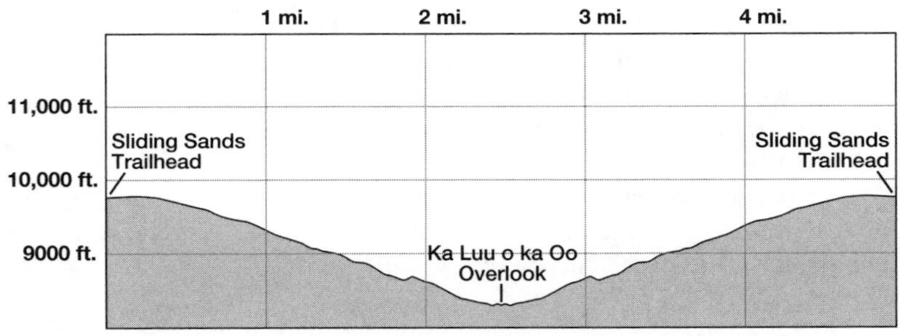

TRAIL 28 Sliding Sands Trail to Ka Luu o ka Oo Elevation Profile

Notice

In the Hawaiian language, *Haleakala* means the "house of the sun." Its name derives from an ancient Hawaiian myth about the demigod Maui. According to legend, Maui originally lifted the island out of the sea using a giant fishhook. Later, his mother pointed out that the days on this island were too short for her to dry her *tapa* (pounded-bark cloth) in the sun. To stop the sun from moving too quickly across the sky, Maui ascended the volcano, hid in a cave until sunrise, and then threw his magical lasso around the sun. Maui only released the sun from being his captive after the heavenly body promised to move more slowly across the sky, granting the island's people longer days in which to get their work done.

MILESTONES

▶1	0.0	Start at summit visitor center parking lot [N 20.71470°, W 156.25064°]
▶2	1.9	Turn left onto Ka Luu o ka Oo spur trail [N 20.71112°, W 156.23369°]
▶3	3.1	Turn right back onto Sliding Sands Trail [N 20.71112°, W 156.23369°]
▶4	5.0	Return to summit visitor center parking lot [N 20.71470°, W 156.25064°]

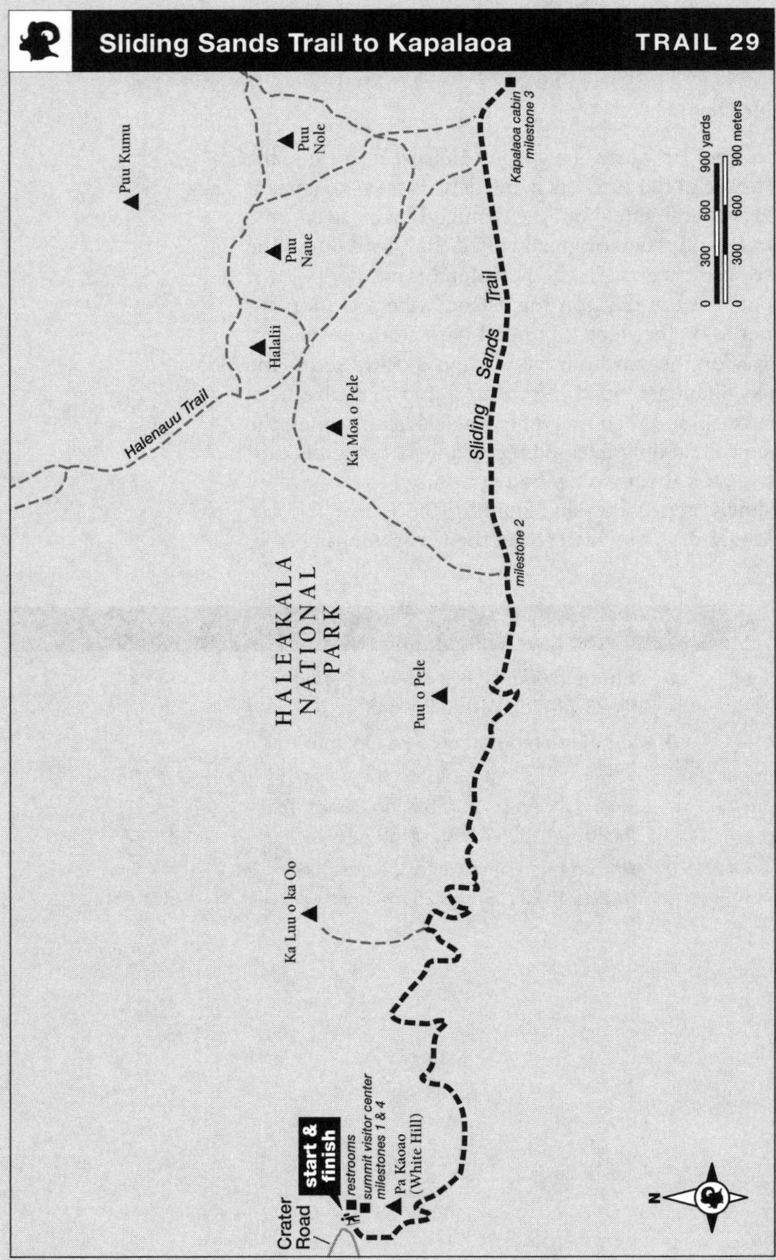

Sliding Sands Trail to Kapalaoa
TRAIL 29
Puu Kumu
Puu Nole
Puu Naue
Halalii
Halenauu Trail
Ka Moa o Pele
Kapalaoa cabin
milestone 3
Sliding Sands Trail
0 300 600 900 yards
0 300 600 900 meters
HALEAKALA NATIONAL PARK
milestone 2
Puu o Pele
Ka Luu o ka Oo
start & finish
restrooms
summit visitor center
milestones 1 & 4
Pa Kaoao (White Hill)
Crater Road
N

Sliding Sands Trail to Kapalaoa

Competing with the shorter Halemauu Trail to Holua (see Trail 25, page 213), the Sliding Sands Trail to Kapalaoa is among the most popular dayhikes around Haleakala's eroded summit region. This colorful cinder path switchbacks down to the volcano floor, then strikes out across ancient lava flows.

TRAIL USE
Dayhike, Backpack

LENGTH
11.8 miles, 5–6 hours

VERTICAL FEET
±5100′

DIFFICULTY
– 1 2 3 4 **5** +

TRAIL TYPE
Out & Back

SURFACE TYPE
Dirt, Grass, Lava, Paved, Sand

START & END
N 20.71470°
W 156.25064°

FEATURES
Lava Flows
Mountain
Birds
Native Plants
Wildlife
Great Views
Geologic Interest
Historic Interest
Steep

FACILITIES
Visitor Center
Restrooms
Picnic Tables
Phone
Water

Best Time

You can hike this trail year-round. Weather in the high-altitude summit region of Haleakala is unpredictable, however; the trail can be hot and sunny one minute, freezing cold and rainy the next. Starting soon after sunrise means that you'll stay ahead of the guided horseback tour groups on the way down. Avoid hiking midday, when the high-altitude sunshine is most intense.

Finding the Trail

From Kahului, follow the Hana Highway (Hwy. 36) southeast past the airport turnoff, then turn right onto the Haleakala Highway (Hwy. 37). Drive uphill for almost 8 miles, then turn left, continuing on the Haleakala Highway (Hwy. 377). Drive about 6 more miles uphill toward Kula, turning left on Hwy. 378, which becomes Crater Road. Continue for a little more than 10 winding, slow-moving miles uphill through open range for grazing livestock to the park's entrance station.

After paying the entrance fee or showing your pass, keep driving uphill for a little more than 10 miles to a stop-sign intersection. Continue straight ahead into the paved parking lot for the summit visitor center (if you turn right, the main park road continues another 0.5 mile uphill to the volcano's actual summit).

If you are staying overnight at Kapalaoa cabin, note that wilderness permits are not available at the summit visitor center. Instead you must pick them up en route to the trailhead at the park headquarters visitor center, less than a mile uphill from the entrance station along the main road. Permits are only available between 8 AM and 3 PM daily.

Trail Description

The panoramic views are peppered with colorful cinder cones, lava flows, and shaggy cliffs covered in vegetation.

The park's summit visitor center (open from 5:15 AM to 3 PM daily) sits at a dizzying elevation of 9740 feet above sea level. Signs advise visitors to walk slowly and not overexert themselves until they become acclimated. Watch for signs of altitude sickness (see page 14). Ask visitor center staff if nonpotable water is available at Kapalaoa cabin. If so, bring a way to purify it. If not, pack in all the water you'll need for this strenuous hike, plus some extra in case of emergencies. Outside the visitor center you'll find restrooms and drinking fountains.

The Sliding Sands Trailhead is on the west side of the **summit visitor center parking lot**. ►1 Walk along the paved sidewalk toward the main park road. The trail passes a metal hitching post used by guided horseback tour groups as it circles the base of Pa Kaoao (White Hill). Reached via a short trail, the top of this cinder cone is a popular perch for sunrise watchers. By the time the ground underfoot turns to cinders, it becomes obvious how the Sliding Sands Trail got its name. But don't worry: The trail is broad enough and compacted by so many hundreds of hikers' feet that your chances of slipping or sliding are quite small.

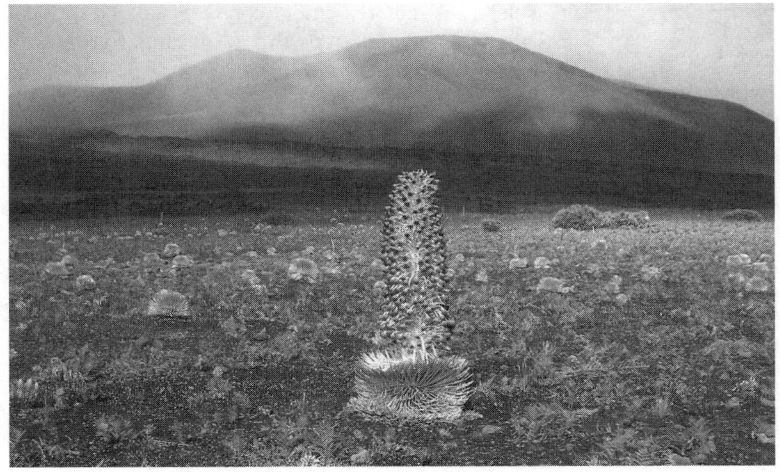

Rare silversword plants *bloom only once in a lifetime before dying.*

The trail's signature switchbacks drop steeply away from the main park road. Equally breathtaking are the panoramic views down into the erosional valley of Haleakala's summit region, peppered with colorful cinder cones, lava flows, and shaggy cliffs covered in vegetation. Plant life is quite sparse along this initial part of the trail, but the farther down the switchbacks you go, the more rare silversword plants you'll notice popping up alongside the path. You may also encounter chukar, a small exotic game bird with distinctive brown and white dorsal body stripes. The larger endangered nene (Hawaiian goose) has a black head, buff-colored cheeks, and a grayish-brown body.

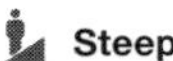

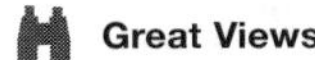

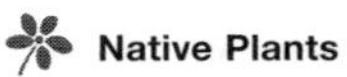

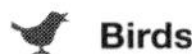

Almost 2 miles from your starting point, the Sliding Sands Trail passes the junction with a spur trail out to Ka Luu o ka Oo cinder cone (see the "Options" box, page 243). Over the next 2 miles, the switchbacks continue descending, but eventually at a more moderate pace. The trail becomes rockier as it passes through crumbly *aa* lava fields, and Puu o

Pony Express Tours leads guided horseback trips along the Sliding Sands Trail. For more information and reservations, call (808) 667-2200 or visit www.ponyexpresstours.com.

Pele, a rust-colored cinder cone, appears off to your left. The trail sidesteps this giant cinder cone and bottoms out on the volcano floor. Nearby is a metal hitching rail used by guided horseback tour groups. Regrettably, the yellow-flowered mamane tree growing here is often littered with aluminum cans, plastic bottles, food wrappers, and toilet paper. Please do your part to leave no trace by packing out all of your trash.

Just past the hitching post, you reach a major signposted trail junction. Turning left here takes you north toward Holua. Instead **continue straight ahead at this Y-junction** ▶**2** toward Kapalaoa, 1.9 miles away. This next long, fairly straight stretch of trail is mostly level and made up of soft gray cinders. More native vegetation, including green ferns and young silversword plants, grow alongside the trail in the moister shadow of the *pali* (cliffs) that rise off to your right. At the next two minor trail junctions, keep hiking straight ahead—do not veer left into the volcano's cinder desert.

Almost 6 miles from the visitor center, the Sliding Sands Trail arrives at **Kapalaoa cabin**, ▶**3** set on a small grassy ledge partly sheltered by the *pali* that serve as a dramatic backdrop. Built in the 1930s by the Civilian Conservation Corps, the Kapalaoa wilderness cabin provides a little shade for hikers

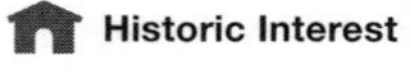

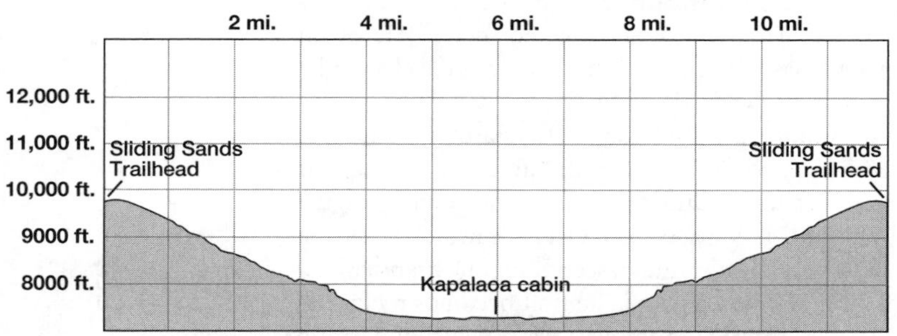

TRAIL 29 Sliding Sands Trail to Kapalaoa Elevation Profile

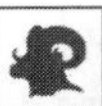

OPTIONS

Alternate Hikes to and from Kapalaoa

For a longer dayhike, add a 1.2-mile side trip out to Ka Luu o ka Oo cinder cone (see Trail 28, page 233). To extend this dayhike into an overnight trip, you could spend the night at Kapalaoa's wilderness cabin. (For details about cabin reservations, permits, and fees, see page 15.)

under its eaves. There's a picnic table out front and a composting toilet nearby. Nene often wander about the cabin, barking and shamelessly begging for food. Help keep these endangered birds wild by not feeding them or letting them drink from the spigot, which provides nonpotable water for hikers (except during times of drought).

When you've rested and had a picnic lunch, retrace your steps all the way west back to the bottom of the switchbacks. Although the climb back to the summit is strenuous, the views on the return trip are just as inspiring as on the way down. Rangers advise that ascending the switchbacks may take up to twice as long as the initial descent, but hikers in good condition will likely arrive back at the **summit visitor center parking lot ▶4** in about two hours or less.

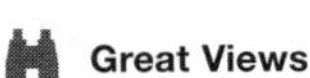

MILESTONES

▶1	0.0	Start at summit visitor center parking lot [N 20.71470°, W 156.25064°]
▶2	4.0	Go straight at Y-junction toward Kapalaoa [N 20.70687°, W 156.21307°]
▶3	5.9	Arrive at Kapalaoa cabin [N 20.70654°, W 156.18402°]
▶4	11.8	Return to summit visitor center parking lot [N 20.71470°, W 156.25064°]

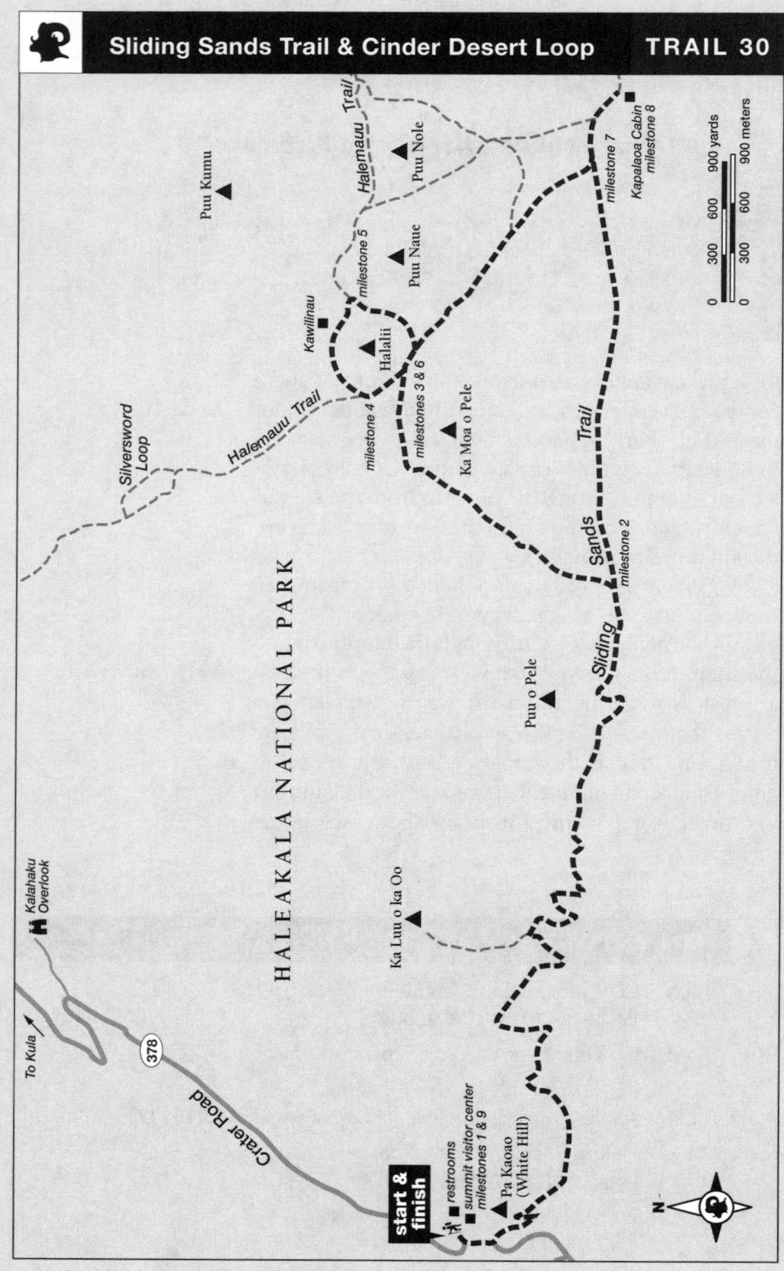

Sliding Sands Trail & Cinder Desert Loop
TRAIL 30
HALEAKALA NATIONAL PARK
Halemauu Trail
Puu Kumu
Puu Nole
Puu Naue
Kawilinau
Halalii
milestone 5
milestone 4
milestones 3 & 6
milestone 7
Kapalaoa Cabin
milestone 8
Ka Moa o Pele
Silversword Loop
Sliding Sands Trail
milestone 2
Puu o Pele
Ka Luu o ka Oo
Kalahaku Overlook
To Kula
378
Crater Road
start & finish
restrooms
summit visitor center
milestones 1 & 9
Pa Kaoao
(White Hill)
N
0
300
600
900 yards
900 meters

Sliding Sands Trail & Cinder Desert Loop

If you've got energy to burn for a strenuous dayhike, this trip tackles the memorable Sliding Sands Trail, starting near Haleakala's summit. Down on the volcano floor, it wanders on crowd-free side trails around towering cinder cones and past Kawilinau, a unique site of archaeological and geologic interest.

TRAIL USE
Dayhike, Backpack

LENGTH
13.6 miles, 6–8 hours

VERTICAL FEET
±5550′

DIFFICULTY
– 1 2 3 4 **5** +

TRAIL TYPE
Semiloop

SURFACE TYPE
Dirt, Grass, Lava, Paved, Sand

START & END
N 20.71470°
W 156.25064°

FEATURES
Lava Flows
Mountain
Birds
Native Plants
Wildlife
Great Views
Geologic Interest
Historic Interest
Archaeological
Steep

FACILITIES
Visitor Center
Restrooms
Picnic Tables
Phone
Water

Best Time

You can hike this trail year-round. Weather in the high-altitude summit region of Haleakala is unpredictable, however; the trail can be hot and sunny one minute, freezing cold and rainy the next. Starting soon after sunrise means that you'll stay ahead of the guided horseback tour groups on the way down. Avoid hiking midday, when the high-altitude sunshine is most intense.

Finding the Trail

From Kahului, follow the Hana Highway (Hwy. 36) southeast past the airport turnoff, then turn right onto the Haleakala Highway (Hwy. 37). Drive uphill for almost 8 miles, then turn left, continuing on the Haleakala Highway (Hwy. 377). Drive about 6 more miles uphill toward Kula, turning left on Hwy. 378, which becomes Crater Road. Continue for a little more than 10 winding, slow-moving miles uphill through open range for grazing livestock to the park's entrance station.

After paying the entrance fee or showing your pass, keep driving uphill for a little more than 10 miles to a stop-sign intersection. Continue straight ahead into the paved parking lot for the summit visitor center (if you turn right, the main park road continues another 0.5 mile uphill to the volcano's actual summit).

If you are staying overnight at Kapalaoa cabin, note that wilderness permits are not available at the summit visitor center. Instead you must pick them up en route to the trailhead at the park headquarters visitor center, less than a mile uphill from the entrance station along the main road. Permits are only available between 8 AM and 3 PM daily.

Trail Description

On clear days, you might even glimpse Mauna Kea and Mauna Loa on the Big Island of Hawaii.

The park's summit visitor center (open from 5:15 AM to 3 PM daily) sits at a dizzying elevation of 9740 feet above sea level. Signs advise visitors to walk slowly and not overexert themselves until they become acclimated. Watch for signs of altitude sickness (see page 14). Ask visitor center staff if nonpotable water is currently available at Kapalaoa cabin. If so, bring a way to purify it. If not, pack in all the water you'll need for this strenuous hike, plus some extra in case of emergencies. Outside the visitor center you'll find restrooms and drinking fountains.

From the west end of the **summit visitor center parking lot**, ▶1 start walking on the paved sidewalk back toward the main park road. The trail passes a metal hitching rail used by guided horseback tour groups as it circles the base of Pa Kaoao (White Hill), a popular perch for sunrise watchers. Soon the Sliding Sands Trail turns to cinders underfoot, but don't be nervous about either slipping or sliding—the trail is broad enough to walk on easily, and passes only a few sheer (and easily avoided) drop-offs.

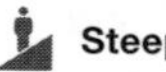

The start of the famous switchbacks may take your breath away—not just because of the trail's high altitude, but also for its sweeping views of

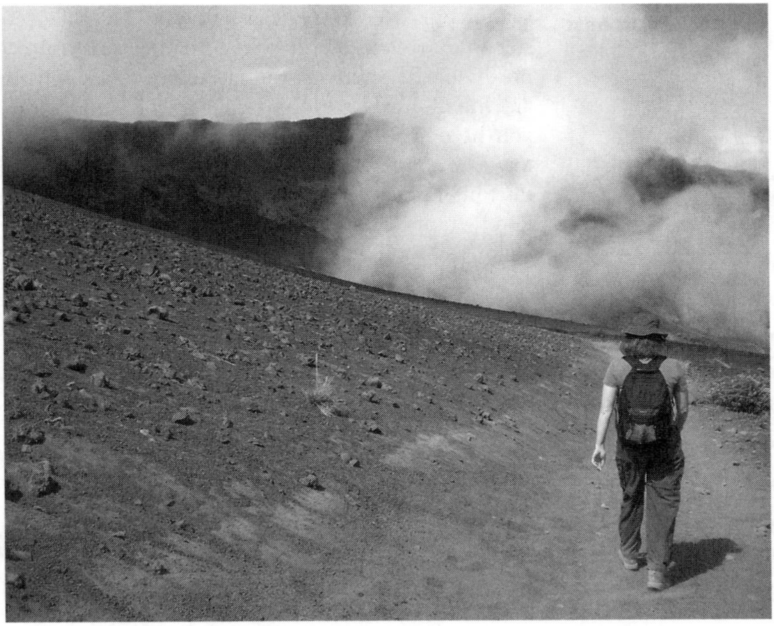

Descending through misty clouds *into Haleakala volcano's cinder desert*

rainbow-colored cinder cones, sprawling lava flows, and rough-edged *pali* (cliffs) flush with green vegetation. On clear days, you might even glimpse the neighborly volcanic peaks of Mauna Kea and Mauna Loa on the Big Island of Hawaii in the distance across Alenuihaha Channel. As you make your way slowly down the switchbacks, look for common yellow-flowering kupaoa plants, as well as the rare and threatened silversword, with its shiny green leaves and flowering stalks of maroon blossoms, hardily growing alongside the trail.

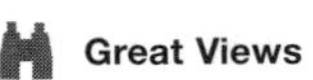

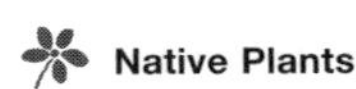

Almost 2 miles from your starting point, you reach a junction with a spur trail leading left out to Ka Luu o ka Oo cinder cone (see the "Options" box, page 251). Past that junction, the main trail keeps descending on switchbacks that become less steep

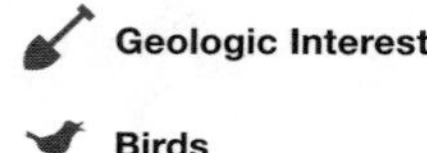

Geologic Interest

Birds

as they pass over rocky *aa* lava flows . The trail sidesteps Puu o Pele, a rust-colored cinder cone to the north. Endangered nene (Hawaiian geese), which are friendly and curious birds, might start tailing you here. The switchbacks finally end near a yellow-flowering mamane tree growing next to a metal hitching rail used by guided horseback tour groups. Food wrappers, empty bottles, and used toilet paper are often found littered about. Please pack out all of your trash.

Ancient Hawaiians once made the trek down into the volcano to drop the umbilical cords of newborn babies into Kawalinau, praying it would give their children strength.

Just beyond the hitching post, approximately 4 miles from the trailhead, **veer left at the signposted Y-junction toward Holua**, ►2 instead of continuing straight ahead toward Kapalaoa. As you walk northeast along a softer cinder trail, you'll notice giant cinder cones looming to your right, while ahead in the distance rises the triangular peak of Hanakauhi (elevation 8907 feet), just east of the volcano's eroded Koolau Gap. The trail reaches a small crest, then rolls downhill to the next major junction. **Turn left at the next four-way junction toward Holua** ►3 and start circling Halalii cinder cone.

After 0.3 mile, **veer right at the Y-junction with Halemauu Trail toward Kawilinau**, ►4 continuing clockwise around the cinder cone. The trail crests a small rise, then passes a spectacular volcanic vent with rainbow-colored cinders. Descending once again, the trail passes over jet-black cinder soil to Kawilinau, about 0.4 mile from the previous trail junction. Nicknamed the "Bottomless Pit," Kawilinau is actually only 65 feet deep. Ancient Hawaiians once made the trek into the volcano to drop the umbilical cords of newborn babies into this pit, praying it would give their children strength.

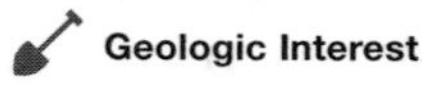

Geologic Interest

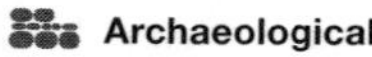

Archaeological

Just past Kawilinau, **turn right at the T-junction toward Kapalaoa**. ►5 Start hiking south across the saddle between Halalii and Puu Naue cinder cones. After just 0.4 mile, you are back where you started circling Halalii. On the south side of the

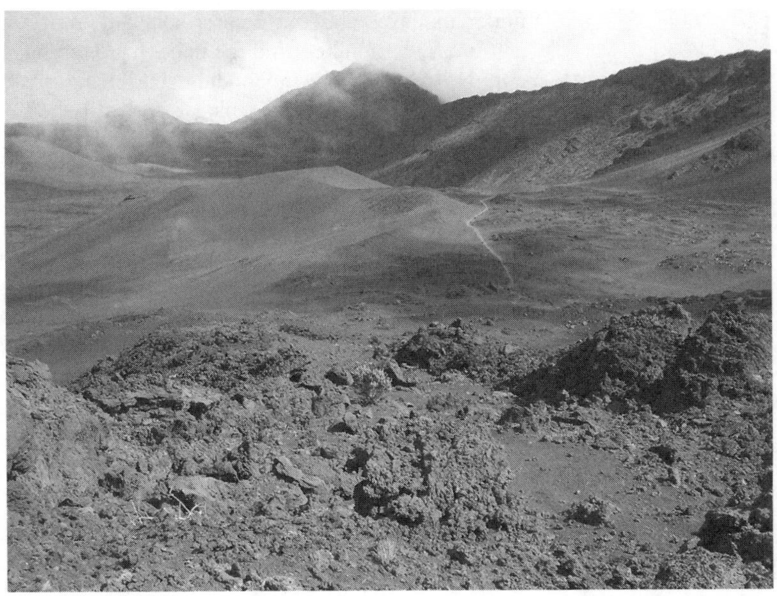

A network of trails *for dayhikers and backpackers beckons in Haleakala's summit area.*

cinder cone, **turn left at four-way junction toward Kapalaoa.** ►6 Gradually dropping through the cinder desert, this spur trail crosses both smooth *pahoehoe* and rocky *aa* lava flows before turning to soft gray-black cinders underfoot. The trail is edged by shrubby ohia lehua plants with red berries often gobbled by nene. Slowly, Kapalaoa cabin comes into view ahead. About 1.1 miles from the previous junction, **turn left at the Y-junction with the Sliding Sands Trail toward Kapalaoa,** ►7 only 0.2 mile away. Ignore the next junction with a side trail that leads back north into the cinder desert.

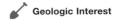

Geologic Interest

Hiking straight ahead, you soon arrive at **Kapalaoa cabin,** ►8 set on a grassy ledge nestled beneath the *pali* (cliffs). This historic wilderness cabin was originally built in the 1930s by the Civilian Conservation Corps (CCC). The shade

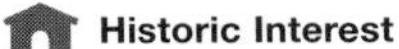

Historic Interest

Birds

under its eaves and the picnic table out front are enjoyed by both hikers and the nene that often hang out. No matter how much these endearing geese may beg, feeding them is illegal and also harms these endangered birds, which need to remain unhabituated to human food to survive in the wild. At the cabin, you'll find a nonpotable water spigot (available except during times of drought) and a composting toilet nearby.

When you're refreshed and ready, start hiking west of Kapalaoa cabin along the Sliding Sands Trail. For the first 2 miles west of the cabin, the trail remains fairly level, passing over gray-black cinders. Covered in vegetation, steep *pali* rise off to your left, with native ferns and silversword plants popping up by your feet. At each of the next three trail junctions, continue straight ahead (do not veer off right toward Holua cabin). From the bottom of the switchbacks, it's a strenuous 4-mile hike back uphill to the summit visitor center. Rangers advise that climbing back

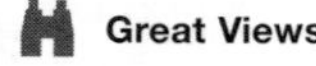

Great Views

up the switchbacks may take twice as long as your initial descent, but hikers in good condition can reach the **summit visitor center parking lot ►9** in two hours or less.

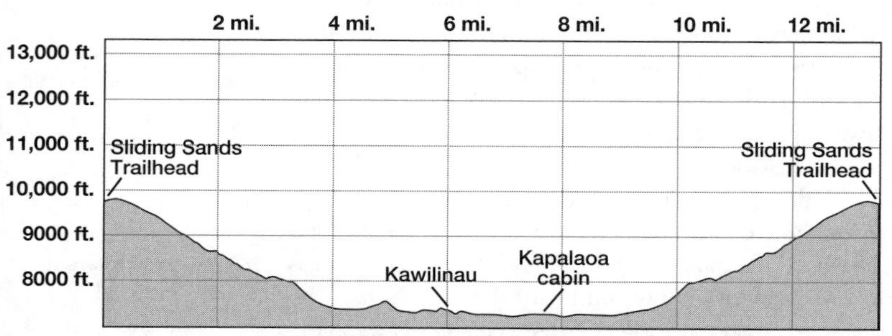

TRAIL 30 Sliding Sands Trail & Cinder Desert Loop Elevation Profile

MILESTONES

▶1	0.0	Start at summit visitor center parking lot [N 20.71470°, W 156.25064°]
▶2	4.0	Veer left at Y-junction toward Holua [N 20.70687°, W 156.21307°]
▶3	5.3	Turn left at four-way trail junction toward Holua [N 20.71775°, W 156.19997°]
▶4	5.6	Veer right at Y-junction toward Kawilinau [N 20.72120°, W 156.20164°]
▶5	6.0	Turn right at T-junction toward Kapalaoa [N 20.72128°, W 156.19638°]
▶6	6.4	Turn left at four-way junction toward Kapalaoa [N 20.71775°, W 156.19997°]
▶7	7.5	Turn left at Y-junction toward Kapalaoa [N 20.70791°, W 156.18807°]
▶8	7.7	Arrive at Kapalaoa cabin [N 20.70654°, W 156.18402°]
▶9	13.6	Return to summit visitor center parking lot [N 20.71470°, W 156.25064°]

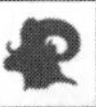

OPTIONS

Alternate Hikes to and from Kapalaoa

For a longer dayhike, add a 1.2-mile side trip out to Ka Luu o ka Oo cinder cone (see Trail 28, page 233). To extend this dayhike into an overnight trip, you could spend the night at Kapalaoa's wilderness cabin. (For details about cabin reservations, permits and fees, see page 15.)

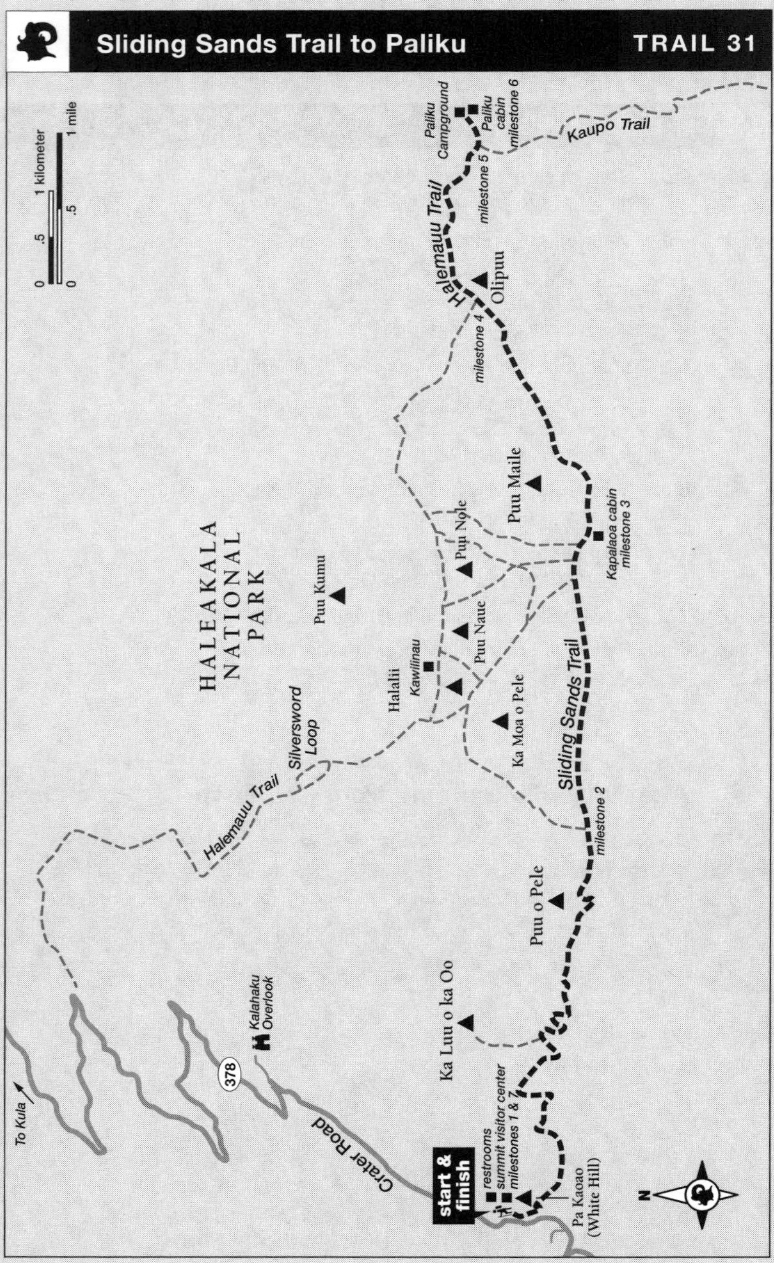

0 .5 1 kilometer
0 .5 1 mile
HALEAKALA NATIONAL PARK
Paliku Campground
Paliku cabin milestone 6
Kaupo Trail
milestone 5
Halemauu Trail
Olipuu
milestone 4
Puu Maile
Kapalaoa cabin milestone 3
Puu Nole
Puu Kumu
Puu Naue
Kawilinau
Halalii
Ka Moa o Pele
Sliding Sands Trail
Silversword Loop
Halemauu Trail
milestone 2
Puu o Pele
Ka Luu o ka Oo
Kalahaku Overlook
378
To Kula
Crater Road
start & finish
restrooms
summit visitor center
milestones 1 & 7
Pa Kaoao (White Hill)
N

Sliding Sands Trail to Paliku

If you're not making a grand loop around Haleakala's summit region (see Trail 33, page 269), this out-and-back trip is the next best thing. Trek past cinder cones and across lava flows to the volcano's lush windward side at Paliku, a peaceful, tucked-away spot.

TRAIL USE
Backpack, Permit Required

LENGTH
18.4 miles, 2 days

VERTICAL FEET
±6900′

DIFFICULTY
– 1 2 3 4 **5** +

TRAIL TYPE
Out & Back

SURFACE TYPE
Dirt, Grass, Lava, Paved, Sand

START & END
N 20.71470°
W 156.25064°

FEATURES
Lava Flows
Mountain
Birds
Native Plants
Wildlife
Great Views
Geologic Interest
Historic Interest
Secluded
Steep

FACILITIES
Visitor Center
Restrooms
Picnic Tables
Phone
Water

Best Time

You can hike this trail year-round. Weather in the high-altitude summit region of Haleakala is unpredictable, however; the trail can be hot and sunny one minute, freezing cold and rainy the next. Starting soon after sunrise means you'll stay ahead of the guided horseback tour groups and avoid the intense midday sun on the way down to Kapalaoa. The final stretch to windward Paliku can be cold and rainy, especially later in the afternoon.

Finding the Trail

From Kahului, follow the Hana Highway (Hwy. 36) southeast past the airport turnoff, then turn right onto the Haleakala Highway (Hwy. 37). Drive uphill for almost 8 miles, then turn left, continuing on the Haleakala Highway (Hwy. 377). Drive about 6 more miles uphill toward Kula, turning left on Hwy. 378, which becomes Crater Road. Continue for a little more than 10 winding, slow-moving miles uphill through open range for grazing livestock to the park's entrance station.

After paying the entrance fee or showing your pass, continue driving uphill for less than a mile to the park headquarters visitor center. Go inside to pick up your wilderness permit for overnight trips (for details about camping and cabins, see page 15). Permits are only available between 8 AM and 3 PM daily.

From the headquarters visitor center, keep driving almost 9.5 miles uphill along the main park road to the stop-sign intersection. Continue straight ahead into the paved parking lot for the summit visitor center. (If you turn right, the main park road continues another 0.5 mile uphill to the volcano's actual summit.)

Trail Description

The atmosphere at Paliku is peaceful, as it's often socked in by rain clouds and mist.

Outside the park's summit visitor center (open from 5:15 AM to 3 PM daily), you'll find restrooms and drinking fountains. Ask the visitor center staff if nonpotable water is currently available at Kapalaoa and Paliku cabins. If so, bring a way to purify it. If not, you must pack in all the water you'll need for your overnight trip, both for drinking and for cooking, plus some extra in case of emergencies.

You'll find the trailhead on the west side of the **summit visitor center parking lot**. ▶1 Follow the sidewalk toward the main park road, passing the metal hitching rail used by guided horseback tour groups. As you circle Pa Kaoao (White Hill), the trail turns to cinders underfoot. Once you're on the south side of the cinder cone, the panoramic views may halt you in your tracks. Ahead, switchbacks dive deep into Haleakala's erosional valley, peppered with cinder cones in a rainbow of hues. It looks as if you'll be walking on another planet.

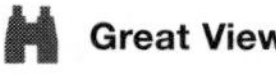
Great Views

Although steep, the switchbacks are broad and the cinders compacted by thousands of hikers' boots. There's little danger of literally slipping or sliding off of the trail, despite its name. As the switchbacks descend, yellow-flowering kupaoa plants and shiny-

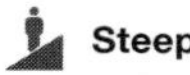
Steep

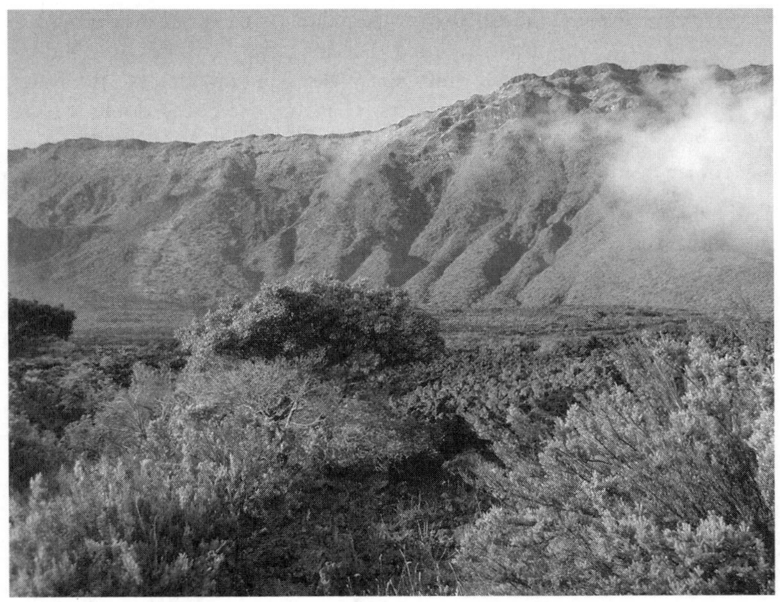

The landscape *becomes lush approaching Paliku on Haleakala's rainier side.*

leafed silversword plants, which send up stalks of maroon blossoms only once in their lifetime, pop up beside the trail. About halfway down the switchbacks, about 2 miles from the summit visitor center, you reach a small junction with a spur trail that leads left toward Ka Luu o ka Oo cinder cone (see the "Options" box, page 259).

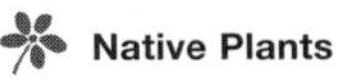

The main Sliding Sands Trail plows straight ahead, switchbacking through rockier lava flows and sidling around Puu o Pele, a prominent rust-colored cinder cone on your left. Finally leveling out, the trail reaches a yellow-flowered mamane tree next to a metal hitching rail used by guided horseback tours. Litter (e.g., aluminum cans, plastic bottles, food wrappers, and toilet paper) is often found around the tree. Please pack out all your trash. **At the next Y-junction, continue straight**

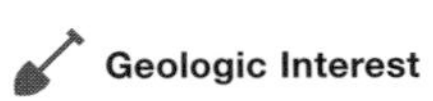

The strenuous climb back up the Sliding Sands Trail is alleviated by the grandeur of the views.

Historic Interest

Birds

Geologic Interest

Native Plants

ahead toward Kapalaoa, ►2 instead of veering left toward Holua. For the next 1.9 miles, the Sliding Sands Trail gently eases its way across lava flows on soft cinders. Giant cinder cones dominate the landscape off to your left, while eroded *pali* (cliffs) rise on your right.

Ignore the next two minor trail junctions that you encounter, where spur trails lead off left (i.e., north) deeper into the volcano's cinder desert. Instead keep hiking straight ahead toward **Kapalaoa cabin**, ►3 nestled on a grassy ledge in the shadow of the steep pali. Built by the Civilian Conservation Corps (CCC) in the 1930s, this rustic wilderness cabin has a picnic table out front, as well as a non-potable water spigot (available except during times of drought) and a composting toilet nearby. You'll often find Haleakala's endangered nene (Hawaiian geese) hanging about the cabin, enjoying the shade. Please do not feed or give any water to these friendly creatures, no matter how persistently they beg. Remaining wild and untamed is the key to this species' survival in the volcano, which is their natural habitat.

Heading east of Kapalaoa cabin, the Sliding Sands Trail drops through fields of jagged *aa* lava. At first Puu Maile cinder cone stays in view off to the left, then disappears into the lava rock landscape. The terrain is not particularly beautiful here, with dry gullies and only a few native shrubs such as white-flowering pukiawe and red-berried ohelo, the latter a favorite food of the nene. Slowly, a round-topped cinder cone partly cloaked by vegetation appears ahead in the distance. About 2 miles from Kapalaoa cabin, you reach the base of **Olipuu cinder cone**. ►4 Veer right toward Paliku at the signposted Y-junction of the Sliding Sands and Halemauu trails.

Continuing east toward Paliku, the landscape becomes more verdant where native plants and trees

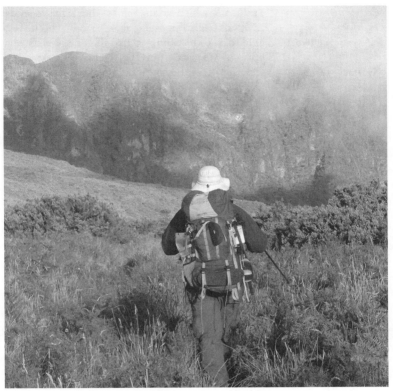

After rainstorms, look for waterfalls *cascading down the cliffs.*

flourish on the rainier windward side of the volcano. Intermittent expanses of smoother *pahoehoe* lava make this downhill part of the hike go faster. But be careful with your footing: There are plenty of chances to twist your ankle in dry washes and gullies. When conditions are foggy, the trail may almost vanish, so pay attention to the National Park Service trail markers and the *ahu* (cairns) left by other hikers.

A little more than a mile from Olipuu, **continue straight ahead at the junction with the Kaupo**

Trail, ▶5 which leads off to the right (see the "Options" box, opposite page). It's only another 0.2 mile to **Paliku cabin**, ▶6 like the one at Kapalaoa, built by the CCC in the 1930s. The cabin is secluded in a grassy meadow among groves of native forest trees. Bird life is abundant here, including the neighborly nene. The atmosphere at Paliku is peaceful, although your chances of seeing the sun are hit-and-miss: It's often socked in by rain clouds and mist. Waterfalls stream down the faces of the stunningly high *pali*.

Historic Interest

Native Plants

Birds

Before reaching the cabin, a short spur leads off left to the designated camping area. A nonpotable water spigot and a composting toilet are nearby. Just uphill east of the wilderness cabin, Paliku's ranger cabin is often unstaffed. If any emergencies arise, be prepared to hike all the way back out of the volcano. If you retrace your steps, it's a 9.2-mile hike back to the trailhead and the **summit visitor center parking lot**. ▶7 The strenuous climb back up the switchbacks of the Sliding Sands Trail is somewhat alleviated by the grandeur of the views along the way. Rangers advise that ascending the switchbacks may take up to twice as long as your initial descent, but experienced backpackers in good shape will likely finish faster.

Camping

Great Views

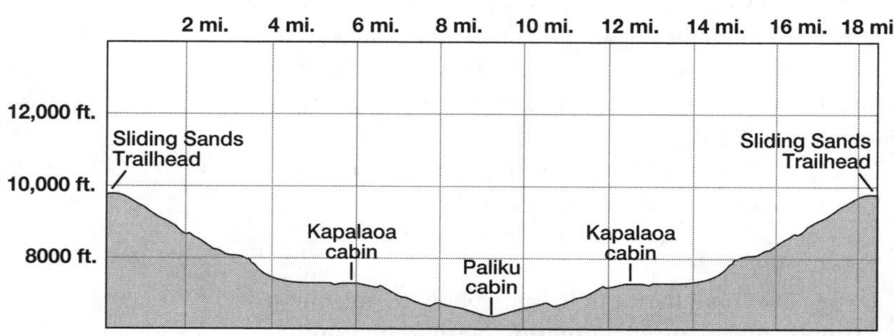

TRAIL 31 Sliding Sands Trail to Paliku Elevation Profile

Notice

Dress in warm, waterproof layers for this hike. You'll pass through different life zones and change elevation significantly, so be prepared for any kind of weather. In the same day, you might experience blistering high-altitude sunshine (wear sunscreen with a high SPF rating) and cold, wet, and windy conditions that can cause hypothermia. It's important to keep the interior of your backpack dry. That way, when you reach Paliku, your tent, sleeping bag, and change of clothes will be warm and dry.

If you're staying in the unheated wilderness cabins, do not rely on the pot-bellied woodstoves, your only external fuel source, to be in working order or stocked with enough fuel to make a fire.

MILESTONES

▶1	0.0	Start at summit visitor center parking lot [N 20.71470°, W 156.25064°]
▶2	4.0	Go straight at Y-junction toward Kapalaoa [N 20.70687°, W 156.21307°]
▶3	5.9	Arrive at Kapalaoa cabin [N 20.70654°, W 156.18402°]
▶4	7.9	Reach Olipuu cinder cone [N 20.71809°, W 156.15982°]
▶5	9.0	Veer left at Kaupo Trail junction [N 20.71657°, W 156.14517°]
▶6	9.2	Arrive at Paliku cabin [N 20.71764°, W 156.14183°]
▶7	18.4	Return to summit visitor center parking lot [N 20.71470°, W 156.25064°]

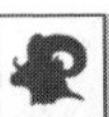

OPTIONS

Alternate Hikes to and from Paliku

You can extend this hike into a three-day backpacking trip by spending the first night at the Kapalaoa cabin before continuing to Paliku. If you have an extra day at Paliku, you could also hike partway down the Kaupo Gap for a strenuous, but beautiful side trip (see Trail 34, page 279).

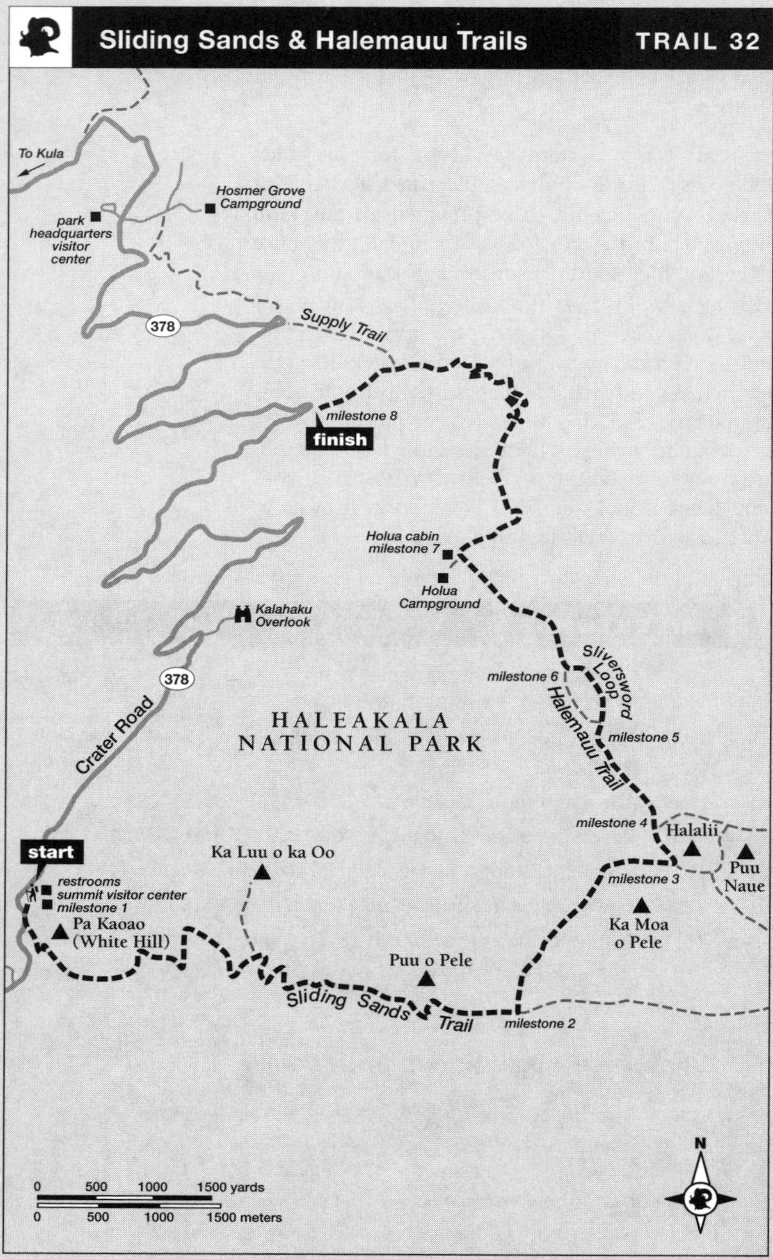

Sliding Sands & Halemauu Trails
TRAIL 32
To Kula
Hosmer Grove Campground
park headquarters visitor center
378
Supply Trail
milestone 8
finish
Holua cabin milestone 7
Holua Campground
Kalahaku Overlook
378
Crater Road
HALEAKALA NATIONAL PARK
milestone 6
Sliversword Loop
Halemauu Trail
milestone 5
milestone 4
Halalii
Puu Naue
milestone 3
Ka Moa o Pele
start
Ka Luu o ka Oo
restrooms
summit visitor center
milestone 1
Pa Kaoao (White Hill)
Puu o Pele
Sliding Sands Trail
milestone 2
N
0 500 1000 1500 yards
0 500 1000 1500 meters

Sliding Sands & Halemauu Trails

If you have only one day in Haleakala's summit region, but you want to see it all, take this trip. Trek through a cinder desert, past colorful volcanic vents and giant cones, then ascend into the volcano's cloud-forest belt. Hitchhiking between trailheads is usually easy, or you can shuttle two cars.

TRAIL USE
Dayhike, Backpack, Run

LENGTH
11.8 miles, 5–7 hours

VERTICAL FEET
±4800′

DIFFICULTY
– 1 2 3 4 **5** +

TRAIL TYPE
Point-to-Point

SURFACE TYPE
Dirt, Grass, Lava, Paved, Sand

START
N 20.71470°
W 156.25064°

END
N 20.75240°
W 156.22845°

FEATURES
Forest, Lava Flows, Mountain, Birds
Native Plants, Wildlife
Great Views, Camping
Geologic Interest
Historic Interest, Steep

FACILITIES
Visitor Center
Restrooms
Picnic Tables
Phone
Water

Best Time

You can hike this trail year-round. Weather in the high-altitude summit region of Haleakala is unpredictable, however; the trail can be hot and sunny one minute, freezing cold and rainy the next. An early morning start allows you enough time to complete the entire hike in one day; it also helps avoid late afternoon clouds and rain that can obscure the views and make the final switchbacks up the cliffs tougher.

Finding the Trail

From Kahului, follow the Hana Highway (Hwy. 36) southeast past the airport turnoff, then turn right onto the Haleakala Highway (Hwy. 37). Drive uphill for almost 8 miles, then turn left, continuing on the Haleakala Highway (Hwy. 377). Drive about 6 more miles uphill toward Kula, turning left on Hwy. 378, which becomes Crater Road. Continue for a little more than 10 winding, slow-moving miles uphill through open range for grazing livestock to the park's entrance station.

After paying the entry fee or showing your pass, continue driving uphill for 4.4 more miles, turning left into the signposted Halemauu Trailhead parking lot. If you need overnight camping or cabin permits (see page 15), stop off en route at the park headquarters visitor center, less than a mile uphill from the entrance along the main road. Permits are only available between 8 AM and 3 PM daily.

After parking your car in the Halemauu Trailhead lot, walk back out onto the main road and head briefly downhill to the officially designated hitchhiking zone on the *mauka* (inland) side of the road. You usually don't have to wait long until someone stops to give you a lift up to the summit visitor center. Alternatively, you can shuttle two vehicles, leaving one at the Halemauu Trailhead and the other at the Sliding Sands Trailhead in the summit visitor center parking lot, 6 miles farther uphill along the main park road.

Trail Description

Be awed by panoramic views into the volcano, dotted with superhero-sized cinder cones in a rainbow of colors and stark lava flows.

The park's summit visitor center (open from 5:15 AM to 3 PM daily) sits at a dizzying elevation of 9740 feet above sea level. Signs advise visitors to walk slowly and not overexert themselves until they become acclimated. Watch for signs of altitude sickness (see page 14). Ask visitor center staff if nonpotable water is available at Holua cabin. If so, bring a way to purify it. If not, you must pack in all the water necessary for this strenuous hike, plus some extra in case of emergencies. Outside the visitor center you'll find restrooms and drinking fountains.

The trailhead is on the west side of the **summit visitor center parking lot.** ▶1 Start walking on the paved sidewalk toward the main park road, passing a metal hitching rail used by guided horseback tour groups. The trail turns to cinders underfoot as you circle the base of Pa Kaoao (White Hill) a small cinder cone that's a popular sunrise-watching perch. As you round the south side of the cinder

 **Great Views**

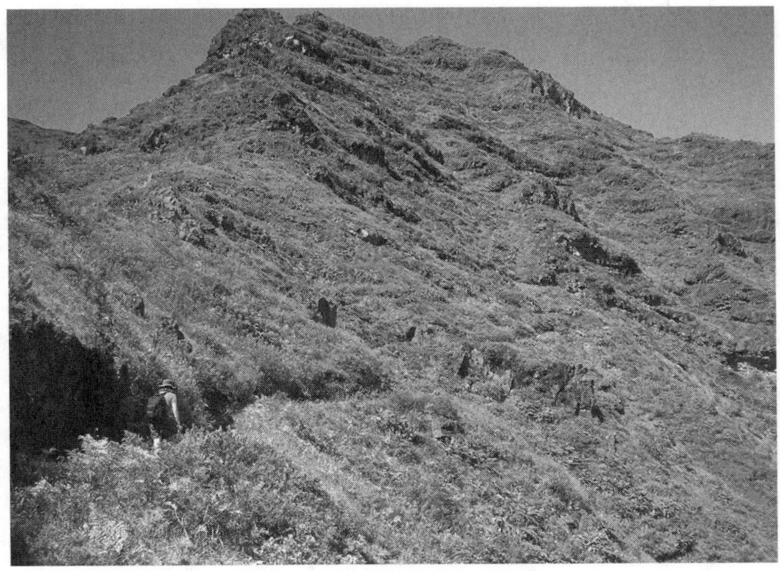

Steep switchbacks *ascend the volcano's* pali *(cliffs), flush with ferns.*

cone, you can't help but be awed by the panoramic views into the volcano, dotted with superhero-sized cinder cones in a rainbow of colors, stark lava flows, and *pali* (cliffs) covered in emerald vegetation. The trail descends on steep, but broad switchbacks. The cinders crunch and shift underfoot, but they're fairly well compacted by thousands of hikers' footsteps daily.

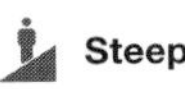

Steep

Almost 2 miles from the trailhead, you reach a junction with the spur trail leading left (i.e., north) out to Ka Luu o ka Oo cinder cone (see the "Options" box, page 267). Staying straight on the main trail, you soon notice more native plants growing alongside the footpath, such as yellow-flowering kupaoa shrubs and the rare and threatened silversword, with its shiny silver leaves that reflect intense high-altitude solar radiation. Keep descending on more gradual switchbacks over rocky *aa* lava flows,

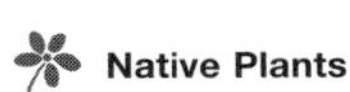

Native Plants

sidestepping Puu o Pele, a rust-colored cinder cone on your left. From there, it's all downhill to the metal hitching rail used by guided horseback tours, standing next to a yellow-flowering mamane tree.

Geologic Interest

Finally, the Sliding Sands Trail levels out about 4 miles from the summit visitor center. **Veer left toward Holua at the signposted Y-junction** ►2 (continuing straight ahead would take you toward Kapalaoa instead). As you head northeast into the volcano's cinder desert, that giant cinder cone off to the right is Ka Moa o Pele, while the strikingly green, triangular peak of Hanakauhi (8907 feet) rises on the distant horizon. After about a mile, the trail contours right around the base of Ka Moa o Pele. **Turn left at the next four-way junction toward Holua**, ►3 unless you'd like to detour to Kawilinau (see the "Options" box, page 267).

Walk clockwise around the base of Halalii cinder cone for 0.3 mile, then **veer left at the next Y-junction onto the Halemauu Trail**. ►4. Heading northwest toward Holua, the Halemauu Trail strikes out across barren-looking *aa* lava flows colored only in shades of gray and black. This stretch of the trail starts out level, gradually gaining in elevation. It traverses perhaps the most alien-looking area of Haleakala's summit region, looking a lot like Mars as it traverses past rust-colored cinders and ancient volcanic rocks.

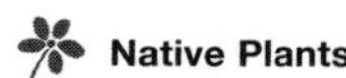

Less than a mile from the previous junction, **detour right onto the signposted Silversword Loop**. ►5 This spur trail rolls through a natural "garden" of silversword plants, which bloom only once in a lifetime when they send up tall stalks of maroon flowers. Don't stray from the trail—the fragile cryptobiotic soil supporting the threatened plants' root systems is easily damaged. After about 0.4 mile, **turn right at the T-junction to rejoin the Halemauu Trail**. ►6 From here, it's a little more than a mile's trek to Holua cabin and campground,

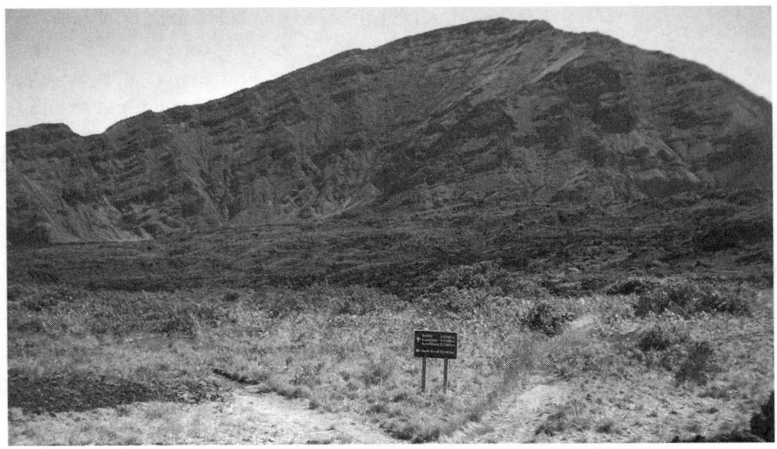

The volcano's summit region *is crisscrossed by hardy trails for dayhikers and backpackers.*

crossing jagged *aa* lava flows partly colonized by hardy native plants, including green ferns and ohelo bushes with red berries that feed nene.

When a rustic wilderness cabin comes into view off to your left, look for a minor T-junction. Turn left onto the spur trail for a short walk over to **Holua cabin**, ►7 built in the 1930s by the Civilian Conservation Corps. Outside the cabin you'll find a picnic table and a nonpotable water spigot (available except during times of drought). Friendly, curious nene often hang out in the shade here, begging for a snack. By not feeding them or giving them any water, you're helping the wild population of these endangered birds thrive. If you're camping overnight at Holua, follow the short use trail directly south of the cabin and uphill, veering left around the ranger cabin (usually unstaffed) and a composting toilet. Already impacted campsites sit on a small ledge beneath the cliffs, partly sheltered from the wind by short lava-rock walls.

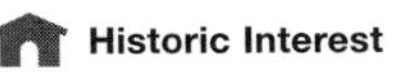

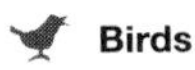

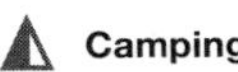

When you're ready, retrace your steps to the small T-junction, turning left back onto the main

Halemauu Trail. It's about a mile's walk across rocky *aa* lava flows with few patches of shade. The trail turns grassy underfoot as you arrive at a wooden gate at the base of the volcano's craggy cliffs. Close the gate securely behind you; it's designed to keep out wild pigs and grazing livestock that would otherwise devastate the volcano's fragile ecosystem. The Halemauu Trail's well-cut switchbacks start out steeply, but soon relax into a more gradual climb. Native Hawaiian ferns cling to the cliffs wherever water seeps through the lava rock. Interestingly, the fringed amauu ferns commonly seen here change color from reddish pink to dark green as they age.

Steep

By the time you've hiked 2 miles from Holua cabin, you're already halfway up the switchbacks. The trail contours around a final ridge to emerge in native shrubland where red-berried ohelo bushes, pink-flowered pukiawe shrubs, and yellow-blooming mamane trees flourish. Hawaiian honeycreepers, such as bright red apapane and iiwi and yellow-green amakihi, flit about the blossoming flowers and trees. Enjoy the breathtaking panoramas at eye level with the clouds, gazing down the volcano's slopes all the way to the ocean. About 0.7 mile before reaching the main park road, you pass the junction with the Supply Trail, which steeply descends toward the Hosmer Grove access road (for details, see the

Hawaiian honeycreepers, such as bright red apapane and iiwi and yellow-green amakihi, flit about the blossoming flowers and trees.

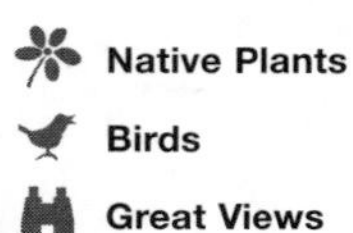

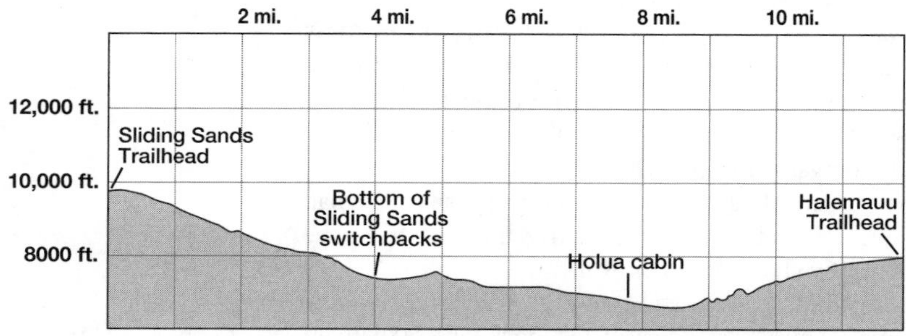

TRAIL 32 Sliding Sands & Halemauu Trails Elevation Profile

"Options" in Trail 24, page 211). Continue straight ahead at this junction, veering left and switchbacking uphill to finish at the **Halemauu Trailhead parking lot**. ►8

MILESTONES

►1	0.0	Start at summit visitor center parking lot [N 20.71470°, W 156.25064°]
►2	4.0	Veer left at Y-junction toward Holua [N 20.70687°, W 156.21307°]
►3	5.3	Turn left at four-way trail junction toward Holua [N 20.71775°, W 156.19997°]
►4	5.6	Veer left at Y-junction toward Holua [N 20.72120°, W 156.20174°]
►5	6.4	Detour right onto Silversword Loop [N 20.73037°, W 156.20615°]
►6	6.8	Turn right back onto Halemauu Trail [N 20.73298°, W 156.20892°]
►7	7.8	Arrive at Holua cabin [N 20.74163°, W 156.21796°]
►8	11.8	Finish at Halemauu Trailhead parking lot [N 20.75240°, W 156.22845°]

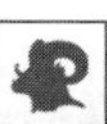

OPTIONS

Detours & Overnight Trips

For a longer dayhike, take the inspiring 1.2-mile detour out to Ka Luu o ka Oo cinder cone (see Trail 28, page 233) or add a side trip to Kawilinau, also known as the "Bottomless Pit" (see the hike description for Trail 30, page 245). To get to Kawilinau, stay straight ahead at the four-way junction (Milestone 3 of this hike), then turn left after 0.4 mile at the T-junction onto the Halemauu Trail. This detour adds 0.5 mile of total distance to your trip.

You could also extend this dayhike into a two-day backpacking trip by staying overnight in the cabin or camping at Holua (for details about backcountry camping and cabins, see page 15).

Haleakala Grand Loop — TRAIL 33

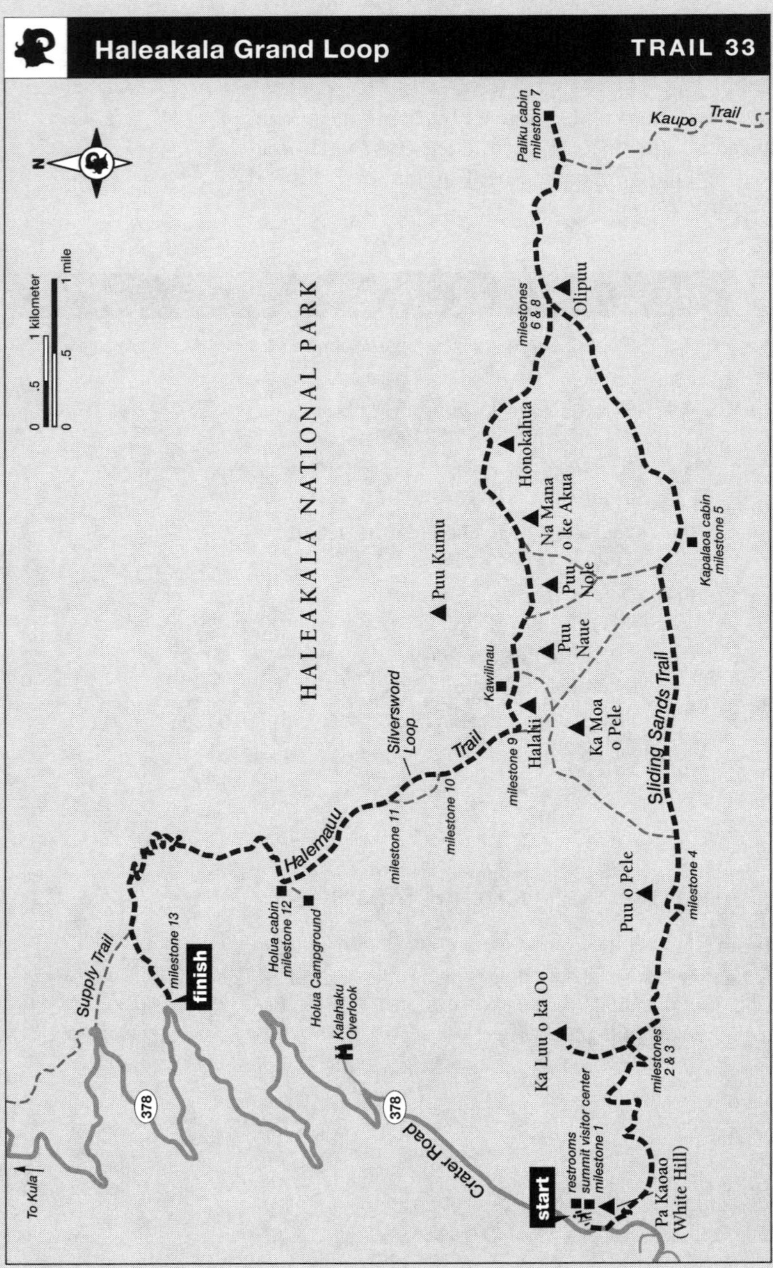
N
0
.5
1 kilometer
0
.5
1 mile
HALEAKALA NATIONAL PARK
Paliku cabin
milestone 7
Kaupo
Trail
Olipuu
milestones
6 & 8
Honokahua
Na Mana
o ke Akua
Kapalaoa cabin
milestone 5
Puu
Nole
Puu Kumu
Puu
Naue
Kawilinau
Halali
Ka Moa
o Pele
Sliding Sands Trail
milestone 9
Silversword
Loop
Trail
milestone 10
milestone 11
Halemauu
milestone 4
Puu o Pele
Holua cabin
milestone 12
Holua Campground
milestone 13
Supply Trail
finish
Kalahaku
Overlook
Ka Luu o ka Oo
milestones
2 & 3
378
378
Crater Road
restrooms
summit visitor center
milestone 1
start
Pa Kaoao
(White Hill)
To Kula

Haleakala Grand Loop

This thrilling high-altitude backpacking trip makes sure hikers see everything that Haleakala's summit area has to offer, from colorful cinder cones between Holua and Kapalaoa to lacy waterfalls pouring over the craggy cliffs at Paliku. Watching the sunrise over the puffy clouds from inside the volcano itself is unforgettable.

Best Time

You can hike this trail year-round. Weather in the high-altitude summit region of Haleakala is unpredictable; the trail can be hot and sunny one minute, freezing cold and rainy the next. Starting soon after sunrise means you'll avoid the intense midday sun on the way to Kapalaoa. The final stretches to windward Paliku and up the cliffs from Holua the next day can be cold and rainy, especially in the late afternoon.

Finding the Trail

From Kahului, follow the Hana Highway (Hwy. 36) southeast past the airport turnoff, then turn right onto the Haleakala Highway (Hwy. 37). Drive uphill for almost 8 miles, then turn left, continuing on the Haleakala Highway (Hwy. 377). Drive about 6 more miles uphill toward Kula, turning left on Hwy. 378, which becomes Crater Road. Continue for a little more than 10 winding, slow-moving miles uphill through open range for grazing livestock to the park's entrance station.

TRAIL USE
Backpack,
Permit Required

LENGTH
20.9 miles, 2–3 days

VERTICAL FEET
±7000′

DIFFICULTY
– 1 2 3 4 **5** +

TRAIL TYPE
Point-to-Point

SURFACE TYPE
Dirt, Grass, Lava,
Paved, Sand

START
N 20.71470°
W 156.25064°

END
N 20.75240°
W 156.22845°

FEATURES
Forest, Lava Flows
Mountain, Birds
Native Plants, Wildlife
Great Views, Camping
Geologic Interest
Historic Interest
Archaeological
Secluded, Steep

FACILITIES
Visitor Center
Restrooms
Picnic Tables
Phone
Water

After paying the entrance fee or showing your pass, continue driving uphill for less than a mile to the headquarters visitor center. Go inside to pick up your wilderness permit for overnight trips (for details about camping and cabins, see page 15). Permits are only available between 8 AM and 3 PM daily.

From the headquarters visitor center, drive 3.5 miles farther uphill along the main park road, turning left into the signed Halemauu Trailhead parking lot. After parking your car, walk back out onto the main park road and head briefly downhill to the officially designated hitchhiking zone on the *mauka* (inland) side of the road. You usually don't have to wait long until someone stops to give you a lift up to the summit visitor center. Alternatively, you can shuttle two vehicles, leaving one at the Halemauu Trailhead and the other at the Sliding Sands Trailhead in the summit visitor center parking lot, 6 miles farther uphill along the main park road.

Trail Description

Outside the park's summit visitor center (open from 5:15 AM to 3 PM daily), you'll find restrooms and drinking fountains. Ask the visitor center staff if nonpotable water is currently available at Kapalaoa, Paliku, and Holua cabins and campgrounds. If so, bring a way to purify the water. During times of drought, you must pack in all the water you'll need for the entire trip, both for drinking and cooking, plus some extra in case of emergencies.

For more in-depth descriptions of the Sliding Sands and Halemauu trails, plus many possible route variations, see the dayhikes described earlier in this chapter.

From the west end of the **summit visitor center parking lot**, ▶1 follow the paved sidewalk toward the main park road as it curls south around Pa Kaoao (White Hill) cinder cone, a quick climb popular with sunrise watchers. The trail soon turns to cinders underfoot and begins dramatically switch-

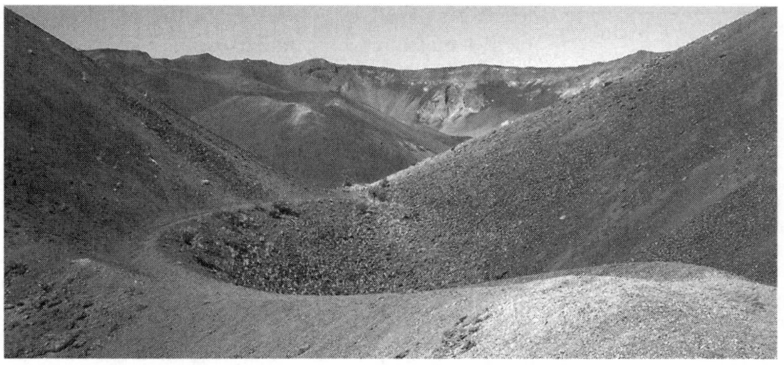

Rainbow-colored vents *await inside the volcano's erosional valleys.*

backing down into the volcano. The panoramic views of giant cinder cones, jagged lava flows, and rugged *pali* (cliffs) blanketed in green vegetation are astonishing. Although steep, the Sliding Sands Trail is fairly broad and handily compacted by thousands of other hikers' feet. Native plants are scarce alongside the trail, except for yellow-flowering kupaoa shrubs and the rare silversword plant, easily recognized by its shiny green leaves and tall stalks with maroon flowers.

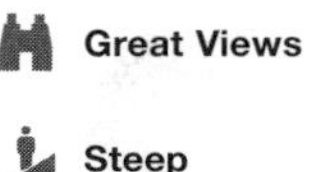

Great Views

Steep

Almost 2 miles from your starting point, **detour left onto the spur trail out to Ka Luu o ka Oo cinder cone.** ►2 After scrambling down a short, but steep slope, this spur trail starts rolling more gently downhill. It then rises again and circles a gaping volcanic vent splashed with a rainbow of colors, including rust-red, emerald, ochre, sand, and chocolate brown. The spur trail ends abruptly at a sweeping viewpoint over the volcano's erosional valley. From the overlook, retrace your steps back to the T-junction, **turning left to rejoin the main Sliding Sands Trail.** ►3

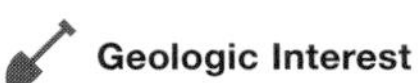

Geologic Interest

Hike another 2 miles downhill, crossing rocky *aa* lava flows and detouring around another remarkable cinder cone, Puu o Pele. The trail eventually

As the trail rounds a final ridge, it emerges into native shrubland habitat where red-berried ohelo, pink-flowered pukiawe, and yellow-blooming mamane all thrive.

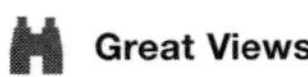

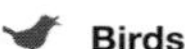

levels and then bottoms out on the volcano floor near a metal hitching rail used by horseback tour groups, set beside a landmark yellow-flowering mamane tree. **Go straight at the next Y-junction**, ►4 following the trail signs toward Kapalaoa cabin. Over the next 1.7 miles, the Sliding Sands Trail is composed mostly of soft gray cinders, bordered by native Hawaiian ferns and scattered silversword plants. At each of the next two trail junctions, continue hiking straight ahead instead of veering left (i.e., north) into the volcano's cinder desert.

Soon you arrive at **Kapalaoa cabin**, ►5 nestled on a grassy ledge partly sheltered from the wind by the steep *pali* (cliffs). Constructed by the Civilian Conservation Corps (CCC) in the 1930s, this wilderness cabin provides a little shade for hikers under its eaves. If you have cabin reservations at Kapalaoa, this is your first night's stop. Camping is prohibited, but there's a picnic table out front and a composting toilet nearby. Friendly nene (Hawaiian geese) often wander about the cabin, begging for food. Remember that you can help these endangered birds by not giving them any food or water, which only tames them and makes their survival in the wild less likely.

From Kapalaoa, the Sliding Sands Trail heads northeast, with Puu Maile cinder cone briefly dominating the landscape off to the left. The trail descends gradually, then more steeply through an arid landscape of jagged *aa* lava flows and dry gullies. The monochrome panoramas are broken up by splashes of color, including red-berried ohelo bushes and white-flowing pukiawe plants. Slowly, round-topped Olipuu cinder cone comes into view in the distance. About 2 miles after leaving Kapalaoa, **veer right at the Y-junction at the base of Olipuu cinder cone** ►6 and follow the signs toward Paliku.

With Olipuu behind you, the trail continues dropping through native shrubland and over rough

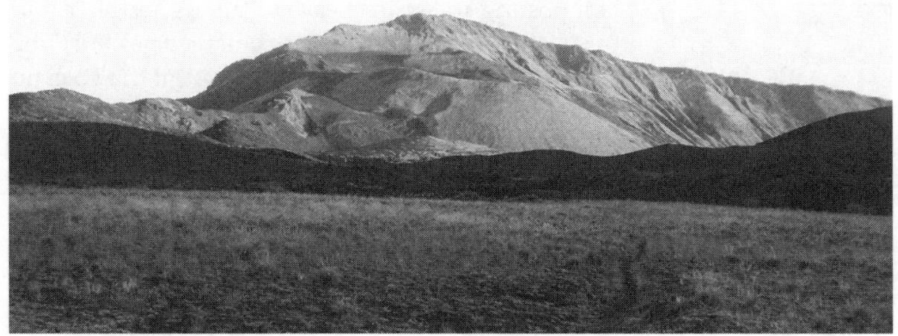

Haleakala's summit region *is a study in contrasts with stark desert-like lava flows beside lush meadows.*

aa and smooth *pahoehoe* lava flows. Native plants and trees flourish here on the windward side of Haleakala's summit area. The trail may almost disappear in the rain, fog, and mist—pay attention to official trail markers and the *ahu* (cairns) left behind by other hikers. Be careful with your footing, because there are plenty of chances to twist your ankle in dry washes and lava gullies.

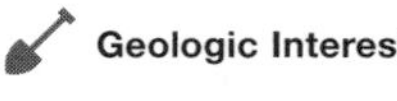

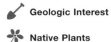

Geologic Interest

Native Plants

A little more than a mile from Olipuu, continue straight ahead at the junction with the Kaupo Trail, which leads off to the right (see the "Options" box, page 277). Another level 0.2 mile brings you to a grassy meadow and **Paliku cabin**, ►7 backed by enormous *pali* down which lacy waterfalls often stream. Compared with the volcano's cinder desert, this lush landscape seems almost miraculous. Paliku cabin was also built by the CCC during the 1930s. Today, it's a peaceful place, where native Hawaiian flora and fauna flourish.

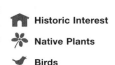

Historic Interest

Native Plants

Birds

The drawback to staying at Paliku is that it's often completely shrouded by mist and clouds. If you're lucky, though, the weather will be warm and sunny. Otherwise, Paliku can be the coldest and wettest place to sleep inside the volcano. A short spur trail before reaching the cabin leads off left to the camping area. A nonpotable water spigot and a

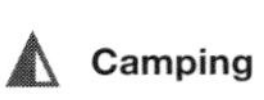

Camping

composting toilet are nearby. Paliku's ranger cabin is usually unstaffed, so if any emergencies arise, be prepared to hike all the way back out of the volcano under your own steam.

Retrace your steps to Olipuu cinder cone, about 1.3 miles west of Paliku. Where the Sliding Sands and Halemauu Trails intersect, **veer right at the Y-junction toward Holua**. ►8 Leaving Olipuu behind, the Halemauu Trail gains steadily in elevation as it rolls through verdant grasslands and a lunar landscape of lava flows. Ignore the next four trail junctions, where spur trails head south across the cinder desert back to Kapalaoa. Instead, keep hiking straight ahead toward Holua, passing several cinder cones on your left.

Archaeological

About 2.6 miles from Olipuu, the trail reaches Kawilinau, nicknamed the "Bottomless Pit," although it's actually only 65 feet deep. In ancient times, some Hawaiians ascended the volcano as a pilgrimage to drop the umbilical cords of newborn infants into this pit, believing it would give their children strength. West of Kawilinau, the Halemauu Trail passes over a small saddle, then gently descends beside a spectacular rainbow-colored volcanic vent on your left. About 0.4 mile from Kawilinau, **veer right at the Y-junction toward Holua**. ►9

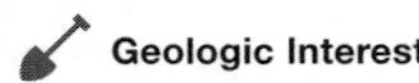

Heading northwest now, this dry stretch of the Halemauu Trail starts off level, then ascends through rocky *aa* lava flows where only a few red-berried ohelo shrubs and other native plants homestead among the cinders. About 0.8 mile from the previous junction, **detour right onto the Silversword Loop**. ►10 A delight for the eyes, this spur trail rolls up and down through a natural "garden" of silversword plants, which bloom only once in a lifetime when they send up stalks of maroon flowers. Be careful not to wander off-trail here, to prevent damage to the fragile cryptobiotic soil that supports these threatened plants' root systems.

Closing the Silversword Loop, **turn right at the T-junction to rejoin the Halemauu Trail.** ►11 It's a little more than a mile's hike across *aa* lava flows to **Holua cabin,** ►12 reached by turning left onto a short spur trail that leads west to the base of the volcano's cliffs. Like the ones at Kapalaoa and Paliku, this historic 1930s wilderness cabin was built by the CCC. Outside you'll find a nonpotable water spigot (available except during times of drought) and a picnic table, underneath which nene often hang out in the shade. If you're camping, follow the short use trail that heads uphill directly south of the cabin, then veer left around the (usually unstaffed) ranger cabin and a composting toilet. Already impacted campsites are set on a small ledge, some with low lava-rock walls that act as partial windbreaks.

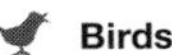

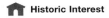

Historic Interest

Birds

Camping

Retrace your steps back to the main Halemauu Trail, turning left to hike another mile across rocky, sun-exposed *aa* lava flows. The ground underfoot becomes grassy as you approach the wooden gate at the base of the cliffs. Close the gate securely behind you, because it's the park's best line of defense against wild pigs and grazing animals that would otherwise devastate the volcano's fragile ecosystem.

Looking up, you can see the Halemauu Trail's well-cut switchbacks, which start out steeply as they make a dramatic ascent up the *pali.* Native ferns grow in some of the shadier spots; look for the fringed amauu, which turns from reddish pink to dark green as it ages. Feeling tired? Don't worry: There are fewer than 2 miles of switchbacks to hike until you're atop the cliffs.

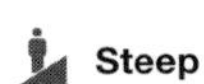

Steep

As the trail rounds a final ridge, it emerges into native shrubland habitat where red-berried ohelo, pink-flowered pukiawe, and yellow-blooming mamane all thrive. Hawaiian honeycreepers such as bright-red apapane and iiwi and yellow-green amakihi, fly about the blossoming flowers and trees. Even more eye-catching are the sweeping

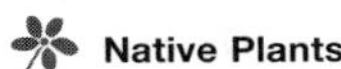

Native Plants

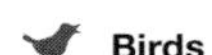

Birds

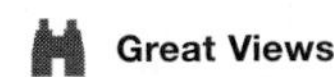

Great Views

views down the volcano's slopes all the way to the Pacific Ocean. About 0.7 mile from the main park road, the Halemauu Trail intersects with the Supply Trail, which doggedly descends toward Hosmer Grove (for details, see the "Options" box for Trail 24, page 211). Ignore this junction, veering left and switchbacking uphill on a rocky dirt trail to finish at the **Halemauu Trailhead parking lot**. ►13

Notice

Dress in warm, waterproof layers for this multiday hike. You'll pass through different life zones and change elevation significantly, so be prepared for any kind of weather. In just one day, you might experience blistering high-altitude sunshine (wear sunscreen with a high SPF rating) and also cold, wet, and windy conditions that can cause hypothermia. It's important to keep the interior of your backpack dry. That way, when you get to Paliku, your tent, sleeping bag, and change of clothes will be warm and dry.

If you're staying in the unheated wilderness cabins, do not rely on the pot-bellied woodstoves to be in working order or stocked with enough fuel to make a fire.

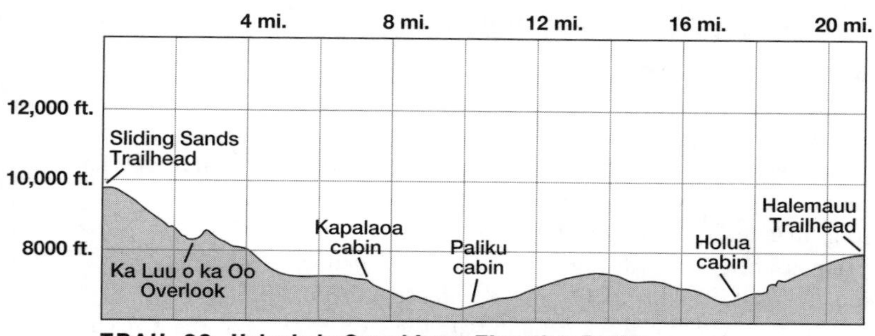

TRAIL 33 Haleakala Grand Loop Elevation Profile

MILESTONES

▶1	0.0	Start from summit visitor center parking lot [N 20.71470°, W 156.25064°]
▶2	2.0	Detour left onto Ka Luu o ka Oo spur trail [N 20.71112°, W 156.23369°]
▶3	3.2	Turn left to rejoin Sliding Sands Trail [N 20.71112°, W 156.23369°]
▶4	5.2	Go straight at Y-junction toward Kapalaoa [N 20.70687°, W 156.21307°]
▶5	7.1	Arrive at Kapalaoa cabin [N 20.70654°, W 156.18402°]
▶6	9.1	Veer right around Olipuu cinder cone [N 20.71809°, W 156.15982°]
▶7	10.4	Arrive at Paliku cabin [N 20.71764°, W 156.14183°]
▶8	11.7	Veer right at Y-junction toward Holua [N 20.71089°, W 156.15982°]
▶9	14.7	Veer right at Y-junction toward Holua [N 20.72120°, W 156.20174°]
▶10	15.5	Detour right onto Silversword Loop [N 20.73037°, W 156.20615°]
▶11	15.9	Turn right to rejoin Halemauu Trail [N 20.73298°, W 156.20892°]
▶12	16.9	Arrive at Holua cabin [N 20.74163°, W 156.21796°]
▶13	20.9	Finish at Halemauu Trailhead parking lot [N 20.75240°, W 156.22845°]

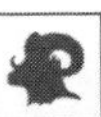

OPTIONS

Detours & Alternate Routes

If you can't get cabin reservations at Kapalaoa for the first night of this trip, plan to hike all the way to Paliku on your first day, maybe skipping the side trip to Ka Luu o ka Oo cinder cone. You could extend this backpacking trip by spending an extra night at Paliku. From there, hiking partway down the Kaupo Gap makes for a challenging, but memorable side trip (see Trail 34, page 279).

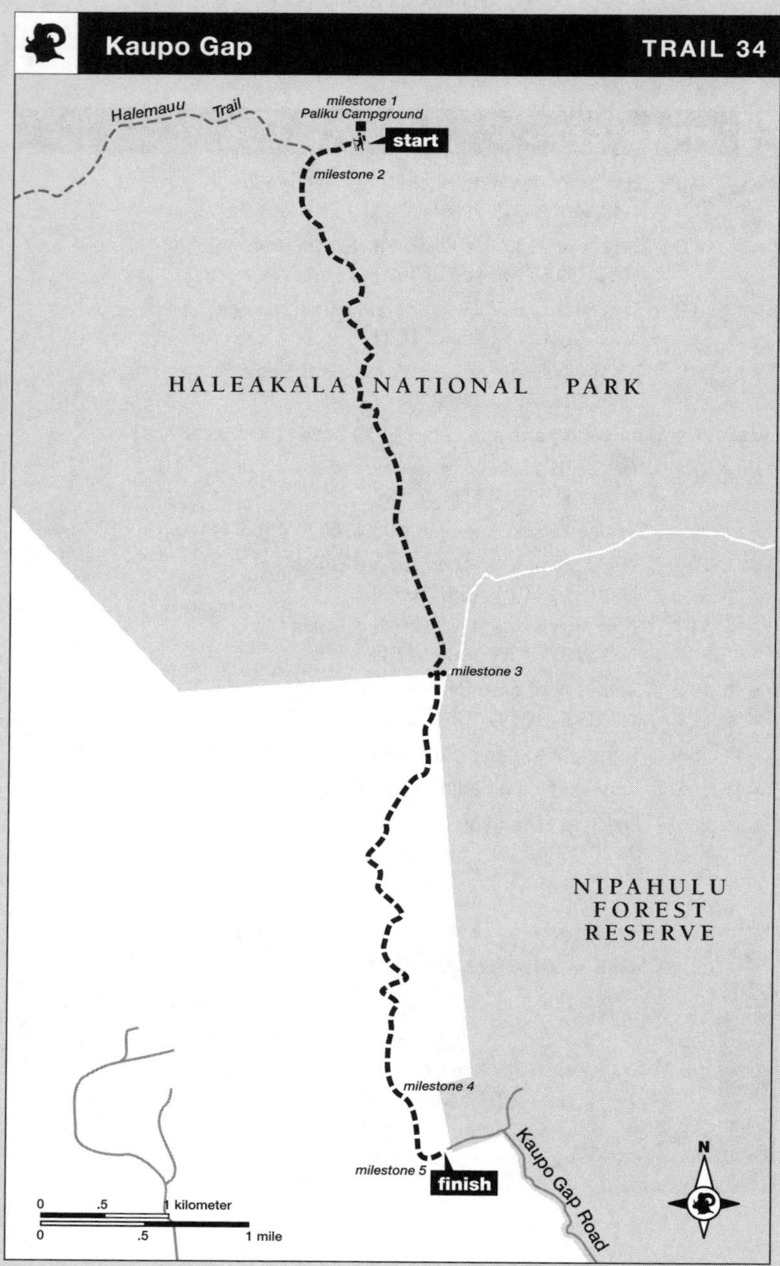
Kaupo Gap
TRAIL 34
Halemauu Trail
milestone 1
Paliku Campground
start
milestone 2
HALEAKALA NATIONAL PARK
milestone 3
NIPAHULU FOREST RESERVE
milestone 4
milestone 5
finish
Kaupo Gap Road
N
0 .5 1 kilometer
0 .5 1 mile

Kaupo Gap

Up for an epic challenge? This rugged trail switchbacks downhill from Paliku on the windward side of Haleakala all the way to Kaupo on Maui's remote south coast. Even hiking partway down this trail is worthwhile for the grand views of the ancient volcano's slopes and the sea.

Best Time

You can hike this trail year-round. Weather in the high-altitude summit region of Haleakala is unpredictable, however. It can be hot and sunny one minute, freezing cold and rainy the next. This trail is almost fully exposed as it runs over rocky lava flows and down a steep 4WD road to Kaupo. Starting soon after sunrise will help you avoid getting dehydrated by the intense heat and humidity.

Finding the Trail

The upper Kaupo Trailhead is located near Paliku, on the eastern side of Haleakala's summit region. There is no road to the trailhead. To get to Paliku, follow the hike directions for Trail 27 (10.5 miles via the Halemauu Trail) or Trail 31 (9.2 miles via the Sliding Sands Trail), described on pages 225 and 253. This is a point-to-point hike, so you'll need to arrange for a pick-up from the lower Kaupo Trailhead outside Kaupo village, or else shuttle two vehicles. Note that if you're tackling this hike in the reverse (uphill) direction, the lower Kaupo Trailhead will be your starting point.

TRAIL USE
Dayhike, Backpack

LENGTH
7.2 miles, 4–5 hours

VERTICAL FEET
-5600′

DIFFICULTY
– 1 2 3 4 **5** +

TRAIL TYPE
Point-to-Point

SURFACE TYPE
Dirt, Grass, Lava

START
N 20.71764°
W 156.14183°

END
N 20.64742°
W 156.13519°

FEATURES
Forest, Lava Flows
Mountain, Birds
Native Plants
Wildlife
Great Views
Camping
Geologic Interest
Historic Interest
Archaeological
Secluded
Steep

FACILITIES
Restrooms
Picnic Tables
Water

To get to the lower Kaupo Trailhead, drive 17 miles southwest of Hana on the Hana Highway (Hwy. 360), which becomes the Piilani Highway (Hwy. 31) around mile marker (MM) 38, west of Kipahulu. This highway is twisting, narrow, and partly unpaved, although it's usually passable by 2WD vehicles; ask at the national park's Kipahulu visitor center about road conditions before heading out. Past MM 35, just 0.1 mile before reaching the usually closed Kaupo Store, turn right onto the rutted, incredibly narrow Kaupo Gap Road, which is usually barely passable by 2WD vehicles (4WD is helpful, however). From the Piilani Highway turnoff, it's about 1.5 miles to the trailhead. Follow the road as it turns left shortly after passing some water tanks on the right. Park safely off the road at the official HALEAKALA NATIONAL PARK sign.

Alternatively, Kaupo is also accessible from Maui's Upcountry via the Piilani Highway (Hwy. 31). Heading west from Kaupo, the Piilani Highway continues for more than 20 miles (mostly paved and normally drivable by 2WD vehicles) to Ulupalakua Ranch, where the road becomes the Kula Highway (Hwy. 37). From the ranch store, it's a 25-mile downhill drive via Pukalani and the Haleakala Highway (Hwy. 37) to Kahului in Central Maui.

Native shrubs and trees crowd alongside the trail, as do tree ferns such as the fringed amauu.

Trail Description

Historic Interest

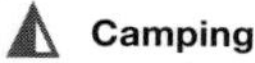

Camping

Built by the Civilian Conservation Corps in the 1930s, historic **Paliku cabin ▶1** is the starting point for this trip. Before setting off from Paliku cabin or its nearby campground, make sure all your water bottles are full. There is absolutely no water available anywhere along this trail. The sunniest, most exposed sections of the trail, including the final stretch along the 4WD road down to Kaupo, can be extremely dehydrating. Consider wearing lightweight, waterproof convertible pants, because the

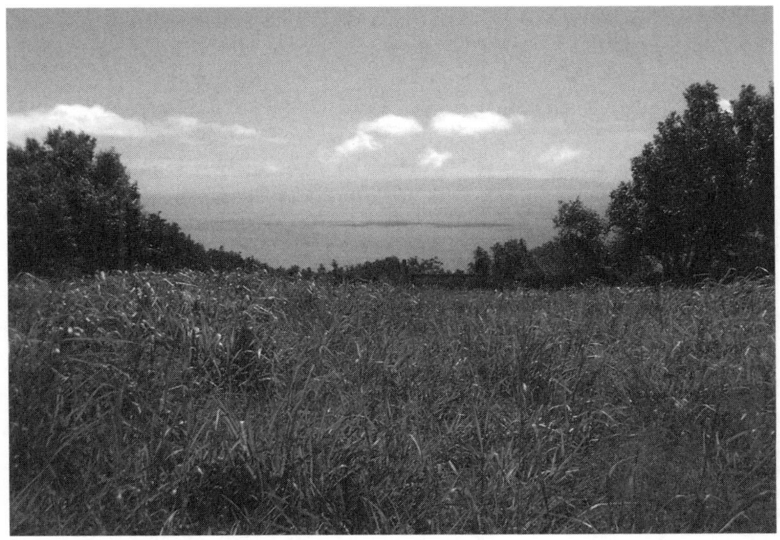

The little-trodden Kaupo Gap Trail *travels the volcano's slopes all the way down to the Pacific Ocean.*

first part of this hike down to the park boundary fence is often muddy and wet, especially with early morning dew, but by the time you reach the sun-baked coast, you'll want to be wearing shorts.

Begin by hiking 0.2 mile west of Paliku cabin, then **turn left at the Y-junction onto the Kaupo Trail**, ►2 which is clearly signposted. The trail, which starts on soft cinders, is partly overgrown by grasses. The trail winds gently downhill through native Hawaiian shrubland that's often dewy until the midday sun dries things out. The well-marked trail begins descending on rockier switchbacks, establishing a repetitive pattern of winding down to a lava bench, then dropping down into shadier forest. Native ohia lehua and mamane shrubs and trees crowd alongside the trail, as do tree ferns like the fringed amauu, which changes color from reddish pink to dark green as the plant ages.

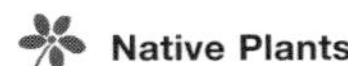

Native Plants

Great Views

Archaeological

Native Plants

Steep

Great Views

Wildlife

Less than a mile after leaving Paliku, the trail grants its first panoramic views down the ancient volcano's eroded slopes to the ocean. On clear days, you can see Hawaii's tallest volcanic peaks, Mauna Kea and Mauna Loa, rising on the Big Island in the distance across the Alenuihaha Channel. Soon the trail starts snaking along beside ancient Hawaiian lava-rock walls splattered with white lichen. Watch out for ankle-twisting sections, especially as the path steepens and becomes rockier. Curving around to the left, the trail passes a small lava-rock outcropping with incredible views of the Kaupo Gap all the way down to the sea. Waterfalls can sometimes be spotted rushing down the volcano's steep *pali* (cliffs) off to the left.

Less than 3 miles from Paliku, the trails winds through a shady grove of koa trees, easily recognized by their silvery, sickle-shaped leaves and pale yellow pom-pom flowers. Although koa is rare today, this once plentiful tropical hardwood was traditionally used by Native Hawaiians to make dugout canoes and surfboards. Next the trail passes through a small clearing, where grasses may be growing up to thigh-high, depending on when the trail was last maintained by park staff and volunteers. Make your way across the grassy clearing and keep following the trail, which drops out of the shady forest to descend more precipitously on rocky lava switchbacks. The views down the volcano's slopes to the ocean are so dreamy that sometimes the line between the blue sea and sky almost disappears.

The switchbacks once again become grassy underfoot as you pass through an area of the national park specially reserved for scientific study. Be careful not to disturb any insect traps hanging on the trees and shrubs that have been set by scientists. The trail winds through another shady grove of koa trees before **reaching the park boundary fence ▶3** at an elevation of 3880 feet, approximately 3.7 miles from Paliku. Close this gate securely behind you—it's the park's best line of defense against wild pigs and grazing livestock that would otherwise harm the volcano's fragile ecosystem. (If you're dayhiking Kaupo Gap as a side trip from Paliku, this is a good turnaround point.)

South of the boundary fence, the Kaupo Trail passes onto private property belonging to the Kaupo Ranch. The trail generally follows the main 4WD road leading steeply downhill toward Kaupo, although smaller dirt spur roads may confusingly head off in other directions—ignore them and stick to the main road. Watch out for loose rocks dangerously rolling underfoot. More than a mile south of the park boundary fence, you will likely have the option of turning left off the 4WD road to keep following the Kaupo Trail, which should be signposted. Growing narrower, the trail passes through both grassy and forested areas that are typically overgrown. Alternatively, you can keep hiking on the dirt 4WD road (unless there are KAPU—NO TRESPASSING signs posted to prevent you from doing so), which passes water tanks on its steep descent.

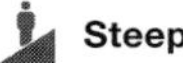

Looking down the volcano's slopes, sometimes the line between the blue sea and sky almost disappears.

In less than another mile, the Kaupo Trail rejoins the main dirt 4WD road, which keeps heading steeply downhill. After hiking for about 1 mile, **turn right off the 4WD road to keep following the trail,** ▶4 which makes its way over a couple of hikers' pass-throughs. Although confusingly laid out and often overgrown, this final 0.5-mile section of trail has been carefully signposted by the park. However, the official trail markers (wooden posts with small white directional arrows painted on them) sometimes fall down, which makes wayfinding extremely difficult. When in doubt, look for small red or faded pink ribbons tied around tree branches at eye level to help point out the trail. If you find yourself bushwhacking for more than a minute, you've probably lost the trail. In that

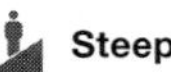

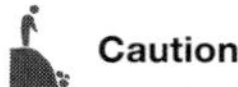

case, backtrack to your last known position and try again.

The trail becomes grassy, but only partly shaded as it rolls modestly downhill to reach the **lower Kaupo Trailhead**, ►5 marked by an official HALEAKALA NATIONAL PARK sign. If you haven't arranged for a shuttle here, it's another 1.4 miles of hiking down the partly paved Kaupo Gap Road to the Piilani Highway. Turning right onto the Pilliani Highway takes you 0.1 mile west to the Kaupo Store, which is often closed. Turning left (east), it's a sunny and exposed 7-mile hike along a narrow, hilly, and only partly paved road to the national park's Kipahulu visitor center, where you'll find a campground. Hitchhiking is difficult along this stretch of highway, as the few passing cars are mostly local.

Notice

This challenging one-way hike, especially if you're going uphill from Kaupo, should only be attempted by those in peak physical condition with no known history of medical problems at altitude. Park rangers advise that anyone with weak knees, a bad back, or heart or lung conditions should avoid hiking this trail, which can be incredibly strenuous, given the change in elevation, the steepness of descent,

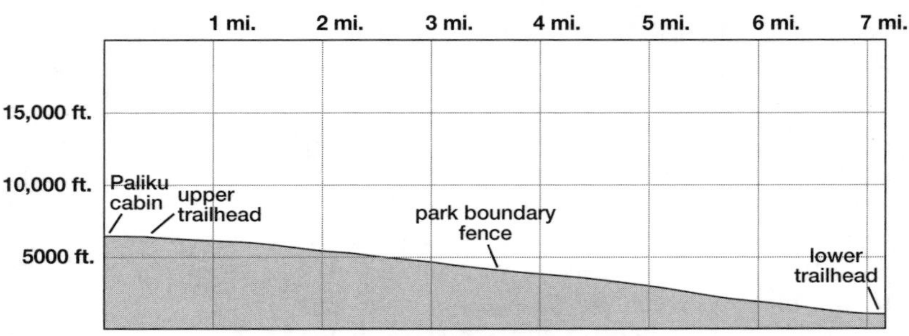

TRAIL 34 Kaupo Gap Elevation Profile

and the blistering sun exposure. You'll also need to bring plenty of water, especially because the lower section of the trail between the park boundary fence and Kaupo is extremely hot, rugged, and exposed. Nonpotable water is usually available at Kapalaoa, Holua, and Paliku cabins and camping areas (except during times of drought), but don't forget to bring a way to treat it.

MILESTONES

▶1	0.0	Start hiking west from Paliku cabin [N 20.71764°, W 156.14183°]
▶2	0.2	Turn left at Y-junction onto the Kaupo Trail [N 20.71657°, W 156.14517°]
▶3	3.7	Reach park boundary fence [N 20.68024°, W 156.13596°]
▶4	6.7	Turn right off 4WD road to keep following footpath
▶5	7.2	Finish at lower trailhead off Kaupo Gap Road [N 20.64742°, W 156.13519°]

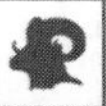

OPTIONS

Alternate Hikes

It's easier to hike this trail downhill from Paliku to Kaupo. As a side trip from Paliku, it's worthwhile just to hike down and back to the park's boundary fence, taking about four or five hours round-trip. Hiking the Kaupo Trail in the uphill direction, some marathoner hikers have successfully made it from Kaupo to Haleakala's summit area in one very long day. But that's a strenuous 16.4-mile (to the Halemauu Trailhead) or 17.7-mile (Sliding Sands Trailhead) hike with an elevation gain of 7000 to 9000 feet. Be aware that the lower part of the Kaupo Trail is much harder to find and follow when you're hiking in the uphill direction, too.

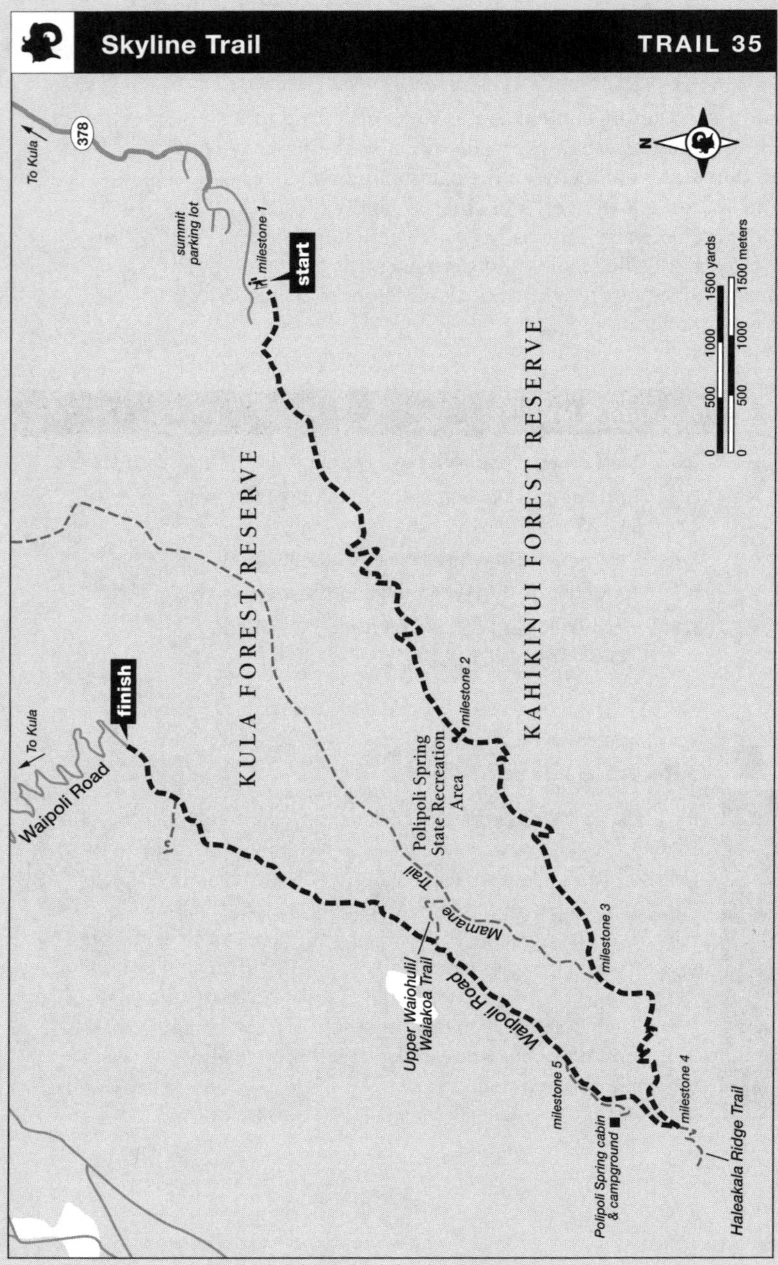
Skyline Trail
TRAIL 35
To Kula
378
summit parking lot
milestone 1
start
KULA FOREST RESERVE
KAHIKINUI FOREST RESERVE
milestone 2
Polipoli Spring State Recreation Area
To Kula
finish
Waipoli Road
Mamane Trail
Upper Waiohuli Waiakoa Trail
Waipoli Road
milestone 3
milestone 5
milestone 4
Polipoli Spring cabin & campground
Haleakala Ridge Trail
N
0 500 1000 1500 yards
0 500 1000 1500 meters

Skyline Trail

Like the Kaupo Trail, this is another seldom-trodden hike down the slopes of Haleakala volcano, this time ending inside remote Polipoli Spring State Recreation Area. This remote one-way hike is among the most adventurous on the island. Be prepared for all kinds of weather and trail conditions.

TRAIL USE
Dayhike, Backpack, Bike

LENGTH
10.5 miles, 5–7 hours

VERTICAL FEET
+200′/-3400′

DIFFICULTY
– 1 2 3 4 **5** +

TRAIL TYPE
Point-to-Point

SURFACE TYPE
Dirt, Grass, Lava, Sand

START
N 20.70594°
W 156.26106°

END
N 20.71411°
W 156.29971°

FEATURES
Forest, Lava Flows
Mountain, Summit
Birds
Native Plants
Wildlife
Great Views
Camping
Geologic Interest
Secluded
Shady
Steep

FACILITIES
Restrooms
Picnic Tables

Best Time

You can hike this trail year-round. Weather in the high-altitude summit region of Haleakala and inside Maui's cloud-forest belt is unpredictable; it can be hot and sunny one minute, freezing cold and rainy the next. Starting soon after sunrise helps avoid the most intense midday sun on the volcano's upper slopes. The latter part of this hike, inside forested Polipoli Spring State Recreation Area, is shady.

Finding the Trail

From Kahului, follow the Hana Highway (Hwy. 36) southeast past the airport turnoff, then turn right onto the Haleakala Highway (Hwy. 37). Drive uphill for almost 8 miles, then turn left, continuing on the Haleakala Highway (Hwy. 377). Drive about 6 more miles uphill toward Kula, turning left on Hwy. 378, which becomes Crater Road. Continue for a little more than 10 winding, slow-moving miles uphill through open range for grazing livestock to the park's entrance station.

After paying the entrance fee or showing your pass, keep driving uphill for a little more than 10 miles to a stop-sign intersection. Instead of

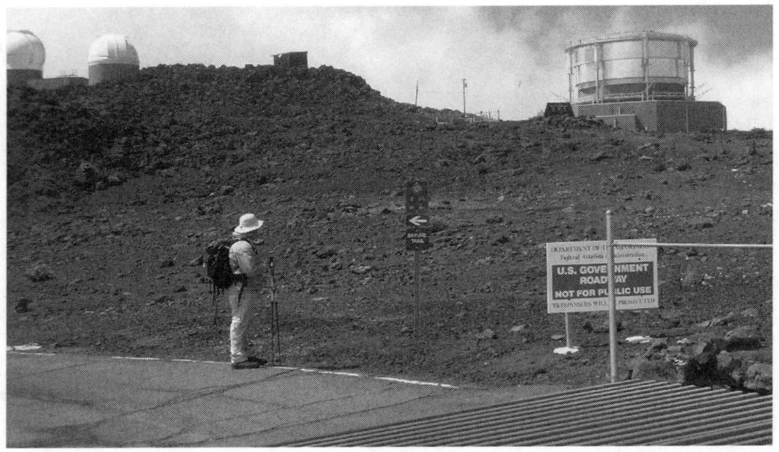
U.S. GOVE NMENT
ROAD AY
NOT FOR PU LIC USE
Government observatories *pop up around the summit area of Haleakala National Park.*

continuing straight ahead into the summit visitor center's parking lot, turn right at this intersection and drive another 0.4 mile uphill. Before reaching the summit parking lot, turn left across a menacing grate onto a paved access road clearly marked as private government property. Follow this road as it curves around toward Science City. After about 0.7 mile, look for the signposted Skyline Trailhead on your left, across the road from a microwave relay station. There's an off-road dirt parking area next to the trailhead. Without a 4WD vehicle, however, you may want to park back alongside the main paved park road, then walk the 0.7 mile along the government road to the trailhead. Alternatively, leave your car in the summit parking lot, 0.1 mile farther uphill along the main park road, then walk 0.8 mile to the trailhead.

To pick up hikers from the end of this hike inside Polipoli Spring State Recreation Area, start by following the same driving directions from Kahului as above. But instead of turning left to continue on Hwy. 377, keep driving on Hwy. 37 for another

6 miles uphill toward Kula, then turn left onto Kekaulike Ave. After only 0.3 mile, make a sharp right onto Waipoli Road. From there, it's a little more than 5 miles of winding slowly uphill along a narrow, switchbacking paved road to the hunter's check station inside Polipoli Spring State Recreation Area. The state recreation area is open for day use from 6 AM to 6 PM daily.

Past the hunters' check station, drive another 0.9 mile uphill into the state recreation area until the pavement ends. You can park cautiously along the road there, as long as you're not blocking traffic. Alternatively, if you have a 4WD vehicle, drive another 3.2 miles along the rough, unpaved access road to the intersection with the side road to Polipoli Spring's campground, saving your hikers from having to walk out to meet you. If your hikers are taking the Mamane and Upper Waiakoa and Waiohuli trails shortcut, drive only 2.2 miles along this 4WD road to where the latter trails are signposted by the roadside.

Trail Description

Although it's possible to hike the Skyline Trail in either direction, hiking downhill is much less exhausting. The upper Skyline Trailhead, near Haleakala's volcano summit, is also easier to find. If you start at Polipoli Spring State Recreation Area instead, you can expect some frustrating route-finding delays at the beginning of your trip. Note that water is *not* available anywhere along this trail, not even if you detour to Polipoli Spring SRA's cabin and campground. En route to the upper Skyline trailhead, the national park's summit visitor center is your last chance for restrooms and drinking fountains.

Watch out for signs of altitude sickness (see page 14) around the upper trailhead, especially if you've driven directly up from the coast.

Start hiking from the upper Skyline Trailhead,
►1 opposite Science City's microwave relay station.

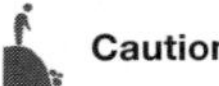
Caution

Park rangers advise walking slowly and taking it easy until you acclimate. The Skyline Trail, which sits at an elevation of nearly 10,000 feet above sea level, can literally take your breath away. Underfoot the crunchy trail is composed of rainbow-colored cinders and jagged *aa* lava that randomly rolls underfoot, so watch your step. Wind around giant cinder cones and past dramatic volcanic vents as the trail heads steadily downhill after cresting a small rise about 0.4 mile from the trailhead. On sunny days, the views can be sensational, with panoramas stretching across West Maui, even to offshore islands.

Geologic Interest

Great Views

A little more than a mile from your starting point, the trail passes near a prominent, but unnamed cinder cone on your left. From there, it veers sharply downhill to the right, continuing through a lunar-looking landscape high on the southwestern slopes of Haleakala. Soon the trail grants broader views of the ever-colorful, changing volcanic terrain. Once you've dropped below the tree line, at an elevation of around 8600 feet, you'll notice native Hawaiian plants colonizing the ancient lava flows. A little more than 2 miles from the upper Skyline Trailhead, the trail borders a grassy area, beyond which white-flowering pukiawe, yellow-blossoming mamane, and other shrubs and trees become more prolific inside the island's Kahikinui Forest Reserve.

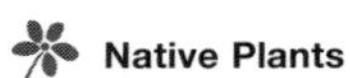
Native Plants

If you plan to bike the Skyline Trail, make sure you're experienced on tricky terrain, wearing full protective gear, and riding a quite well-maintained, full-suspension mountain bike.

Keep winding downhill along the Skyline Trail, which now feels like a wider 4WD road. Although private vehicles are not allowed on this upper part of the trail, you may hear the sounds of ATVs from the forest below. Approximately 3.4 miles from the upper Skyline Trailhead, the trail **passes through the lower Skyline Trail gate ►2** at an elevation of a little above 8000 feet. Beyond this gate, you'll be hiking on Polipoli Spring State Recreation Area's network of 4WD roads and hiking and mountain-biking trails. Watch out for feral pigs, wild goats,

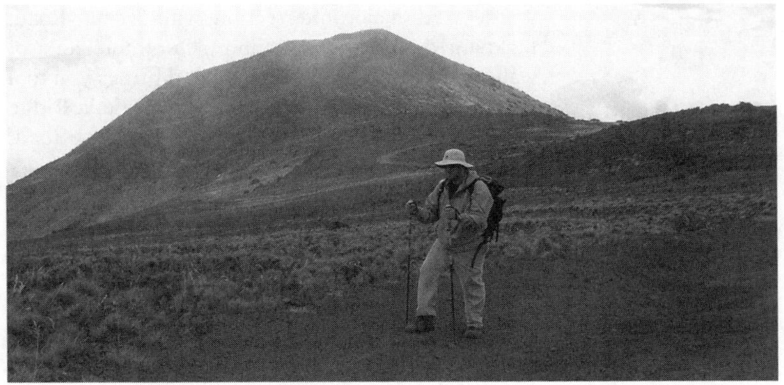

Remote Skyline Trail *starts in Haleakala's high-altitude volcanic summit region.*

and exotic game birds, as well as hunting parties with weapons, especially on weekends. Wearing bright colors (e.g., safety orange) will help alert hunters to your presence and avoid unfortunate accidents.

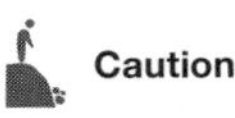

Caution

After hiking about 2 more miles downhill, **an intersection with the Mamane Trail ▶3** appears on your right. If you're up for a challenging shortcut, you can try hiking this single-track mountain biking trail, named for the common native tree that grows alongside it. After about 1.2 miles, the Mamane Trail connects with the Upper Waiohuli and Waiakoa Trail. Turning left, the Upper Waiakoa and Waiohuli Trail leads steeply down the mountainside for 0.7 mile to meet the state recreation area's unpaved access road. This shortcut saves you a little more than 1 mile of hiking. However, these side trails may be in almost impassable condition and not clearly signed. Some hikers will find it pretty tough going, even if they manage to follow the trails all the way down to Polipoli's access road.

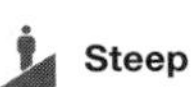

Steep

Although it takes longer, it's much easier (at least, navigationally speaking) to keep walking downhill along Skyline Road for almost a half mile

Great Views

to the next major intersection with Kahua Road, nicknamed “Ballpark Junction.” One more mile of walking downhill along Kahua Road brings you to **a signposted intersection with the Haleakala Ridge Trail** ▶4 on your left. From this bend in the road, you may enjoy views of offshore islands, if Polipoli's normally thick layer of clouds don't obscure the horizon. Keep hiking along the main road, which curves to the right and continues downhill for a half mile to the **junction with the side road to Polipoli Spring campground**, ▶5 leading off to your left. This 4WD-only side road heads downhill for about 0.5 mile to a backcountry campground and house-keeping cabin (see the “Options” box, facing page).

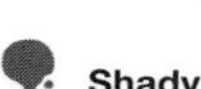
Shady

Dayhikers should continue straight ahead along the bumpy, often muddy and gloomy pine-shaded 4WD road for approximately 3.2 miles to **finish where the 4WD road meets the paved road** ▶6 inside Polipoli Spring State Recreation Area, less than a mile uphill from the hunter's check station.

Notice

This challenging one-way hike should only be attempted by people in good physical condition with no known medical problems at altitude. You'll

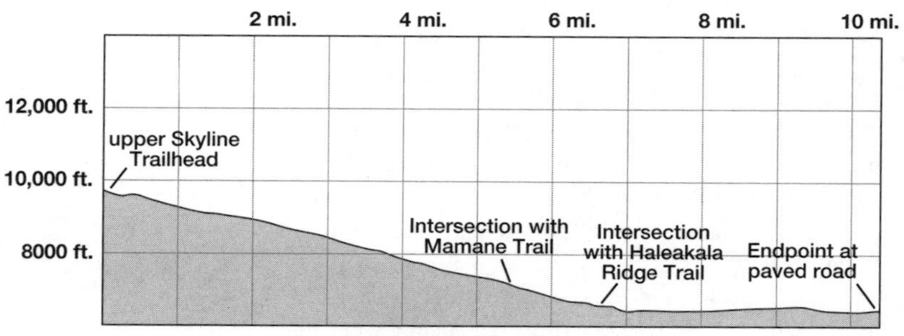

TRAIL 35 Skyline Trail Elevation Profile

need to bring plenty of water, as water is *not* available anywhere along this trail. Dress in warm, waterproof layers for this hike—you'll pass through different life zones and change elevation significantly. During the course of one day, you might experience blistering high-altitude sunshine and cold, wet, and windy conditions that can hasten the onset of hypothermia. It's best not to hike alone, because of the trail's remoteness.

MILESTONES

▶1	0.0	Start at upper Skyline Trailhead [N 20.70594°, W 156.26106°]
▶2	3.4	Reach lower Skyline Trail gate
▶3	5.4	Pass intersection with Mamane Trail
▶4	6.8	Pass intersection with Haleakala Ridge Trail
▶5	7.3	Pass side road to Polipoli Spring SRA campground
▶6	10.5	Finish at paved road inside Polipoli Spring SRA [N 20.71411°, W 156.29971°]

OPTIONS

Overnight Trips

If you want to extend this dayhike into a backpacking trip, you can stay overnight inside Polipoli Spring State Recreation Area. This approach adds a little more than a mile of total distance to your trip, but the lonely campground and housekeeping cabin are rarely used by hikers. The cabin and campground are usually either occupied by hunters or else they're deserted. You'll need to carry in all of your water; water is *not* available inside Polipoli SRA. For details about permits, fees, and reservations for overnight stays, see page 16. For an explanation of why other trails inside Polipoli Spring State Recreation Area have not been included in this hiking guide, see page 11.

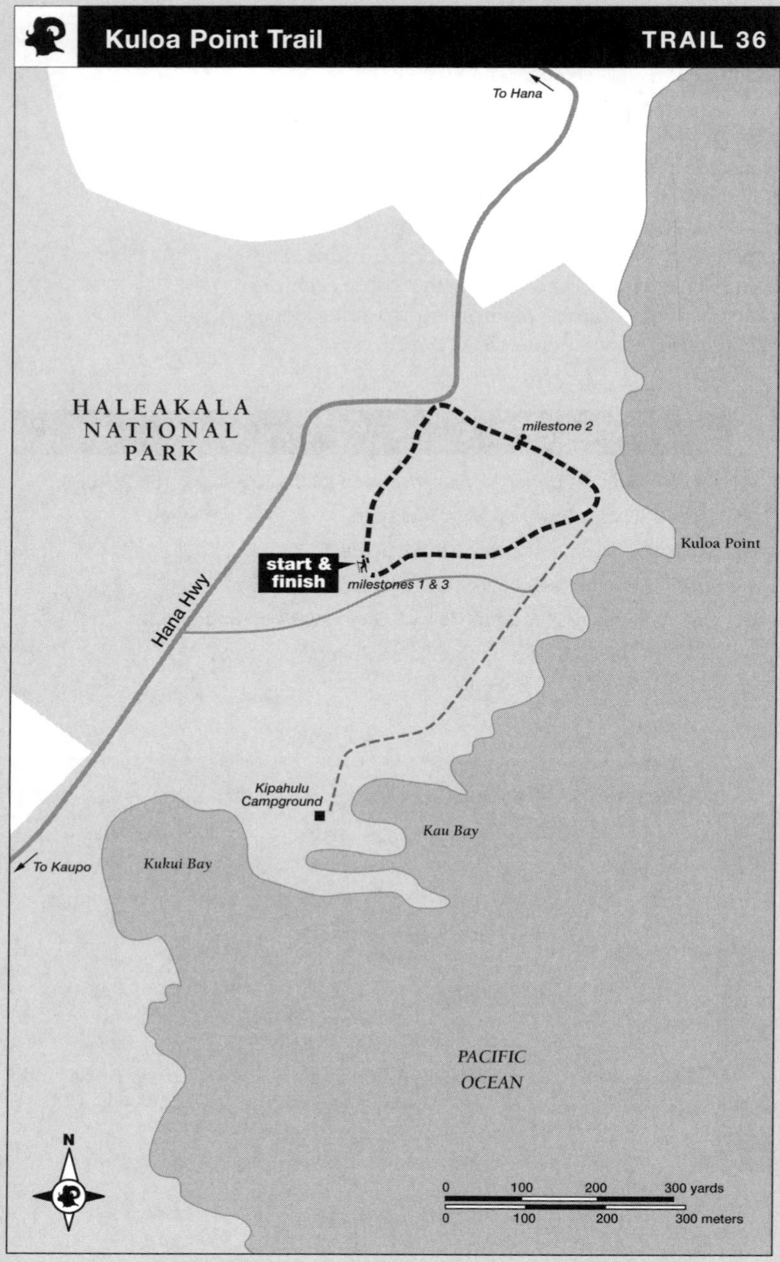
Kuloa Point Trail
TRAIL 36
To Hana
HALEAKALA
NATIONAL
PARK
milestone 2
Kuloa Point
start &
finish
milestones 1 & 3
Hana Hwy
Kipahulu
Campground
Kau Bay
To Kaupo
Kukui Bay
PACIFIC
OCEAN
N
0
100
200
300 yards
0
100
200
300 meters

Kuloa Point Trail

In the national park's coastal Kipahulu area, tumbling waterfall pools and ancient Hawaiian archaeological sites await beyond the ranch town of Hana on Maui's rural south coast. If you decide to take a dip in Oheo Gulch's pools, watch out for flash floods, which can be fatal.

TRAIL USE
Dayhike, Child Friendly
LENGTH
0.5 mile, 15–30 mins.
VERTICAL FEET
±200′
DIFFICULTY
- **1** 2 3 4 5 +
TRAIL TYPE
Loop
SURFACE TYPE
Dirt, Grass
START & END
N 20.66178°
W 156.04453°

FEATURES
Stream
Waterfall
Birds
Native Plants
Wildlife
Great Views
Swimming
Archaeological

FACILITIES
Visitor Center
Restrooms
Picnic Tables
Phone

Best Time

You can hike this trail year-round. Arrive before noon to avoid the biggest crowds of daytrippers. Ask about current conditions at the visitor center before taking a swim. Do not enter the Oheo Gulch pools if rain is forecast or there are dark clouds in the sky overhead or farther upstream (i.e., inland). Flash floods are always a possibility here.

Finding the Trail

From Hana town in East Maui, drive 10 miles southwest along the paved Hana Highway (Hwy. 360) toward Kipahulu. This stretch of highway is twisting and narrow, with one-lane bridges and blind curves and hills. Past mile marker (MM) 42, look for the national park entrance fee station and parking lot on your left.

Trail Description

Your last chance to stock up on food and water is in Hana town, though a few roadside vendors along the highway toward Kipahulu sell fresh fruit-smoothies, plate lunches, island barbecue,

A few roadside vendors along the highway toward Kipahulu sell fresh fruit smoothies, plate lunches, island barbecue, and more.

and more. At the national park's entrance station, pay the fee or show your pass, then proceed to the signed parking lot. Nearby are portable restrooms but there is *no* drinking water. From the parking lot, it's a short walk over to the visitor center (open 9 AM to 5 PM daily), which has nature displays and offers ranger talks and guided walks. Call (808) 248-7375 to check current program schedules.

Start at the **signposted trailhead**, ▶1 a short stroll east of the visitor center and parking lot on the far side of a grassy clearing. Turning left takes you on the Pipiwai Trail (see Trail 37, page 301), a beautiful dayhike up on the southern slopes of Haleakala volcano to Waimoku Falls, passing Makahiku Falls and through musical bamboo groves. Turning right onto the Kuloa Point Trail takes you instead to Oheo Gulch's famous waterfall pools, this trip's destination.

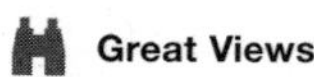
Great Views

Archaeological

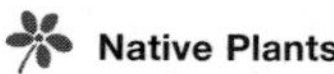
Native Plants

The trail starts off wide and grassy as it rolls gently downhill toward the sea. Past a few picnic tables set up for visitors, panoramic ocean views open up ahead. On clear days, you might glimpse the twin volcanic peaks, Mauna Kea and Mauna Loa, over on the Big Island of Hawaii across the Alenuihaha Channel. Alongside the trail, look for lava-rock walls and other evidence of the ancient Hawaiian village that once stood here along the coast. Hala (screwpine, or pandanus) trees, with their thick prop roots and triangular orange seed pods, grow beside the path. Traditionally in Hawaii, the bladelike green leaves of these trees are dried into fibrous strips that are then used for weaving, called *lauhala*.

Waterfall

The trail curves left along the coast, then starts ascending beside the gorgeous waterfall pools for which Oheo Gulch is famous. The views alone fulfill almost every fantasy of a tropical paradise, with jungly cascades tumbling downhill into frothy surf. Looking back downhill, you can see the ocean crashing against the jet-black lava rocks that border

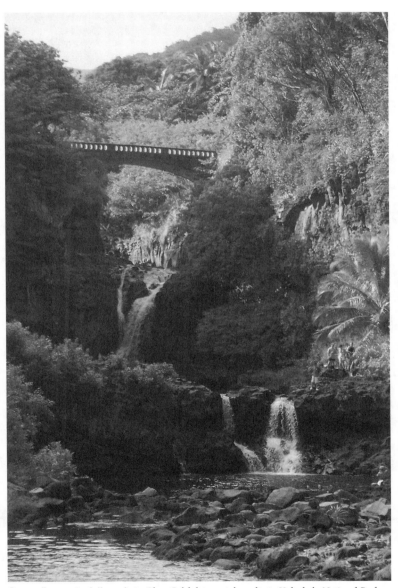

Cascading waterfall pools *in Oheo Gulch let you take a dip in Haleakala National Park.*

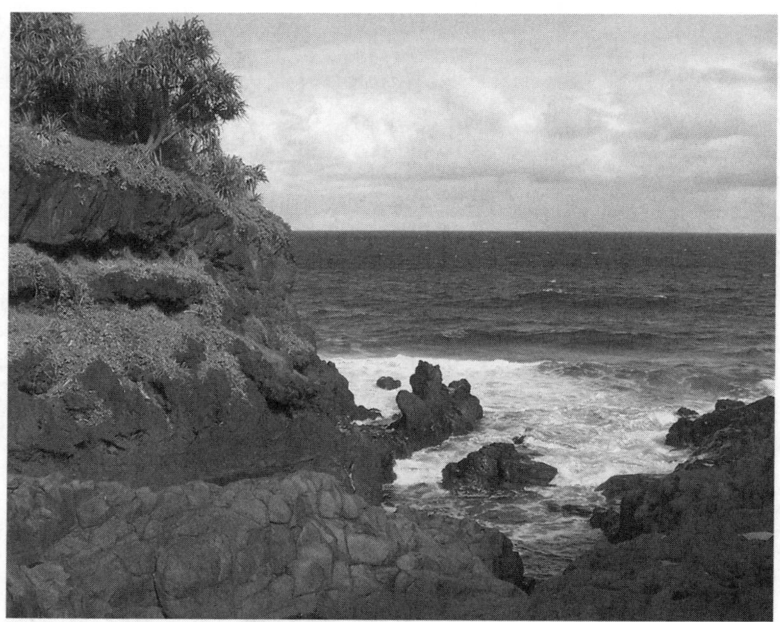

The national park's coastal Kipahulu section *is backed by stormy surf.*

Swimming

and encircle the lowest pools. Heading uphill, look for **a gated stairway down to the pools** ▶2 on your right. Remember that swimming in this area is entirely at your own risk; there are no lifeguards on duty.

It fulfills almost every fantasy of a tropical paradise, with jungly cascades tumbling downhill into frothy surf.

When you've soaked up the scenery and perhaps taken a dip (see "Notice," opposite page), rejoin the main trail and start walking up a stone staircase. For shutterbugs, there's a better overlook of the waterfall pools from the railings farther uphill. At the top of the stairs, the trail briefly continues upward, then circles around to the left and descends back downhill to the **signposted trailhead** ▶3 where you started.

Notice

If the level of water in the pools at Oheo Gulch starts to rise (e.g., because of rainfall or an approaching flash flood), get out immediately. Remember that flash floods can occur without warning any time, even if rain is *not* falling in the immediate area. Entering the ocean below the pools is foolhardy because of high surf and the presence of sharks. Jumping from the cliffs or the bridge above into the pools is also prohibited, for safety's sake.

MILESTONES

►1	0.0	Start at signposted trailhead [N 20.66178°, W 156.04453°]
►2	0.3	Reach gated stairway down to the pools
►3	0.5	Arrive back at signposted trailhead [N 20.66178°, W 156.04453°]

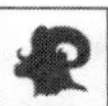

OPTIONS

Detours & Overnight Trips

For a longer coastal walk, detour along the 0.5-mile round-trip trail leading southwest along the coast from Kuloa Point to the park's primitive campground, high atop the *pali* (cliffs). For more details about free camping here (reservations *not* accepted), see page 15.

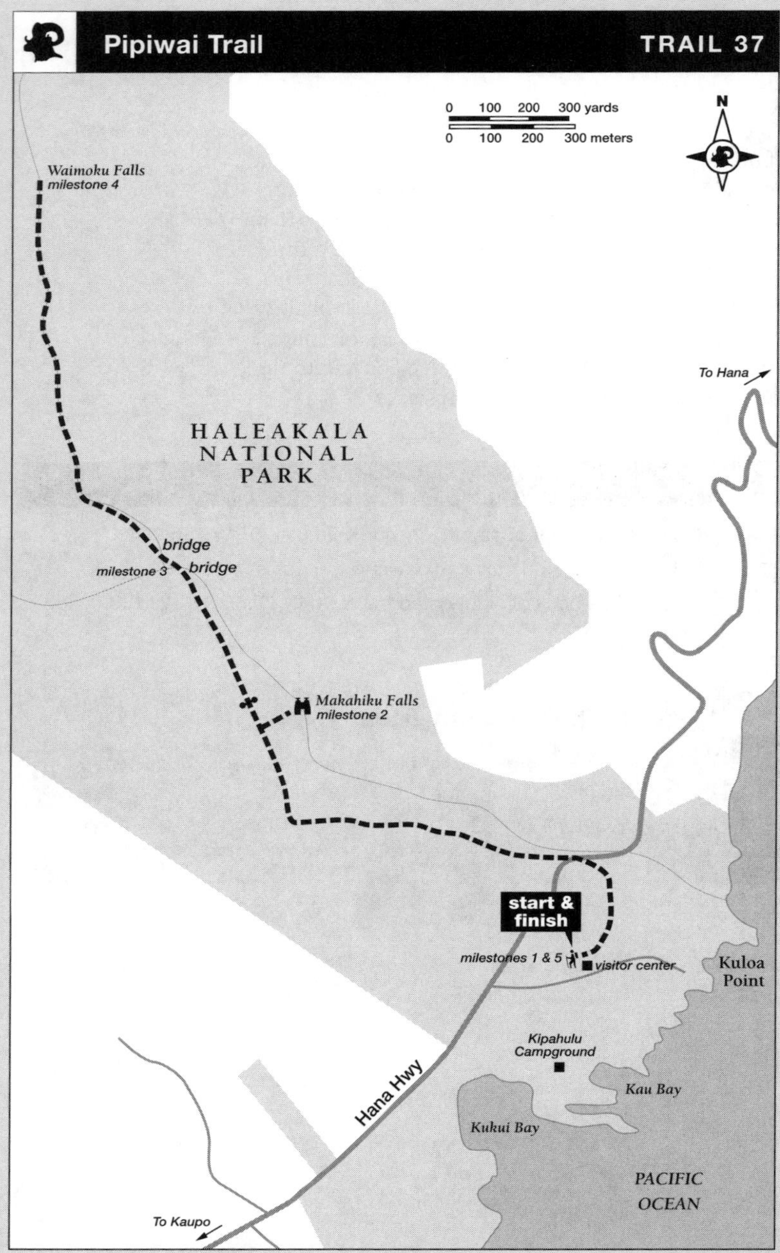
Pipiwai Trail
TRAIL 37
0 100 200 300 yards
0 100 200 300 meters
N
Waimoku Falls
milestone 4
HALEAKALA
NATIONAL
PARK
To Hana
bridge
milestone 3
bridge
Makahiku Falls
milestone 2
start &
finish
milestones 1 & 5
visitor center
Kuloa
Point
Kipahulu
Campground
Kau Bay
Hana Hwy
Kukui Bay
PACIFIC
OCEAN
To Kaupo

Pipiwai Trail

Seeing fewer crowds than the coastal Kuloa Point Trail, this family-friendly hike ascends through South Maui's jungly terrain, over bridges, and through a musically windblown bamboo forest, to reach beautiful Waimoku Falls. Because of the dangers of rockfall and flash floods, swimming is unsafe anywhere along this trail, unfortunately.

TRAIL USE
Dayhike, Run, Child Friendly

LENGTH
4.0 miles, 2–3 hours

VERTICAL FEET
±2000′

DIFFICULTY
– 1 2 **3** 4 5 +

TRAIL TYPE
Out & Back

SURFACE TYPE
Boardwalk, Dirt, Grass

START & END
N 20.66178°
W 156.04453°

FEATURES
Forest
Stream
Waterfall
Birds
Native Plants
Wildlife
Great Views
Shady

FACILITIES
Visitor Center
Restrooms
Phone

Best Time

You can hike this trail year-round. Starting early in the morning (say, before 10 AM) will help you avoid the biggest crowds of daytrippers. Although the trail is partly shaded, the midday sun can be quite hot and the tropical humidity severe. This trail is usually busiest on weekends, when locals join the tourist crowds visiting the national park.

Finding the Trail

From Hana town in East Maui, drive 10 miles southwest along the paved Hana Highway (Hwy. 360) toward Kipahulu. This stretch of highway is twisting and narrow, with one-lane bridges and blind curves and hills. Past mile marker (MM) 42, look for the national park entrance fee station and parking lot on your left.

Trail Description

Your last chance to stock up on food and water is in Hana town, though a few roadside vendors along the highway toward Kipahulu sell fresh fruit

Don't forget to bring insect repellent. The mosquitoes can be voracious, especially near the streams and waterfall pools.

smoothies, plate lunches, island barbecue, and more. At the national park's entrance station, pay the fee or show your pass, then proceed to the signed parking lot. Nearby are portable restrooms but there is *no* drinking water available.

From the parking lot, it's a short walk over to the visitor center (open 9 AM to 5 PM daily), which has nature displays and offers ranger talks and guided walks. Call (808) 248-7375 to check current program schedules. A short walk east of the visitor center, look for the **signposted trailhead ▶1** on the far side of a small, grassy clearing. Turning right takes you past ancient Hawaiian archaeological sites and to Oheo Gulch's famous waterfall pools (see Trail 36, page 295).

To follow the Pipiwai Trail, turn left and walk uphill on a rocky dirt path with tangled tree roots. The trail quickly crosses the paved highway at a pedestrian crossing (but watch out for passing traffic, which doesn't stop). On the north side of the highway, the trail heads to the right, paralleling the road for a short distance, then sharply turns left. Now you begin ascending under a forest canopy, thick with strawberry guava trees,whose smashed, sweet-smelling fruit makes the dirt trail—often muddy and twisted with tree roots—even more slippery.

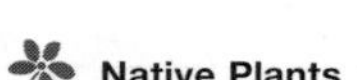

Several large red warning signs posted by the national park along the Pipiwai Trail warn visitors not to venture off-trail, cross the stream, or clamber down the cliffs to get a closer look at any of the waterfalls you'll soon be seeing. A few visitors have died after being swept away in flash floods, while hiking on crumbling cliffs, from being hit by falling rocks under waterfalls, and after diving into submerged rocks hidden below the surface of streams. Be safe and stick to the trail, no matter how tempting those waterfalls might look.

Less than 0.5 mile from the trailhead, a lava-rock wall appears on your right at the signposted

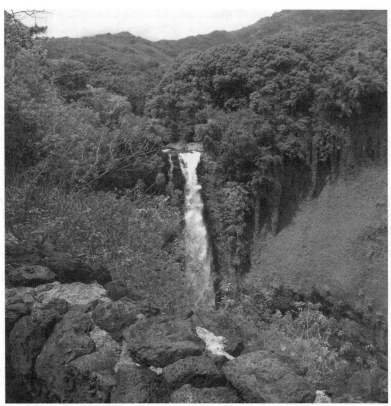

Look, but don't approach *powerful Makahiku Falls, which have fatally swept some away.*

Makahiku Falls Overlook. ►2 If it has been raining recently, Pipiwai Stream will be raging along like a mighty river as it drops almost 200 feet over distant cliffs. Beyond the overlook, the trail continues uphill, passing through a small gate. Close the gate securely behind you, to prevent wild pigs and grazing animals from entering the park's protected ecosystem. As you hike uphill, you pass several use trails leading off to your right. Because they're dangerous to follow, ignore them. The park asks all

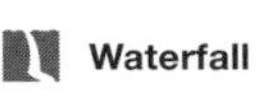

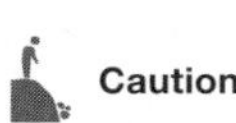

The shorter coastal Kuloa Point Trail (see Trail 36, page 295) leads to waterfall pools where swimming is usually permitted.

hikers to STAY ON TRAIL using arrowed signs. Another five minutes' walk brings you to an officially signposted spur trail on your right, which leads down to a safer close-up look at Makahiku Falls.

A little more than a mile from the trailhead, the Pipiwai Trail **crosses a stream via two metal bridges ▶3** that appear in quick succession. If it has been raining recently, water will be thundering through this narrow gulch, spraying hikers above who have stopped on the bridges to take photos. After crossing the second bridge, the trail climbs a few flights of stone steps, then levels out after rising and entering a shady bamboo forest. Take a few minutes to stop and listen to the wind blowing on the bamboo stalks, which creak and knock against each other, sounding almost like xylophones.

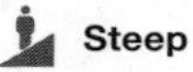

Steep

As it passes through the bamboo forest, the trail alternates between dirt sections (often muddy and slick, but bordered by flat rocks) and sections of wooden boardwalk elevated above the muck. Because of its thick forest cover, the trail rarely dries out completely. If you haven't been bothered by mosquitoes yet on this hike, they'll probably start biting here. The trail winds through the bamboo forest for more than 0.5 mile, emerging at a small stream crossing. If water levels are low, you can probably hopscotch across the rocks. But if the

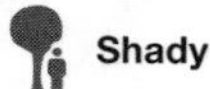

Shady

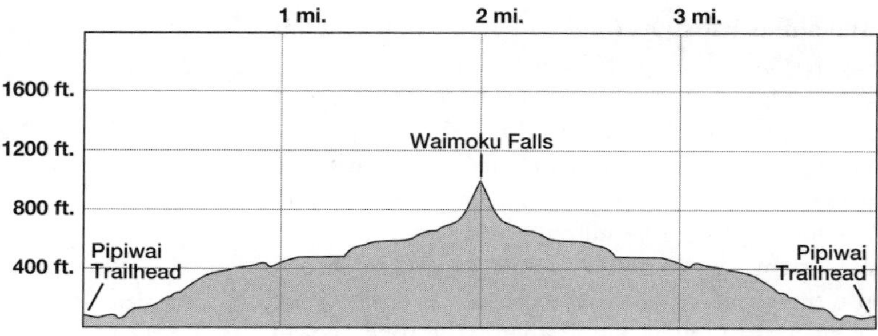

TRAIL 37 Pipiwai Trail Elevation Profile

stream suddenly starts to rise, get out of the water immediately. Flash floods are always possible here.

Once you're safely across the stream, it's a short walk to **Waimoku Falls**, ▶4 clearly visible ahead. The Pipiwai Trail ends at a large pool right at the base of the spectacular falls, which drop almost 400 feet. The waterfall is idyllic, with lacy cascades streaming down the verdant cliffs covered in mosses and ferns. Although you may see other people venturing into the water, the park strongly discourages it, because of the serious dangers of rockfalls and flash floods. Smart hikers will be satisfied with the views alone. After a restful break and perhaps a picnic lunch, turn around and retrace your steps for 2 miles (almost entirely downhill) to the **signposted trailhead**. ▶5

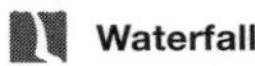

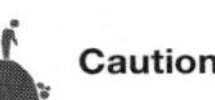

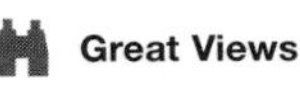

Notice

For Native Hawaiian cultural tours of the Kipahulu area, including traditionally farmed *loi kalo* (taro fields), call the Kipahulu Ohana at (808) 248-8558 or visit www.kipahulu.org. At press time, the 3-mile guided morning hike (taking approximately 2 hours) cost from $49 per person, while the 4.5-mile guided afternoon hike (3½ hours, from $79) visited Waimoku Falls.

MILESTONES

▶1	0.0	Start at signposted trailhead [N 20.66178°, W 156.04453°]
▶2	0.4	Reach Makahiku Falls Overlook [N 20.66701°, W 156.05122°]
▶3	1.2	Cross two metal bridges over stream [N 20.67103°, W 156.05359°]
▶4	2.0	Arrive at Waimoku Falls [N 20.67894°, W 156.05694°]
▶5	4.0	Return to signposted trailhead [N 20.66178°, W 156.04453°]

Appendix 1

Top-Rated Trails

Chapter 1: West Maui
Trail 5: Maunalei Arboretum & Honolua Ridge
Trail 6: Mahana Ridge
Trail 10: Waihee Ridge
Trail 11: Waihee Valley

Chapter 2: Central & South Maui
Trail 17: Hoapili Trail

Chapter 3: East Maui & Upcountry
Trail 19: Twin Falls
Trail 23: King's Highway South

Chapter 4: Haleakala National Park
Trail 26: Halemauu Trail & Silversword Loop
Trail 28: Sliding Sands Trail to Ka Luu o ka Oo
Trail 32: Sliding Sands & Halemauu Trails
Trail 33: Haleakala Grand Loop
Trail 34: Kaupo Gap
Trail 37: Pipiwai Trail

Appendix 2

Major Public Agencies & Nonprofit Organizations

National Parks & Wildlife Refuges

Haleakala National Park

www.nps.gov/hale
P.O. Box 369
Makawao, HI 96768
General park information: (808) 572-4400
Kipahulu visitor center: (808) 248-7375

Hawaiian Islands Humpback Whale National Marine Sanctuary

http://hawaiihumpbackwhale.noaa.gov/
726 S. Kihei Road
Kihei, HI 96753
(808) 879-2818 or (800) 831-4888

Kealia Pond National Wildlife Refuge

www.fws.gov/kealiapond
P.O. Box 1042
Kihei, HI 96753
(808) 875-1582

State Parks, Monuments & Recreation Areas

Division of State Parks

www.hawaiistateparks.org
54 S. High Street
Wailuku, HI 96793
(808) 984-8109

Halekii–Pihana Heiau State Monument

End of Hea Place, off Kuhio Place, off Waiehu Beach Road (Hwy. 340)
Wailuku, HI 96793

Iao Valley State Monument

End of Iao Valley Road (Hwy. 32)
Wailuku, HI 96793

Makena State Park

End of Wailea Alanui Road
Makena, HI 96753

Polipoli Spring State Recreation Area

Waipoli Road, off Kekaulike Avenue (Hwy. 377)
Kula, HI 96790

Waianapanapa State Park

Off the Hana Highway (Hwy. 360), near mile marker (MM) 32
Hana, HI 96713
(808) 248-4844

Other State Agencies & Programs

Department of Land and Natural Resources (DLNR)

http://hawaii.gov/dlnr
54 S. High Street
Wailuku, HI 96793
(808) 984-8109

Division of Forestry and Wildlife (DOFAW)

http://hawaii.gov/dlnr/dofaw
54 S. High Street
Wailuku, HI 96793
(808) 984-8100

Na Ala Hele (Hawaii Trail & Access System)

https://hawaiitrails.ehawaii.gov/
54 S. High Street
Wailuku, HI 96793
(808) 873-3508

County Parks & Permit Offices

Maui County Parks & Recreation

www.co.maui.hi.us/parks
War Memorial Complex
700 Halia Nakoa Street
Wailuku, HI 96793
(808) 270-7230

Central District Permit Office

Kahului Community Center
275-D Uhu Street
Kahului, HI 96732
(808) 270-7389

Hana District Permit Office

5101 Uakea Road
Hana, HI 96713
(808) 248-7022

East District Permit Office

931 Makawao Avenue
Makawao, HI 96768
(808) 572-8122

South District Permit Office

Kihei Community Center
303 E. Lipoa Street
Kihei, HI 96753
(808) 879-4364

West District Permit Office

Lahaina Civic Center
1840 Honoapiilani Highway
Lahaina, HI 96761
(808) 661-4685

Nonprofit Organizations

Friends of Haleakala National Park

www.fhnp.org
P.O. Box 322
Makawao, HI 96768

Hawaii Audubon Society (Oahu)

www.hawaiiaudubon.com
850 Richards Street
Honolulu, HI 96813
(808) 528-1432

Hawaii Wildlife Fund

http://wildhawaii.org
P.O. Box 790637
Paia, HI 96779
(808) 280-8124

Maui Coastal Land Trust

www.mauicoastallandtrust.org
2371 Vineyard Street
P.O. Box 965
Wailuku, HI 96793
(808) 244-5263

The Nature Conservancy (TNC)

www.nature.org/hawaii
Pukalani Square
81 Makawao Ave., Suite 203-A
P.O. Box 1716
Makawao, HI 96768
(808) 572-7849

Sierra Club: Hawaii Chapter (Maui Group)

www.hi.sierraclub.org/maui
P.O. Box 791180
Paia, HI 96779

Surfrider Foundation: Maui Chapter

www.surfrider.org/maui
P.O. Box 790549
Paia, HI 96779

Appendix 3

Maps, Books & Internet Resources

You can buy island maps and Hawaiiana books at tourist shops and major chain bookstores like Borders (808-877-6160; 270 Dairy Rd., Kahului), near the airport in central Maui, or Barnes & Noble (808-662-1300; 325 Keawe St., Lahaina) in West Maui. Smaller nonprofit bookstores inside visitor centers at Haleakala National Park also stock a good selection of maps and books.

Maps

The simple maps included in this book are sufficient for most dayhikes. Consult the introductory "Permits & Maps" sections at the beginning of each regional hiking chapter earlier for details. Developed hiking trails in coastal resort areas, such as Kapalua, Wailea, and Kihei, feature map signboards along the trails, and resorts may offer free map brochures for hikers. Hawaii's Department of Land and Natural Resources (DLNR) distributes the *Maui Recreation Map*, a shaded relief map that shows many of the island's public parks, trails, and campgrounds. You can pick up a free copy of this map from the Division of Forestry and Wildlife (DOFAW) office in Wailuku (see Appendix 2). If you're planning any overnight or backcountry trips on Maui, topographic maps may be helpful, especially for following less traveled and infrequently maintained island trails. Be aware that handheld GPS devices do not always function on Maui, especially in dense forest cover or in cloudy weather, so consider bringing a compass, too. Every hike described in this book lists GPS coordinates for the start and end points of the trail, as well as waypoints for some milestones along the trail that are likely to be useful to hikers. All coordinates are listed in decimal degrees.

National Geographic's TOPO! series offers digital topographic maps scaled at 1:24,000, 1:100,000 and 1:500,000 on CD-ROM. The TOPO!

Hawaii mapping product ($49.95) includes National Geographic's outdoor recreation mapping software, which lets you customize and print your own trail maps. This mapping software is compatible with both Macs and PCs. It also allows maps to be uploaded to most handheld GPS receivers. You'll probably need to purchase this mapping product before your trip to Maui, as it is rarely stocked at bookstores or by outdoor outfitters either in Hawaii or on the U.S. mainland. To order any National Geographic mapping product, visit www.natgeomaps.com or call (800) 437-5521.

The US Geological Survey (USGS) publishes 7.5-minute topographic quadrangle maps at a scale of 1:24,000. Although USGS quad maps ($8 each) comprehensively cover the entire island, you may need to buy multiple maps for just one hike, which quickly becomes expensive. Also, the survey information tends to be outdated; newer trails may not appear at all, while some artificial features shown on the maps no longer exist. Unless you're exploring the backcountry, the level of detail on these maps is probably more than you'll need. Besides, quad maps are bulky to carry on the trail and printed on paper that is neither waterproof nor rip-resistant. More conveniently, the USGS website now allows you to download its digital topo maps for *free* as printable PDFs. Otherwise, you can still order print copies of these maps online at http://store.usgs.gov or by calling (888) 275-8747.

While driving around Maui, free tourist-oriented maps will rarely help you navigate to island hiking trailheads. Alternatively, the University of Hawaii's full-color, topographic *Map of Maui: The Valley Isle* ($4.95), 8th edition (2008), is an inexpensive fold-out map showing some campgrounds, trails, and other points of interest. It is widely available at local bookstores, or you can order it directly from the University of Hawaii Press at www.uhpress.hawaii.edu or by calling (808) 956-8255 or (888) 847-7737. For a more detailed road atlas with a comprehensive street index, but lacking any topographic details or features, Odyssey Publishing's black-and-white *Ready Mapbook of Maui County* ($11) is sold at island bookstores and some gas stations.

Recommended Reading

Benson, Sara, et al. *Hawaii*. Oakland, CA: Lonely Planet Publications, 2011.

Crowe, Ellie. *Exploring Lost Hawaii*. Waipahu, HI: Island Heritage, 2008.

Daws, Gavin. *Shoal of Time: A History of the Hawaiian Islands*. Honolulu: University of Hawaii Press, 1989.

Decker, Barbara, and Robert Decker. *Road Guide to Haleakala and the Hana Highway*. Mariposa, CA: Double Decker Press, 1999.

Grant, Kim. *Hawaii: An Explorer's Guide*. Woodstock, VT: Countryman Press, 2009.

Hall, John. *A Hiker's Guide to Trailside Plants in Hawaii*. Honolulu: Mutual Publishing, 2008.

Harden, M. J. *Voices of Wisdom: Hawaiian Elders Speak*. Miilani, HI: Booklines Hawaii, 1997.

Hawaii Audubon Society. *Hawaii's Birds*. Honolulu: Hawaii Audubon Society, 1997.

Hazlett, Richard W., and Donald W. Hyndman. *Roadside Geology of Hawaii*. Missoula, MT: Mountain Press Publishing Company, 1996.

James, Van. *Ancient Sites of Maui, Molokai, and Lanai*. Honolulu: Mutual Publishing, 2002.

Kalakaua, David. *Legends and Myths of Hawaii*. Honolulu: Mutual Publishing, 1990.

Kane, Herb Kawainui. *Ancient Hawaii*. Captain Cook, HI: Kawainui Press, 1998.

Kepler, Angela K. *Haleakala: From Summit to Sea*. Miilani, HI: Booklines Hawaii, 2005.

———. *Hawaii's Floral Splendor*. Honolulu: Mutual Publishing, 2001.

———. *Trees of Hawaii*. Honolulu: University of Hawaii Press, 1990.

Kirch, Patrick Vinton. *Feathered Gods and Fishhooks: An Introduction to Hawaiian Archaeology and Prehistory*. Honolulu, HI: University of Hawaii Press, 1998.

———. *Legacy of the Landscape*. Honolulu: University of Hawaii Press, 1996.

Krauss, Beatrice H. *Plants in Hawaiian Culture*. Honolulu: University of Hawaii Press, 2001.

Merlin, Mark. *Hawaiian Forest Plants*. Honolulu: Pacific Guide Books, 1999.

Pratt, H. Douglas. *A Pocket Guide to Hawaii's Birds*. Honolulu: Mutual Publishing, 2002.

———. *A Pocket Guide to Hawaii's Trees and Shrubs*. Honolulu: Mutual Publishing, 1999.

Simonson, Douglas. *Pidgin to da Max*. Honolulu: Bess Press, 2005.

Valier, Kathy. *Ferns of Hawaii*. Honolulu: University of Hawaii Press, 1995.

Walther, Michael. *A Guide to Hawaii's Coastal Plants*. Honolulu: Mutual Publishing, 2004.

Internet Resources

Government & Public Agencies

Hawaii Visitors & Convention Bureau
www.gohawaii.com

Maui County Parks & Recreation
www.co.maui.hi.us/parks

Maui Natural Area Reserves
http://hawaii.gov/dlnr/dofaw/nars/reserves/maui

Maui State Parks
www.hawaiistateparks.org/parks/maui/

Maui Visitors Bureau
www.visitmaui.com

Na Ala Hele (Hawaii Trail & Access System)
https://hawaiitrails.ehawaii.gov

National Park Service: Hawaii
www.nps.gov/state/hi/index.htm

Media

Akaku: Maui Community Television
www.akaku.org

Honolulu Star-Advertiser
www.honoluluadvertiser.com

Honolulu Star-Bulletin
www.starbulletin.com

Maui News
www.mauinews.com

Maui Time Weekly
www.mauitime.com

Maui TV News
www.mauitvnews.com

Maui Weekly
www.mauiweekly.com

Other Helpful Resources

Alternative Hawaii
www.alternative-hawaii.com

Environment Hawaii
www.environment-hawaii.org

Hawaii Agritourism Association
www.hiagtourism.org

Hawaii Audubon Society
www.hawaiiaudubon.com

Hawaii Bicycling League
www.hbl.org

Hawaii Conservation Alliance
http://hawaiiconservation.org

Hawaii Ecosystems at Risk Project (HEAR)
www.hear.org

Hawaii Ecotourism Association
www.hawaiiecotourism.org

Malama Hawaii
www.malamahawaii.org

Maui Tomorrow Foundation
www.maui-tomorrow.org

Out in Hawaii
www.outinhawaii.com

Appendix 4

Local Guides, Tour Operators & Hiking Clubs

Haleakala National Park

www.nps.gov/hale
P.O. Box 369
Makawao, HI 96768
(808) 572-4400

Hike Maui

www.hikemaui.com
P.O. Box 330969
Kahului, HI 96733
(808) 879-5270 or (866) 324-6284

Kipahulu Ohana

www.kipahulu.org
P.O. Box 454
Hana, HI 96713
(808) 248-8558

Maui Hiking Safaris

www.mauihikingsafaris.com
P.O. Box 11198
Lahaina, HI 96761
(808) 573-0168 or (888) 445-3963

Pony Express Tours

www.ponyexpresstours.com
P.O. Box 535
Kula, HI 96790
(808) 667-2200

Sierra Club

www.hi.sierraclub.org/maui
P.O. Box 791180
Paia, HI 96779

Appendix 5

Outdoor Gear, Supplies & Food

If you'll be camping or backpacking on Maui, it's best to bring your own gear from home. When available (which is not often), rental camping equipment on Maui is usually geared toward outdoor parties or hunting trips, not individual backpackers or car campers. Equipment tends to be too heavy to hike with (e.g., 20-person canvas tents, dual-burner propane stoves) and often of the same quality as army-navy surplus stores.

If you're planning to buy any camping equipment on Maui, your options are limited. Your best bet for finding backpacking and hiking gear and trail food supplies is at the Sports Authority (808-871-2558, 270 Dairy Road, Kahului), which sells everything from freeze-dried meals to small fuel canisters designed for portable campstoves. The latter are especially difficult to find and may not be sold anywhere else on the island. Remember that you may not transport these fuel canisters on planes, either as checked baggage or as carry-on luggage, so you'll need to buy them here before hitting the trail or setting up camp anywhere on the island.

Mega-chain stores such as Walmart, Kmart, and Costco have branches in central Maui, not far from the main island airport. Walmart (808-871-7820, 101 Pakaula St., Kahului) and Kmart (808-871-8553, 424 Dairy Road, Kahului) both carry limited camping equipment, but it's mostly designed for large hunting parties. Costco (808-877-5248, 540 Haleakala Highway, Kahului) doesn't carry much, if any camping gear, but it does sell trail-ready food in bulk (e.g., beef jerky, power bars, and granola); if you already have a Costco membership, food prices are typically lower here than at supermarket chains such as Foodland or Safeway. Island health-food stores are another good source of trail food supplies for hiking and backpacking. Try the following places:

Central Maui: Down to Earth

(808) 877-2661
305 Dairy Road, Kahului

South Maui: Hawaiian Moons

(808) 875-4356
2411 S. Kihei Road, Kihei

East Maui: Mana Foods

(808) 579-8078
49 Baldwin Avenue, Paia

For more details about campgrounds on Maui and the required permits and fees, consult the "Camping, Cabins & Permits" section of the "Introduction to Maui" chapter earlier in this book (see page 15).

Index

T

U

V

W

Author

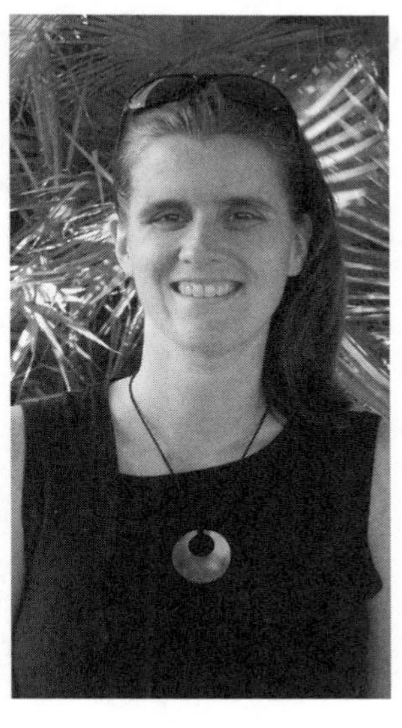

Sara Benson

Sara Benson is a prolific travel journalist whose career has taken her skipping across the Pacific from California to Japan and back, including stints living on Maui, the Big Island of Hawaii, and Oahu. Her first backpacking experience in Hawaii was at Haleakala National Park on Maui, to which she has returned countless times over the last 15 years. Sara has worked as a national park ranger and is an avid hiker everywhere she travels. For this guide, she rehiked every trail on Maui described in this book, racking up well more than 100 miles on all types of terrain, from jagged lava flows and cinder deserts to misty cloud forests and muddy waterfall paths.

Sara is the author of dozens of travel and outdoor activity guidebooks, including for Lonely Planet and Fodor's. She has traveled to every continent except Antarctica and has visited over 30 countries. Her writing regularly appears in newspapers and magazines around the world, including the *Honolulu Star-Advertiser* and *Backpacker*, as well as on popular travel and news websites. Keep up with Sara's latest adventures online at:

www.indietraveler.blogspot.com
www.twitter.com/indie_traveler
www.indietraveler.net

Future updates for this book will be posted online at www.toptrailsmaui.blogspot.com, where feedback and comments from enthusiastic hikers like you are always welcome.